T0354615

The Ethics of Inheritable Genetic Modification
A Dividing Line?

"For who is harmed by the genetic supermarket? The parents are not harmed by having the healthier, handsomer, and more intelligent children that they want. Are the children harmed?"

From the Foreword by Peter Singer: *Shopping at the Genetic Supermarket.*

These provocative questions, and their possible answers from biomedical science, ethics, sociology and philosophy, are the subject of this searching investigation. In seeking to establish whether inheritable genetic modification is the new dividing line in gene therapy, the editors, themselves representing clinical medicine, public health and biomedical ethics, have brought together a distinguished team of scientists and scholars to address the issues from the perspectives of biological and social science, law and ethics. Their purpose is to consider how society might deal with the ethical concerns raised by inheritable genetic modification, and to re-examine prevailing views about whether these kinds of interventions will ever be ethically and socially justifiable. The book also provides background to define the field, and discusses the biological and technological potential for inheritable genetic modification, its limitations and its connection with gene therapy, cloning, and other reproductive interventions.

For scientists, bioethicists, clinicians, counsellors and public commentators, this is an essential contribution to one of the critical debates in current genetics.

John E.J. Rasko holds a personal chair in the Faculty of Medicine, Centenary Institute, University of Sydney and practises as a hematologist at Royal Prince Alfred Hospital, where he is Director of Cell and Molecular Therapy.

Gabrielle M. O'Sullivan is a scientist who specialized in biochemistry and immunology at the Universities of Dublin, London, and Sydney. Her current work focuses on genetics, gene technology, ethics, and public health.

Rachel A. Ankeny is Senior Lecturer in the Unit for History and Philosophy of Science at the University of Sydney where she teaches and does research in bioethics, and the history and philosophy of biomedical sciences.

"This thoughtful and stimulating book will excite a vision of the likely future of the human species or give you nightmares about the brave new world. It is timely, readable and very important. Despite the puzzles it presents, the book affirms that human intelligence can think these issues through and come to rational and moral decisions about them. The book shows how exciting it is to live in an age when technology, moral philosophy and values are suddenly the stuff of politics and a global civic debate. The puzzles will not go away because we ignore them. To look the other way is to make a decision to do nothing."

Justice Michael Kirby, AC CMG, Justice of the High Court of Australia and Member of the International Bioethics Committee of UNESCO.

"The time to think clearly about germline gene therapy is now. The distinguished group of scholars contributing to this volume have much to offer readers who want to reflect seriously on animal research in genetic modification, and on the prospect of human germline genetic alteration."

Thomas H. Murray, PhD, President, The Hastings Center, New York, U.S.A.

"I think this is a rather wonderful collection. It is put together exactly as these things should be, but rarely are – with a good mix of science, social science, law, and ethics. Anyone seriously interested in the issues around germline gene therapy (inheritable genetic modification, human genetic engineering) will find this the most helpful and insightful resource. I think any of these papers could be published in a good peer-reviewed journal. There is no wasted material or lightweight material. Ethicists may find some of the science hard going, but there is nothing there that cannot be understood (as I judge it!) and ethicists ought to understand the scientific issues properly before wading in to pronounce on the ethics."

Richard Ashcroft, Reader in Biomedical Ethics, Imperial College, London, U.K.

"This is a very high quality work in at least two senses. First, it is scientifically sophisticated. This is important, because there is too much discussion of the ethics of genetics that is not accurately anchored in an understanding of the scientific situation of research. Second, it is conceptually quite advanced. I could easily see using this text in a graduate seminar. The work coheres very well, which is often missing in some edited works."

George Agich, Department of Bioethics, Cleveland Clinic, Cleveland, U.S.A.

The Ethics of Inheritable Genetic Modification

A Dividing Line?

Edited by

John E. J. Rasko
University of Sydney and Royal Prince Alfred Hospital

Gabrielle M. O'Sullivan
University of Sydney and Royal Prince Alfred Hospital

Rachel A. Ankeny
University of Sydney

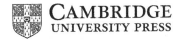
CAMBRIDGE
UNIVERSITY PRESS

CAMBRIDGE
UNIVERSITY PRESS

University Printing House, Cambridge CB2 8BS, United Kingdom

One Liberty Plaza, 20th Floor, New York, NY 10006, USA

477 Williamstown Road, Port Melbourne, VIC 3207, Australia

314-321, 3rd Floor, Plot 3, Splendor Forum, Jasola District Centre, New Delhi - 110025, India

103 Penang Road, #05-06/07, Visioncrest Commercial, Singapore 238467

Cambridge University Press is part of the University of Cambridge.

It furthers the University's mission by disseminating knowledge in the pursuit of education, learning and research at the highest international levels of excellence.

www.cambridge.org
Information on this title: www.cambridge.org/9780521529730

© Cambridge University Press 2006

First published 2006

A catalogue record for this publication is available from the British Library

ISBN 978-0-521-82277-0 Hardback
ISBN 978-0-521-52973-0 Paperback

Cambridge University Press has no responsibility for the persistence or accuracy of URLs for external or third-party internet websites referred to in this publication, and does not guarantee that any content on such websites is, or will remain, accurate or appropriate.

....

Every effort has been made in preparing this book to provide accurate and up-to-date information which is in accord with accepted standards and practice at the time of publication. Although case histories are drawn from actual cases, every effort has been made to disguise the identities of the individuals involved. Nevertheless, the authors, editors and publishers can make no warranties that the information contained herein is totally free from error, not least because clinical standards are constantly changing through research and regulation. The authors, editors and publishers therefore disclaim all liability for direct or consequential damages resulting from the use of material contained in this book. Readers are strongly advised to pay careful attention to information provided by the manufacturer of any drugs or equipment that they plan to use.

JEJR: To three generations of my tolerant family connected by shared genes and joy: Helen, Simone, Nathalie, and Adam.

GMO'S: To my beloved courageous parents, Margaret and James, who have cherished me boundlessly. To Dermot, Emmet, Caoimhe, Eimear, and Eoin who make my world shine.

RAA: To my extended family, near and far.

Contents

Contributors

Rachel A. Ankeny received a master's in philosophy, a master's in bioethics, and a PhD in the history and philosophy of science, all from the University of Pittsburgh. She was an Assistant Professor of History and Philosophy of Science at Pittsburgh, and Class of '43 Assistant Professor of Philosophy of Science at Connecticut College before becoming Director of the Unit of History and Philosophy of Science at the University of Sydney in 2000, where she is now Senior Lecturer. Her research and teaching examines issues at the intersection of the history and philosophy of biomedical sciences and bioethics.

Françoise Baylis is Canada Research Chair in Bioethics and Philosophy at Dalhousie University, Halifax, Nova Scotia, Canada. Her research involves exploring fundamental philosophical questions concerning our obligations to future generations in the development of specific technologies. Of particular interest are issues of justice, community, and identity. Major recent publications are available at www. noveltechethics.ca. Her biography is included in *Who's Who in Black Canada* (2002) and in *Canadian Who's Who* (2004, 2005).

Roberta M. Berry, JD, PhD (History and Philosophy of Science), is Associate Professor of Public Policy and Director of the Law, Science and Technology Program at the Georgia Institute of Technology, Atlanta, Georgia, U.S.A. She is a co-editor of *A Health Law Reader* and has published a number of articles and book chapters on the legal, ethical, and policy implications of life sciences research and biotechnological innovation. Her book comparing the adequacy of utilitarian, deontological, and virtue-based ethical and political theories in addressing the issues posed by the possible advent of germ-line genetic engineering of human beings will be published by Routledge in 2006.

Rudolf Jaenisch, a founding Member of the Whitehead Institute and Professor of Biology at Massachusetts Institute of Technology, has made fundamental contributions to our knowledge of genome function and regulation. In 1996, he was awarded the Boehringer Mannheim Molecular Bioanalytics Prize, and was named the first recipient of the Peter Gruber Foundation Award in Genetics in 2001. Professor Jaenisch received the 2002 Robert Koch Prize for Excellence in Scientific Achievement;

in 2003, he was awarded the Charles Rodolphe Brupbacher Prize for basic research in oncology and was elected a member of the National Academy of Sciences, U.S.A.

Douglas J. Jolly is a leading figure in gene technology in the U.S.A. He is currently President of Advantagene Inc. For the last 16 years, as a senior biotechnology executive, he has been involved in moving gene based products from research through clinical development in the biotechnology industry, at Viagene Inc., Chiron Corporation, BioMedica Inc., and Advantagene Inc. Dr Jolly has published over 90 scientific articles and is an inventor on 40 issued patents. He is also on the editorial board of several professional journals, and is on the steering committee of the National Gene Vector Laboratories. He has advised the U.S. National Institutes of Health and the FDA on science and regulation and the International Olympic Committee on gene-enhancement technologies in relation to sport.

Eric T. Juengst is Associate Professor of Bioethics and Director of the Center for Genetic Research Ethics and Law at the Case Western Reserve University School of Medicine, Cleveland, Ohio, U.S.A. He was Chief of the Ethical, Legal, and Social Implications (ELSI) Branch of the National Center for Human Genome Research at the U.S. National Institutes of Health from 1990 to 94. His research interests and publications have focused on the conceptual and ethical issues raised by new advances in human genetics and biotechnology. He currently serves on the U.S. National Council for Human Genome Research, the Ethics Committee of the American Society for Human Gene Therapy, and the editorial boards of *Community Genetics*, the *Journal of Medicine and Philosophy*, and *Human Gene Therapy*.

Isabel Karpin is a Senior Lecturer in the Faculty of Law at the University of Sydney, specializing in feminist legal theory, health law, law and culture, and constitutional law. Her research has been concerned with rethinking legal and medical approaches to the body, as well as legal responses to developments in genetic technologies and the challenges posed by these new technologies to legal understandings of individuality, identity, and family. One of her most significant contributions to this area has been her conceptualization of the pregnant woman as not-one-but-not-two adopted by the Australian Medical Association in its major 1995 Fetal Welfare and the Law Report. Recent publications include Genetics and the Legal Conception of Self in Roxanne Mykitiuk and Margrit Shildrick (eds.), *Ethics of the Body: Postconventional Challenges* (MIT Press, out in June 2005).

Denis Kenny was a 1997 Templeton Award winner and is the former Dean of Humanities and Social Sciences at Royal Melbourne Institute of Technology (RMIT) University, and Former Director of Liberal and General Studies at the University of New South Wales, Australia. He is a moral philosopher who has taught at universities in Australia and the U.S.A., and is now an independent scholar based in Sydney, Australia.

Roxanne Mykitiuk is Associate Professor of Law at Osgoode Hall Law School, York University, Toronto, Canada. She has published widely on the legal regulation and construction of the body and about the legal implications of new reproductive and genetic technologies. She is the co-editor (with Margrit Shildrick) of *Ethics of the Human Body: Challenging the Conventions* (Boston: MIT Press, 2005). Her research interests include health law, bioethics, and feminist theory and focus on the legal construction and regulation of the human body. She was senior legal researcher for the Royal Commission on New Reproductive Technologies from 1990 to 1992.

Gabrielle M. O'Sullivan (PhD, University of London) is a Senior Scientist at Royal Prince Alfred Hospital, Sydney and a research associate at the Unit for History and Philosophy of Science at the University of Sydney. She has worked in the areas of genetics, gene technology, ethics, and public health and co-edited *Goodbye Normal Gene* (Pluto Press, 1999), a popular exploration of the impact of gene technology on society and culture.

John E.J. Rasko completed his medical degree at the University of Sydney and specialized in clinical hematology. He received a PhD from research undertaken in Professor Donald Metcalf's Cancer Research Unit at the Walter and Eliza Hall Institute followed by 3 years at the Fred Hutchinson Cancer Research Center in Seattle, U.S.A. in Professor Dusty Miller's Laboratory. He has published widely in the biomedical literature, recently reporting the discovery of the long-sought gene for Hartnup disease in humans. He holds a Personal Chair in the Faculty of Medicine, University of Sydney and practises as a hematologist at Royal Prince Alfred Hospital, where he is Director of Cell and Molecular Therapy. Professor Rasko contributes to national gene technology policy and leads the Gene and Stem Cell Therapy Program at the Centenary Institute in Sydney, Australia.

Christoph Rehmann-Sutter is Head of the Unit of Ethics in Biosciences at the University of Basel, Switzerland. His research interests include foundations and methods of bioethics, technical-ecological risks, the philosophical interpretation of developmental genetics, the ethics of gene therapy, and genome analysis. He was a Research Fellow in the Department of Environmental Science, Policy, and Management (ESPM) at the University of California, Berkeley, U.S.A. Since 2001 he has been Chairman of the Swiss National Advisory Commission on Biomedical Ethics.

Jason Scott Robert is Assistant Professor in the School of the Life Sciences at Arizona State University. His research currently spans conceptual, methodological, and ethical issues in developmental biology (including stem cell biology and regenerative medicine) and psychiatric genetics. His book, *Embryology, Epigenesis, and Evolution: Taking Development Seriously*, was published in 2004 by Cambridge University Press.

Joan A. Scott is the Deputy Director of the Genetics and Public Policy Center at Johns Hopkins University. She is a board certified Genetic Counselor with more than 25 years of experience encompassing clinical genetic services, professional education, and the policy implications of advances in genetics. She is Past President of the National Society of Genetic Counselors and was instrumental in setting certification standards for genetic counselors. Her research interests include reproductive genetic technologies and public attitudes.

Jackie Leach Scully is Senior Research Associate in the Department of Bioethics, Institute for Medical History and Ethics, at the University of Basel, Switzerland. Trained in Britain in biochemistry and molecular biology, her scientific research was in the molecular biology of cancer and of neurodegeneration. Her bioethical research interests are in feminist ethics, disability, marginalized ethical standpoints, and moral psychology. Recent research projects have investigated variations in ethical attitudes to gene therapy between different groups, especially people with disabilities; patients' genetic testing decisions; and lay processes of moral evaluation.

Peter Singer is Ira W. DeCamp Professor of Bioethics in the University Center for Human Values at Princeton University, and Laureate Professor in the Centre for Applied Philosophy and Public Ethics at the University of Melbourne. His books include *Animal Liberation, Practical Ethics, Rethinking Life and Death, One World,* and *Pushing Time Away.*

Rosemarie Tong is the Distinguished Professor in Health Care Ethics at the Center for Professional and Applied Ethics of The University of North Carolina at Charlotte, U.S.A., the first faculty member to hold the position. She teaches in the Department of Philosophy and directs the University's Center for Professional and Applied Ethics. She is a former national professor of the year as named by the Carnegie Foundation for the Advancement of Teaching. She has written numerous books and articles on her research interests, which include feminist ethics, reproductive ethics, global bioethics, death and dying, and law, among other topics.

Foreword: shopping at the genetic supermarket

Peter Singer

Consider ... the issue of genetic engineering. Many biologists tend to think the problem is one of *design*, of specifying the best types of persons so that biologists can proceed to produce them. Thus they worry over what sort(s) of person there is to be and who will control this process. They do not tend to think, perhaps because it diminishes the importance of their role, of a system in which they run a "genetic supermarket," meeting the individual specifications (within certain moral limits) of prospective parents ... This supermarket system has the great virtue that it involves no centralized decision fixing the future of human type(s).[1]

The genocide of deaf culture?

Robert Nozick's genetic supermarket has arrived on the wings of angels brought to us by Ron Harris, the founder of ronsangels.com, "the only website that provides you with the unique opportunity to bid on eggs from beautiful, healthy, intelligent women."[2] How should we respond to this and other options that will soon be beckoning? To assist us in answering these questions, I shall begin by considering a technique that has been with us for some time, but that has the effect of changing the nature of children. Understanding the basis on which this technique can be supported may help us to grapple with the more difficult question of what we should do about newer options that also change the nature of our children. It is not, however, my aim here to deal with all the objections that could be urged against these options. My purpose is the narrower one of developing a clear understanding of the central values at stake.[3]

In the deaf community there has, for some years now, been a debate over attempts to alleviate some of the effects of deafness by the provision of cochlear ear implants in children. Although this is not a technique that makes use of genetics, the issues raised are in many respects similar to those that would be raised by the discovery of a genetic marker for congenital deafness. Cochlear implants do not restore normal hearing; instead they transform speech and other sounds into electrical impulses, and transmit these impulses to auditory nerve fibers in the inner ear. When implanted in children below the age of 3 years, they make it possible for them to grow up "hearing" speech and thus to be able to take part in the speaking community as if they could hear.[4] In children who have been deaf from birth, the implants are less successful when implanted at a later age.

The scientists who first developed cochlear implants assumed that they would be enthusiastically embraced by the deaf community, and especially by the parents of congenitally deaf infants. Some parents of deaf children do have exactly this response. But others have a very different response, as the following statement indicates:

THE GENOCIDE OF DEAF CULTURE
FACT: The law says that genocide is the destruction of an ethnic group.
FACT: The law says that an ethnic group is "a set of individuals whose identity is distinctive in terms of common cultural traditions or heritage."
FACT: Deaf people are "a set of individuals whose identity is distinctive in terms of common cultural traditions or heritage."
Cochlear implants are an attempt to eliminate the trait of Deafness.
Eliminating the trait of Deafness will destroy "a set of individuals whose identity is distinctive in terms of common cultural traditions or heritage." (That "set" of individuals will no longer exist.)
THEREFORE – COCHLEAR IMPLANTS ARE GENOCIDE.[5]

Though extreme in its language, this is not an isolated point of view. A significant number of deaf parents are refusing to allow their deaf children to have the implants. They argue that the implants will cut them off from the Deaf community and from Deaf culture, which survives because of its distinctive language and its separation from the world of hearing people. The Deaf community expresses the idea that it has a distinctive culture by the use of capitalization. To be Deaf is to be part of a culture (like being French or Jewish) whereas to be deaf is to be unable to hear. As one parent said: "If somebody gave me a pill to make me hear, would I take it? No way. I want to be deaf."[6]

Something similar is happening among people with the short, stocky body shape known as achondroplasia, or dwarfism, since the discovery of the gene for this condition raised the prospect of prenatal diagnosis and selective termination. Little People of America, an association for those with short stature, has issued a position statement asserting that some of its members fear "genetic tests such as these will be used to terminate affected pregnancies and therefore take the opportunity for life away from children such as ourselves and our children." In response, they remind the rest of us that they are productive members of society who "face challenges, most of them are environmental (as with people with other disabilities)" and "value the opportunity to contribute a unique perspective to the diversity of our society …" They have "a common feeling of self-acceptance, pride, community and culture."[7]

For a final example, consider the contrasting views taken of Down syndrome. In both the U.S.A. and the U.K., at least 90% of women tested will terminate a pregnancy after prenatal diagnosis shows that they are carrying a child with Down syndrome.[8] Yet others have described people with Down syndrome as "stars in an increasingly materialistic world," "without exception magic children," and capable of "unconditional love." One parent has said:

Those of us with a Down syndrome child (our son, Robert, is almost 24) often wish that all our children had this extraordinary syndrome which deletes anger and malice, replacing them with humour, thoughtfulness, and devotion to friends and family.[9]

Consistent with this view, Diane Beeson has opposed present practices of prenatal diagnosis on the grounds that:

The central assumption behind the deployment of prenatal diagnosis is that life with a disability is not worthwhile and is primarily a source of suffering … From a disability-rights perspective, prenatal testing for fetal anomalies gives a powerful message that we seek to eliminate future persons with disabilities, fails to recognize the social value of future persons with disabilities, and conveys a devaluation of those now living with disability … By focusing so many resources on the elimination of potential persons with disability, we are drifting toward a eugenic resurgence that differs only superficially from earlier patterns. In the process we are seriously distorting the historical purpose of medicine as healing. We are creating a society in which disability is becoming increasingly stigmatized, with the result that human imperfection of all kinds is becoming less tolerated and less likely to be accepted as normal human variation.[10]

The cochlear ear implant, the discovery of the gene for achondroplasia, and the use of selective abortion to prevent the birth of children with Down syndrome serve to test the outer limits of our support for the politics of equality and diversity. We say that we believe that all humans are equal, and we value diversity. Does our belief in equality go so far that we hesitate to say that it is better not to have a disability than to have one? Does the value we place on diversity mean that we should oppose any measures that might weaken Deaf culture, or reduce the number of people born with Down syndrome or achondroplasia? Should we stop the use of public funds for prenatal diagnosis or cochlear ear implants?

To assess these criticisms of prenatal diagnosis, it will help to think for a moment about two related questions. First, how important is it to most parents to give their child the best possible start in life? Second, how serious a reason does a woman need in order to be justified in ending her pregnancy?

The answer to the first question is that, for most parents, giving their child the best possible start in life is extremely important. The desire to do so leads pregnant women who have smoked or drunk heavily to struggle to kick the addiction; it sells millions of books telling parents how to help their child achieve her or his potential; it causes couples to move out to suburbs where the schools are better, even though they then have to spend time in daily commuting; and it stimulates saving so that later the child will be able to go to a good college.

The answer to the second question must begin with the fact that, in accordance with the decision in *Roe v. Wade*, a woman in the U.S.A. can, in the first and second trimesters, or at least until the fetus is viable, terminate her pregnancy for any reason whatsoever. This does not, of course, mean that she is ethically justified in doing so. Some say that she is *never* ethically justified in terminating her pregnancy, and others that she is justified in doing so only to save her own life, or in cases of rape and incest. Beeson and many others who are concerned about prenatal diagnosis, however, do not rest their argument on opposition to abortion. So rather than argue this point in detail here, I shall simply state that, as I have argued elsewhere, I do not think that a fetus is the kind of being that has a right to life.[11] Hence it is not hard to justify terminating a pregnancy. For example, suppose that a couple plan to have children, but an unplanned pregnancy has occurred before they feel ready to do so – let us say that at present they are sharing a studio apartment and cannot afford anything larger, but in 5 years they will be able to move to a larger home. In my view, they would not be acting unethically if they decide to obtain an abortion.

Now think about a couple who are told that the child the woman is carrying will have a disability, say Down syndrome. Like most parents, the couple think it important to give their child the best possible start in life, and they do not believe that having Down syndrome is the best possible start in life. Is it true that this couple must be making the assumption that "life with a disability is not worthwhile and is primarily a source of suffering"? There is no more reason to believe that these parents make that assumption, than there is to believe that parents who terminate a pregnancy because they cannot afford a larger apartment believe that "life as a child in one room with one's parents is not worthwhile and is primarily a source of suffering." In both cases, all that the parents need assume is that it would be *better* to have a child without Down syndrome, or to have a child who can have a room of her own. After all, in neither case are the parents choosing whether or not to have a child at all. They are choosing whether to have *this* child or another child that they can, with reasonable confidence, expect to have later, under more auspicious circumstances.[12]

Thus it is possible to justify abortion in these circumstances while accepting Beeson's claims that people with congenital disabilities "often achieve the same high levels of life satisfaction as non-disabled persons." A couple may reasonably think that "often" is not good enough. They may also accept – as I do – that people with Down syndrome often are loving, warm people who live happy lives. But they may still think that this is not the best they can do for their child. Perhaps they just want to have a child who will, eventually, come to be their intellectual equal, someone with whom they can have good conversations, someone whom they can expect to give them grandchildren, and to help them in their old age. Those are not unreasonable desires for parents to have.

What of the "powerful message that we seek to eliminate future persons with disabilities" that Beeson tells us is sent by prenatal diagnosis and abortion to people with disabilities? Her concern seems highly selective. She has surely noticed that every bottle of alcoholic beverage sold in the U.S.A. bears the words:

GOVERNMENT WARNING: (1) ACCORDING TO THE SURGEON GENERAL, WOMEN SHOULD NOT DRINK ALCOHOLIC BEVERAGES DURING PREGNANCY BECAUSE OF THE RISK OF BIRTH DEFECTS.

Does not that warning – much more visible to ordinary Americans than prenatal diagnosis – send out a "powerful message" that we should prevent the birth of children with defects? What about the message sent by programs that immunize girls against rubella? Is anyone seriously proposing to withdraw such government warnings, or end such immunization programs?

The Surgeon General's desire that women should not, through alcohol consumption, give birth to people with disabilities, does not in any way imply that he has less concern for the interests of people living with disabilities than he has for those without disabilities. As I have argued elsewhere, we can and should have equal consideration for the interests of all beings that have interests.[13] Although this is, in my view, the fundamental basis of equality both within our own species and between our species and beings of other species that have interests, for that very reason it may not satisfy the advocates of people with disabilities. But what other defensible sense can we give to the idea of equal worth?

Ani Satz has argued that measures to prevent the birth of people with disabilities are compatible with regarding people with disabilities as having equal worth, because these practices do not imply any judgments about the value of life with a disability:

The obese are not devalued by overweight individuals who join Jenny Craig on the belief that obesity detracts from quality of life ... Organizations actively try to prevent workplace, automobile, household, and sporting accidents, contributors to disabling conditions. These precautions do not judge the moral worth of disabled individuals. To argue otherwise would be to assume, reductio absurdum, that industrial workers or rock concert-goers who wear earplugs are indicating that membership in the deaf community would be of less value than membership in the hearing community.[14]

We should distinguish two different kinds of judgment that are in danger of being conflated in this passage: judgments about "the moral worth of disabled individuals" and judgments about the general quality of life, or even the value of life, with a given disability. The moral worth of individuals is not dependent on their abilities, except where they have very limited intellectual capacities; but the reductio with which Satz ends her argument in the passage quoted above is, in my view, not at all absurdum. If I take precautions to prevent deafness, I do so on the grounds that I think life with the ability to hear is, in general, better than life without the ability to hear. Is this perhaps just because I have been able to hear for the first 50 years of my life, and would have difficulty in making the adjustment to being a member of the Deaf community? That may be part of the story, but it is not the whole story. Imagine that shortly after the birth of our child, a doctor tells us that it has an ear infection, which unless treated will cause deafness. Fortunately, the doctor adds, there is an antibiotic that will clear up the infection in a few days. Would we contemplate for a moment saying: "Wait a minute, Doctor, we need to think about whether we value membership of the hearing community more highly than membership of the Deaf community"? Obviously not: but the reason we would not is not that we are judging membership in the Deaf community to be less desirable than membership in the hearing community, but because we take it for granted that it is less desirable.

To make this point correctly, we need to be very precise in our language. Jonathan Glover has said: "Medical treatment presupposes that health is better than sickness, but those who believe in it are able to treat sick people as their equals."[15] That is true, of course, but the sense in which the sick are our equals needs to be specified. As Glover himself has pointed out, if we do not have enough resources to treat all the sick, we have to decide who to treat. He has supported the view that in making this decision we should take into account both the expected life-span of the sick person, and the quality of that person's life, at least when it is clear that it is not worth living.[16] So while we treat the sick as our equals, socially, morally, and politically, when it comes to tough decisions about saving their lives, some of the sick are less equal than others.

The same point applies to a claim made by Allen Buchanan:

We devalue disabilities because we value the opportunities and welfare of the people who have them – and it is because we value people, all people, that we care about limitations on their welfare and opportunities. We also know that disabilities, as such, diminish opportunities and welfare, even when they are not so severe that the lives of those who have them are not worth living. Thus, there is nothing incoherent or disingenuous in our saying that we devalue the disabilities and wish to reduce their incidence *and* that we value all *existing* persons with disabilities – and value them equally to those who are not disabled.[17]

The argument of this passage is compelling, until we get to the word "equally" in its final clause. Suppose that there are two infants in the neonatal intensive care unit, and we have the resources to save only one of them. We know nothing about either of them, or their families, except that one infant has no disabilities, and the other has one of the disabilities that Buchanan mentions – a disability that will limit the child's "welfare and opportunities." In these circumstances, it seems rational, for precisely the reasons Buchanan gives, to save the life of the child without disabilities – but this shows that there is a clear sense in which we do not value both children equally.[18]

In our very commendable concern to give equal consideration and respect to every member of our community, and to avoid the least appearance of bias against those with disabilities, we are in danger of going to what is a truly absurd conclusion: that the abilities we have – to hear, to see, to walk, to speak, to understand, and reflect upon information given to us – are of no value. We must not deny the obvious truth that most people, disabled or not, would prefer to be without disabilities, and would prefer to have children without disabilities. There may be some members of the Deaf community and some people with achondroplasia who disagree, and of course there are many people with intellectual disabilities who are incapable of expressing an opinion, but to the best of my knowledge advocates for people in wheelchairs accept that they would be better off if they could walk; at least I am not aware of them ever calling for governments to stop wasting their taxes by supporting research into ways of overcoming paralysis.

If the use of cochlear implants means that there are fewer Deaf people, is this "genocide"? Does our acceptance of prenatal diagnosis and selective abortion mean that we are "drifting toward a eugenic resurgence that differs only superficially from earlier patterns"? If the use of the term "genocide" is intended to suggest a comparison with the Holocaust, or Rwanda, it overlooks the crucial fact that cochlear implants do not have victims. On balance, it seems that they benefit the people who have them; if this judgment is contestable, it is at least not clear that they are worse off for having the implant. Imagine a minority ethnic group in which all the parents reach separate decisions that their children will be better off if they marry a member of the majority group, and hence urge them to do so. Is this encouraging "genocide"? If so, it is genocide of such a harmless form that the term should be divorced from all its usual moral associations.

Similarly, if Beeson's reference to "earlier patterns" of eugenics is a veiled reference to Nazi policies that led to the murder of tens of thousands of disabled people, she is guilty of overlooking the vast moral gulf between what happened then and what is happening now. No state is ordering anyone's death; no one who wants to go on living is being murdered; no children whose parents want them to survive are being killed. The Nazi program was based on the interests of the *Volk*, and utter indifference to the interests of the individuals most involved, including both the victim and his or her family. Even if Beeson has in mind not Nazism but American eugenics in the first half of the present century, the differences are profound. That eugenics movement used compulsory sterilization of criminals, introduced an immigration policy based on belief in the superiority of the Northern European races, and became, as Dan Kevles puts it, a facade for "advocates of race and class prejudice, defenders of vested interests of church and state, Fascists, Hitlerites, and reactionaries generally."[19] There is no comparison between such state-sponsored, coercive policies, and the use of prenatal diagnosis and selective abortion by couples who choose to avail themselves of this option.

Even if cochlear implants are not genocidal, and prenatal diagnosis combined with selective abortion is not at all like past eugenic practices, they might be considered wrong. But consider the following principle:

For any condition X, if it would be a form of child abuse for parents to inflict X on their child soon after birth, then it must, other things being equal, at least be permissible to take steps to prevent one's child having that condition.

I propose this not as a self-evident truth, nor as a derivation from any particular moral foundation, but as something that might appeal to many people, irrespective of the foundations of their moral views. The "preventive principle," as I shall call it, requires us to reject the view that the fact that something is the outcome of the genetic lottery is enough to make it right. Why would anyone believe that? Only, I suggest, if somewhere deep down, they think of the genetic lottery as no lottery at all, but rather the workings of a divine Providence. If that were the case, then we might think it wrong to interfere with the natural order of things. But let us put that view aside, for lack of supporting evidence, and assume that the genetic lottery really is a lottery. Then, if there is no moral barrier that says we must not interfere with the way things are, the preventive principle seems sound.

Now let us apply the preventive principle to the cases we have been considering. Suppose that a Deaf couple give birth to a daughter who can hear normally. As they value very highly their membership of the Deaf community, and they fear that their daughter will not be a part of the Deaf community, they make arrangements with a sympathetic surgeon to destroy the child's hearing. The operation, performed under general anesthesia, causes the child no pain, but achieves its goal. The child will now be permanently deaf. Is this a case of child abuse? I suggest that it is. What the parents have done ensures that their child will never be able to hear Beethoven, or a babbling brook, or listen to lectures and debates delivered in spoken languages, except in translation. The child will also be at a disadvantage in countless other ways in getting through life. Admittedly, we must also take into account the benefits that the child will get from being part of the Deaf community, especially when being a part of the Deaf community means that the child grows up in the community to which her parents already belong. But that does not justify what they have done.

If you respond to this example in the way I do, and accept the principle I stated above, it follows that it must at least be permissible, other things being equal, for parents to take steps to ensure that their child will not be deaf. This argument does raise the difficulty of where to draw the line. Strictly, I could avoid this difficulty by pointing out that the preventive principle simply says that prenatal diagnosis and selective termination are permissible if they are a way of avoiding a condition that it would be child abuse to inflict on one's child. So the question could be answered with another question: would it be child abuse for a couple to ensure that their child would be a homosexual? In whatever way you answer that question, you should also answer the question whether the couple should be allowed to terminate a pregnancy on the basis of prenatal diagnosis that the child will be homosexual.

I will, however, say a little more on this topic. Andrew Solomon has written:

Being Deaf is a disability and a culture in modern America; so is being gay; so is being black; so is being female; so even, increasingly, is being a straight white male.

So is being paraplegic, or having Down syndrome. What is at issue is which things are so "cultural" that you would not think of "curing" them, and which things are so "disabling" that you must "cure" them – and the reality is that for some people each of these experiences is primarily a disability experience while for others it is primarily a cultural one.[20]

Is being black a disability? Is being gay a disability? The racial case is easy to distinguish from the case of deafness, because although it may be true deaf people must contend with some socially constructed barriers, it is also indisputable that they lack the ability to hear. African-Americans do not lack any ability that people of other races possess. There are only patterns of discrimination or prejudice. Hence being black is not a disability.

What about being gay? While gays and lesbians lack the ability to be sexually attracted to the opposite sex, straight people lack the ability to be sexually attracted to their own sex. This line of argument implies that unless we are bisexual we are suffering from an erotic disability. Is it possible to argue that homosexuals are disabled because they cannot enjoy "normal" sexual intercourse, involving a penis and a vagina? That would require an argument to the effect that this mode of sexual intercourse is superior to others that are available to gays and lesbians, and I do not know how, in the absence of an argument from "natural law," such an argument could be grounded. Nor do I think that an argument based in natural law would be satisfactory.[21]

Stephen Macedo has suggested a more plausible ground for seeing homosexuality as a disability:

Even if we were to wipe away all the prejudice in the world and even if homosexuals had all of the same opportunities as heterosexuals – including marriage and adoption – homosexuality would still be a misfortune: a misfortune resembling marriage to a sterile partner. Sterility is properly regarded as a misfortune (though *not*, it should be stressed, an especially grave one) and homosexuality can likewise be regarded as one, insofar as some of the great goods of marriage – the shared participation in pregnancy and new life – are not fully available to homosexual couples.

In a footnote, Macedo adds:

... because some gays and lesbians are likely to take (unjustified, I believe) offense on this score, I should emphasize that to the extent that there is misfortune here, it is a misfortune that I share.[22]

If infertility is a disability, it is one that seems in principle soluble for lesbians at least, once we learn how to mix gametes from same sex partners and inject them into a denucleated egg. Male homosexuals would still have to find a surrogate willing to carry the child for them. But perhaps at present, infertility within the relationship does mean that homosexuality remains a disability, though as Macedo says, not an especially grave one.

Shopping for beauty and brains

In February 1999, advertisements in newspapers in some of America's most prestigious universities offered $50,000 to an egg donor who was athletic, had scored extremely well in scholastic aptitude tests, and was at least 5′10″ tall.[23] Later in the same year Ronsangels.com opened with a splash of publicity. It featured eight "models," offering "beauty and brains to the highest bidder." Visitors to the site can see a photograph of each model, together with her vital statistics, the ages of her mother and grandmother, a brief biography, and an indication of the minimum bid required to obtain an egg, which ranges from $15,000 to $90,000. To provide some gender balance, the site also has a "sperm auction" featuring a well-muscled man in a brief bathing suit. His sperm is available for a minimum bid of $15,000.

The "Ron" in Ron's Angels is Ron Harris, no mere egg and sperm auctioneer but also something of a philosopher, as an "Editorial" that he has added to the site reveals:

It is human nature to strive to improve everything. From fruits and vegetables, to medicine, and even to plant and animal genes, we modify everything to produce the best we can. Now, modern science presents the miraculous possibility of improving ourselves. Currently, our means is *in vitro* fertilization, wherein your eggs or sperm are combined with the eggs or sperm of superior genetic background ... Of course, there are no guarantees that the children produced from superior genes combined with your own will result in similarly superior children – but our striving reflects the determination to pass every advantage possible along to our descendants.

It is not our intention to suggest that we make a super society of only beautiful people. This site simply mirrors our current society, in that beauty usually goes to the highest bidder. There are of course many other attributes that impart an advantage in our increasingly competitive society: intelligence, talent, personality, and social skills ... This is the first society to truly comprehend how important beautiful genes are to our evolution. Just watch television and you will see that we are only interested in looking at beautiful people. From the network anchors, to supermodels that appear in most advertisements, our society is obsessed with youth and beauty. As our society grows older, we inevitably look to youth and beauty ... If you could increase the chance of reproducing beautiful children, and thus giving them an advantage in society, would you?

Any gift such as beauty, intelligence, or social skills, will help your children in their quest for happiness and success.

Some may, admittedly, have their suspicions about ronsangels.com. The models and bids went unchanged for months. Bids were listed, but none exceeded the specified minimum. When I began work on this paper, the auctions had closing dates, some of which had already passed. Subsequently the closing dates disappeared from the site, and later the models offering their eggs became accessible only to subscribers. A clue to why this may be the case could be found in a link, no longer present, that once took you, in two clicks, to another Ron Harris site, where the interest in women was explicitly sexual rather than reproductive. Another click took you to Harris's very candid advice on "how to make money with an adult web site." Prominent here is the injunction to: "Get traffic, any way you can! ... do whatever you have to do to get traffic. Traffic is the e-porn industries' currency. The more you have the more money you will make."

Even if his egg sales are just a way of getting people to visit his porn site, Ronsangels.com is a test case for the view that the market knows best. The U.S.A. is exceptional among the industrialized nations in allowing a free market in human gametes. There are already other commercial operations selling gametes, and there can be little doubt that, unless such activities are prohibited, there will soon be more, offering couples ever more technologically sophisticated ways of improving their odds of having tall, slim children with above-average beauty, health, intelligence, and athletic, musical, and artistic talent.

There are many grounds on which we might find the ideas behind Ron's Angels distasteful, or worse. We could argue that they indicate a warped sense of how to think about one's future child, a sense shaped by a society that puts too high a premium on beauty and success. That may be, but what should we do about it? There is credible evidence suggesting that many of the things that parents look for in their children have a genetic component: physical appearance, including height and body shape, intellectual aptitude, many athletic skills, and longevity.

As we have already noted, parents already do their best to influence the environmental factors that undoubtedly also play a part in shaping these characteristics. They can now influence genetic factors as well as environmental ones, in one of three ways. By using *in vitro* fertilization, they can have the embryo screened before implantation; they can use prenatal diagnosis and selective abortion; and they can obtain eggs, sperm, or embryos from people they regard as genetically superior. All of these techniques have disadvantages. The first is costly, inconvenient, and does not always lead to a pregnancy. The second involves an abortion, which is not a pleasant procedure for a woman, irrespective of her views about the moral status of the fetus. The third means that the child will not be a biological child of the couple, but will carry the genes of at least one other person. Probably within the next two decades, however, we will have a fourth option: genetic enhancement of our own embryos.

Harris asks: "If you could increase the chance of reproducing beautiful children, and thus giving them an advantage in society, would you?" He is doubtless correct in his assumption that most of us will answer that question affirmatively. We go to so much effort to shape our children's environment to give them the best possible start in life, that once we gain the ability to select their genes, we are unlikely to reject it. What might restrain some potential parents are factors like risk, cost, and whether the children will still be their own children, in a biological sense. The last of these has up to now been a constraint on the number of couples willing to use donor eggs and sperm. But our rapidly increasing knowledge of human genetics will soon make it possible for us to have children who are genetically our own, and yet who are genetically superior to the children we would produce if we left it to the random process of normal reproduction. This will come initially through increasingly sophisticated genetic screening of *in vitro* embryos. Before very long, however, it will become possible to insert new genetic material safely into the *in vitro* embryo. Both of these techniques will enable couples to have a child whose abilities are likely to be superior to those offered by the natural lottery but who will be "theirs" in the sense of having their genes, not the genes of only one of them, or the genes of a third person, except (when genetic modification rather than simply genetic selection is used) to the extent necessary to produce the specific desired characteristics.

Many people say that they accept selection against serious diseases and disabilities, but not for enhancement above what is normal. There is, however, no bright line between selection against disabilities and selection for positive characteristics. From selecting against Huntington disease it is no great step to selecting against genes that carry a significantly elevated risk of breast or colon cancer, and from there it is easy to move to giving one's child a better than average genetic health profile. Similarly, if almost all of us are willing to abort a fetus that has Down syndrome, most of us will also be willing to abort one with genes that indicate other intellectual limitations, for example genes that correlate with IQ scores below 80. But why stop at 80? Why not select for at least average IQ? Or a bit above average? The existing market in human eggs suggests that some people will also select for height, which in turn correlates to some extent with income. Then, as Harris points out, there is beauty, and we will not reject the opportunity to ensure that our children are beautiful.

Choices, private and public

How should we react to the scenario that extrapolates beyond Ron's Angels? We could treat it as a slippery slope argument, one that proves that we must act now to stop prenatal screening, because otherwise we are heading toward a nightmarish future in which children are made to order, and wanted for their specifications, not loved for what they are. But taking the argument that way forces us either to reject something – current practices of prenatal diagnosis – that most people regard as a great boon, or to show that we can stop somewhere short of permitting the choices I have described. Neither is a convincing option. A second possibility is to say that the future just sketched is no nightmare, but a better society than we now have, one full of healthier, more intelligent, taller, better-looking – perhaps even more ethical? – people. There is, therefore, no "slippery slope," because the slope does not lead down to an abyss, but upward to a higher level of civilization than we have achieved so far.

Nozick's words cited at the start of this essay suggest a third possible answer: it is not up to us to judge whether the outcome of this process will be better or worse. In a free society, all we can legitimately do is make sure that the process consists of freely chosen individual transactions. Let the genetic supermarket rule – and not only the market, but also altruistic individuals, or voluntary organizations, anyone who wishes, for whatever reason, to offer genetic services to anyone who wants them and is willing to accept them on the terms on which they are offered.

That the U.S.A. should allow a market in eggs and sperm which goes some way towards fulfilling Nozick's prophecy is no accident. In other countries a practice that threatens to turn the child of a marriage into an item of commerce would meet powerful opposition from both conservative "family values" politics and from left of center groups horrified at the idea of leaving to the market something as socially momentous as the way in which future generations are conceived. In the U.S.A., however, that leftist attitude is restricted to groups on the margins of political life, and the conservatives who dominate Congress show their support for family values merely by preventing the use of federal funds for ends that they dislike; in all other respects, they allow their belief that the market always knows best to override their support for traditional family values.

There are strong arguments against state interference in reproductive decisions, at least when those decisions are made by competent adults. If we follow John Stuart Mill's principle that the state is justified in interfering with its citizens only to prevent harm to others, we could see such decisions as private ones, harming no one, and therefore properly left to the private realm.[24] For who is harmed by the genetic supermarket?

The parents are not harmed by having the healthier, handsomer, and more intelligent children that they want. Are the children harmed? In an article on the practice of buying eggs from women with specific desired characteristics like height and intelligence, George Annas has commented:

What's troubling is this commodification, this treating kids like products. Ordering children to specification cannot be good for the children. It may be good for adults in the short run, but it is not good for kids to be thought of that way.[25]

But to say that this is "not good" for these children forces us to ask the question: not good compared with *what*? The children for whom this is supposed not to be good could not have existed by any other means. If the egg had not been purchased, to be fertilized with the husband's sperm, that child would not have been alive. Is life going to be so bad for this child that he or she will wish never to have been born? That hardly seems likely. So on one reading of what the standard of comparison should be, it is clearly false that the purchase of these eggs is not good for the kids.[26]

Suppose that we read "not good for kids" as meaning "not the best thing for the next child of this couple." Then whether the purchase of the egg is or is not good for the kid will depend on a comparison with other ways in which the couple could have had a child. Suppose, to make the comparison easier, they are not infertile – they bought an egg only in order to increase their chances of having a tall, athletic child who would get into a very good university. If they had not done so, they would have had a child in the normal way, who would have been their genetic child. Was it bad for their child to buy the egg? Their child may have a more difficult life because he or she was "made to order," and perhaps will disappoint his or her parents. But perhaps their own child would have disappointed them even more, by being less likely to be any of the things that they wanted their child to be. I do not see how we can know which of these outcomes is more likely. So I do not think we have grounds for concluding that a genetic supermarket would harm either those who choose to shop there, or those who are created from the materials they purchase.

If we switch from an individualist perspective to a broader social one, however, the negative aspects of a genetic supermarket become more serious. Even if we make the optimistic assumption that parents will select only genes that are of benefit to their children, there are at least three separate grounds for thinking that this may have adverse social consequences. The first is that some of the traits that people seek to ensure for their children will be advantageous for them only in comparative, not absolute terms. To increase one's children's longevity is good for them, whether or not everyone else's longevity has been increased by a similar amount. To increase one's children's height, however, is beneficial only if it also moves them up relative to the height of others in their society. There would be no disadvantage in being 5′ tall, if the average height in the community were 4′9″ and there will be no advantage in being 6′3″ if the average height is 6′6″. Arguably, it would be better if everyone were shorter, because we would require less food to sustain us, could live in smaller houses, drive smaller, less powerful cars, and make a smaller impact on the environment. Thus being able to select for height – something couples are already doing, on a small scale, by offering more for the eggs of tall women – could start the human equivalent of the peacock's tail – an escalating "height race" in which the height that distinguishes "tall" people from those who are "normal" increases year by year, to no one's benefit, at considerable environmental cost, and perhaps eventually even at some health cost to the children themselves.[27]

The second ground for objecting to a genetic supermarket is the fear that it would mean less diversity among human beings. Not all forms of diversity are good. Diversity in longevity is greater when there are more people with genes that doom them to an early death. The loss of this diversity is welcome. But what about the loss of the merely unusual, or eccentric? Antony Rao, a specialist in behavioral therapy in children, finds that many middle and upper class parents come to him when their children behave in unusual ways, wanting them to be medicated, because "they fear that any deviation from the norm may cripple their child's future."[28] If this is true of behavioral abnormalities that for many children are merely a passing phase, it is likely to be even more true of genetic abnormalities. It is easy to imagine genetic screening reports that indicate that the child's genes are unusual, although the significance of the abnormality is not well understood (usually medical shorthand for "we do not have a clue"). Would many parents decide to terminate the pregnancy in those circumstances, and if so, would there be a loss of diversity that would leave human society a less rich place, and perhaps even, in the long run, reduce the species' capacity to adapt to changing circumstances?

The third and in my view most significant ground for objecting to a genetic supermarket is its threat to the ideal of equality of opportunity. John Schaar has written: "No policy formula is better designed to fortify the dominant institutions, values, and ends of the American social order than the formula of equality of opportunity, for it offers *everyone* a fair and equal chance to find a place within that order."[29] It is, of course, something of a myth to believe that equality of opportunity prevails in the U.S.A., because wealthy parents already give their children enormous advantages in the race for success. Nevertheless, the Ron's Angels slogan of "beauty and brains to the highest bidder" points to a future in which the rich have beautiful, brainy, healthy children, while the poor, stuck with the old genetic lottery, fall further and further behind. Thus inequalities of wealth will be turned into genetic inequalities, and the clock will be turned back on centuries of struggle to overcome the privileges of aristocracy. Instead, the present generation of wealthy people will have the opportunity to embed their advantages in the genes of their offspring. These offspring will then have not only the abundant advantages that the rich already give their children, but also whatever additional advantages the latest development in genetics can bestow on them. They will most probably therefore continue to be wealthier, longer-lived, and more successful than the children of the poor, and will in turn pass these advantages on to their children, who will take advantage of the ever more sophisticated genetic techniques available to them.

Will this lead to a *Gattaca* society in which "Invalids" clean toilets while "Valids" run the show and get all the interesting jobs?[30] Lee Silver has pictured a United States a millenium hence in which the separation between "Gene-enriched" humans and "Naturals" has solidified into separate species.[31] That is too far in the future to speculate about, but Maxwell Mehlman and Jeffrey Botkin may well be right when they predict that a free market in genetic enhancement will widen the gap between the top and bottom strata of our society, undermine belief in equality of opportunity, and close the "safety valve" of upward mobility.[32]

Suppose that we do not wish to accept this situation: what choices do we have? We can ban all uses of genetic selection and genetic engineering that go beyond the elimination of what are clearly defects. There are some obvious difficulties with this course of action.

First, are we violating Mill's principle, and if so, can we justify doing so? We could claim that although individual reproductive decisions appear only to affect the parties to the decision, and the child who develops from it, this appearance is deceptive. Reproduction of the kind described will change the nature of society by taking away the age-old dream that anyone can make it to the top. This is, arguably, a "harm to others" serious enough to justify the intervention of the state.

Second, who will decide what clearly is a defect? Presumably, a government panel will be assigned the task of keeping abreast with relevant genetic techniques, and deciding which are lawful and which are not. This allows the government a role in reproductive decisions, which some may see as even more dangerous than the alternative of leaving them to the market.

Third, there are serious questions about whether a ban on genetic selection and engineering for enhancement purposes could be made to work across the U.S.A., given that matters regulating conception and birth are in the hands of the states, rather than the federal government. In the case of surrogacy, attempts by various states of the U.S.A. to make the practice illegal, or to make surrogacy contracts void, have had little effect because Arkansas, California, and Ohio are more friendly to surrogacy. Couples seeking a surrogate to bear a child for them are prepared to travel to achieve what they want. As Silver remarks: "What the brief history of surrogacy tells us is that Americans will not be hindered by ethical uncertainty, state-specific injunctions, or high costs in their drive to gain access to any technology that they feel will help them achieve their reproductive goals."[33]

Fourth, assuming that we could get the U.S. Congress to ban genetic selection and engineering when used for enhancement, persuade the Supreme Court that the legislation violates neither the rights of the states to legislate in this area nor any constitutional rights to privacy in reproduction, and effectively enforce the ban within the U.S.A., we would still have to deal with the fact that we now live in a global economy. A small impoverished nation might be tempted to allow enhancement genetics, thus setting up a niche industry serving wealthy couples from the U.S.A. and other countries that have banned enhancement. Moreover, in view of the competitive nature of the global economy, it may even pay industrialized nations to encourage enhancement genetics, thus giving them an edge on those that do not. On Singapore's National Day, in 1983, Prime Minister Lee Kuan Yew gave a speech about the heritability of intelligence, and its importance for Singapore's future. Shortly afterwards, the government introduced measures explicitly designed to encourage university graduates to have more children.[34] Had genetic enhancement been available to Lee Kuan Yew at the time, he might well have preferred it to the government-sponsored computer dating services and financial incentives on which he was then forced to rely.

If a ban in the U.S.A. turns out to be unattainable, ineffective, or contrary to the vital interests of the U.S. economy, a bolder strategy could be tried. Assuming that the objective is to avoid a society divided in two along genetic lines, genetic enhancement services could be subsidized, so that everyone can afford them. But could society afford to provide everyone with the services that otherwise only the rich could afford? Mehlman and Botkin propose an ingenious solution: the state should run a lottery in which the prize is the same package of genetic services that the rich commonly buy for themselves. Tickets in the lottery would not be sold; instead every adult citizen would be given one. The number of prizes would relate to how many of these packages society could afford to pay for, and thus would vary with the costs of the genetic services, as well as with the resources available to provide them. To avoid placing a financial burden on the state, Mehlman and Botkin suggest, the use of genetic technologies could be taxed, with the revenue going to fund the lottery.[35] Clearly universal coverage would be preferable, but the use of a lottery would at least ensure that everyone has some hope that their children will join the ranks of the elite; and taxing those who are, by their use of genetic enhancement for their own children, changing the meaning of human reproduction seems a fair way to provide funds for it.

Thus shopping at the genetic supermarket has taken us to the surprising conclusion that the state should be directly involved in promoting genetic enhancement. The justification for this conclusion is simply that it is preferable to the most probable alternative – leaving genetic enhancement to the marketplace.

NOTES

1 Robert Nozick, *Anarchy, State and Utopia*. New York: Basic Books (1974), p. 315n.

2 Ron's Angels, www.ronsangels.com/index2html (last accessed 16 September 2005).

3 For further discussion of other objections, see Allen Buchanan, Choosing who will be disabled: genetic intervention and the morality of inclusion, *Social Philosophy and Policy* 13 (1996), 18–45; Christian Munthe, *The Moral Roots of Prenatal Diagnosis*, Royal Society for Arts and Sciences in Gothenburg, Studies in Research Ethics No. 7 (Gothenburg, Sweden, 1996); Dena Davis, Genetic dilemmas and the child's right to an open future, *Hastings Center Report* 27 (1997), 7–15; Lynn Gillam, Prenatal diagnosis and discrimination against the disabled, *Journal of Medical Ethics* 25 (1999), 163–71; Rosemarie Tong, Traditional and feminist bioethical perspectives on gene transfer: is inheritable genetic modification really *the* problem (Chapter 9, this volume); and Jackie Leach Scully, Inheritable genetic modification and disability: normality and identity (Chapter 10, this volume).

4 U.S. National Institutes of Health, Cochlear implants in adults and children, *NIH Consensus Statement Online* 13 (1995, 15–17 May), 1–30.

5 Brice Alden, The genocide of deaf culture, http://hometown.aol.com/scarter11/gdc.htm (last accessed 21 March 2000 and no longer available in 2005).

6 Sally Weale, Hearing both sides, *The Guardian* 6 October 1999, 10.

7 Ruth E. Ricker, Do we really want this? Little People of America Inc. comes to terms with genetic testing, July 1995, http://home.earthlink.net/~dkennedy56/dwarfism_genetics.html (last accessed 16 September 2005).

8 Arie Drugan, Anne Greb, M.P. Johnson, *et al.*, Determinants of prenatal decisions to abort for chromosome abnormalities, *Prenatal Diagnosis* 10 (1990), 483–90; Eva

Alberman, David Mutton, Roy G. Ide, *et al.*, Down's syndrome births and pregnancy terminations in 1989 to 1993: preliminary findings, *British Journal of Obstetrics and Gynaecology* 106 (1995), 445–7; cited by Rayna Rapp, *Testing Women, Testing the Fetus: The Social Impact of Amniocentesis in America.* London: Routledge (1999), p. 223.

9 Quoted from Ann Bradley, Why shouldn't women abort disabled fetuses? *Living Marxism* 82 (September 1995).

10 Diane Beeson, Social and ethical challenges of prenatal diagnosis, *Medical Ethics Newsletter* (Lahey Clinic) Winter (2000), 2; for similar claims, see Adrienne Asch, Prenatal diagnosis and selective abortion: a challenge to practice and policy, *American Journal of Public Health* 89 (1999), 1649–57, especially 1650; Christopher Newell, Critical reflections on disability, difference and the new genetics. In: Gabrielle O'Sullivan, Everlyn Sharman and Stephanie Short (eds.), *Goodbye Normal Gene: Confronting the Genetic Revolution.* Annandale, NSW: Pluto Press (1999).

11 See Peter Singer, *Practical Ethics*, 2nd edn, Cambridge: Cambridge University Press (1993), (Chapter 5).

12 Allen Buchanan makes the same point, using the example of a woman who postpones having a child because she is living in a refugee camp, in his Choosing who will be disabled: genetic intervention and the morality of inclusion, *Social Philosophy and Policy* 13 (1996), 18–45, 29.

13 Peter Singer, *Animal Liberation*, 2nd edn, New York: New York Review/Random House (1990), (Chapter 1).

14 Ani Satz, Prenatal genetic testing and discrimination against the disabled: a conceptual analysis, *Monash Bioethics Review* 18 (1999), 11–22, 16.

15 Jonathan Glover, Gene mapping, gene therapy and equality of respect. In: *Advances in Biotechnology: Proceedings of an International Conference organized by the Swedish Council for Forestry and Agricultural Research and the Swedish Recombinant DNA Advisory Committee* (Sollentuna, Sweden), 11–14 March 1990, p. 2.

16 Jonathan Glover, *Causing Death and Saving Lives.* Harmondsworth, Middlesex: Penguin (1977), see especially pp. 220–4.

17 Buchanan, Choosing who will be disabled, p. 33.

18 The World Health Organization is currently attempting to measure the global burden of disease. Its analysis holds that it is equally valuable to extend life by a finite period – say one year – irrespective of whether the person whose life is saved has a disability – say blindness – and that it can be justifiable to spend health care resources to prevent a disability such as blindness, even at the cost of not extending some lives that could be extended by those resources. It seems doubtful that these positions can be reconciled. Information from Dan Wikler, Measuring the global burden of disease: are all lives of equal worth? (lecture presented to the DeCamp Bioethics Seminar, Princeton University, April 18, 2000).

19 Daniel Kevles, *In the Name of Eugenics: Genetics and the Uses of Human Heredity.* New York: Knopf (1985), p. 164.

20 Andrew Solomon, Defiantly deaf, *The New York Times Magazine* 28 August 1994, p. 38.

21 See Peter Singer and Deane Wells, *Making Babies.* New York: Scribner (1985), pp. 24–9.

22 Stephen Macedo, Homosexuality and the conservative mind, *The Georgetown Law Journal* 84 (1995) 261–300, especially p. 269 and Note 122 at 292.

23 Gina Kolata, $50,000 offered to tall, smart egg donor, *The New York Times* 3 March 1999, A10.

24 John Stuart Mill, *On Liberty*, 3rd edn, London: Longmans, Green, Reader, and Dyer (1864).

25 Lisa Gerson, Human harvest, *Boston Magazine*, May 1999.

26 On the difficult issue of whether we can benefit a child by bringing it into existence, see Derek Parfit, *Reasons and Persons*. Oxford: Clarendon Press (1984), and Peter Singer, *Practical Ethics*, pp. 123–5.

27 Helena Cronin, *The Ant and the Peacock*. Cambridge: Cambridge University Press (1991), Chapter 5.

28 Jerome Groopman, The doubting disease, *New Yorker* 10 April 2000, p. 55.

29 John Schaar, *Legitimacy in the Modern State*. New Brunswick, NJ: Transaction Books (1981), p. 195; cited in Maxwell Mehlman and Jeffrey Botkin, *Access to the Genome: The Challenge to Equality*. Washington, DC: Georgetown University Press (1998), p. 100.

30 Andrew Niccol (director), *GATTACA* (film), Sony Pictures, 1997.

31 Lee Silver, *Remaking Eden*. New York: Avon (1998), p. 282.

32 Mehlman and Botkin, *Access to the Genome*, Chapter 6.

33 Silver, *Remaking Eden*, p. 177.

34 Chan Chee Khoon and Chee Heng Leng, Singapore 1984: breeding for big brother. In: Chan Chee Khoon and Chee Heng Leng, *Designer Genes: I.Q., Ideology and Biology*. Selangor, Malaysia: Institute for Social Analysis (Insan) (1984).

35 Mehlman and Botkin, *Access to the Genome*, see pp. 126–8.

List of Abbreviations

AAV:	adeno-associated virus (vector)
ADA:	adenosine deaminase
ARTs:	assisted reproductive technologies
AV:	adenoviral (vector)
CF:	cystic fibrosis
CVS:	chorionic villus sampling
DNA:	deoxyribonucleic acid
EG cell:	embryonic germ cell
ES cell:	embryonic stem cell
GLGT:	germ-line gene transfer
HD:	Huntington disease
HSC:	hematopoietic stem cell(s)
IGM:	inheritable genetic modification
IVF:	*in vitro* fertilization
IVONT:	*in vitro* oocyte nuclear transplantation
mRNA:	messenger RNA
MS:	multiple sclerosis
mtDNA:	mitochondrial DNA
NK cell:	natural killer cell
NT:	nuclear transplantation
PGD or PIGD:	preimplantation genetic diagnosis
PKU:	phenylketonuria
RNA:	ribonucleic acid.
SCGT:	somatic cell gene transfer
SCID:	severe combined immune deficiency
SCNT:	somatic cell nuclear transfer

Acknowledgments

We wish to thank Dr Richard Barling, Cambridge University Press, for his forbearance in seeing this project through; Fiona Mackenzie, Unit for History and Philosophy of Science, University of Sydney for indexing the book and for willingly assisting us, especially with pulling the project together at the end; our authors for their contributions and their contemplations; the staff at Cambridge University Press: Betty Fulford, Athena Horsten and Jayne Aldhouse; and the Project Management staff at Charon Tec for their help in finalizing the book. JEJR wishes to thank the National Health and Medical Research Council of the Australian Government for funding.

Is inheritable genetic modification the new dividing line?

John E.J. Rasko, Gabrielle M. O'Sullivan, and Rachel A. Ankeny

1.1 Slow but clear progress in achieving gene therapeutics

The promise of gene transfer as a way to cure or ameliorate a range of genetic and acquired human diseases dates back over 40 years.[1] "Gene therapy" can be defined as the introduction of new genetic information to achieve a therapeutic goal, for instance to replace, correct, or augment parts of the recipient's genome. Generally the use of wild-type or attenuated-virus vaccines is excluded from the purview of gene therapy, although their applications may be regarded technically as forms of gene-based prevention. Gene therapeutics include gene-based immunization strategies designed to prevent or treat cancers and autoimmune disorders, which are relatively non-controversial applications that are likely to prove successful. For over 30 years, the molecular biology revolution has steadily provided tools that allow us to manipulate, synthesize, and sequence DNA, culminating in the publication of the human genome sequence in 2000.[2] There has been an accelerating rate of discoveries since the earliest sequencing of mutated genes revealed the genetic basis of many human diseases. Nowadays a month rarely passes without a new disease-causing gene being linked to one of over 4000 human diseases that have been described. But besides providing new diagnostic genetic tests and some insights into disease causation, the discovery of disease-causing genes in itself has not generally led directly to therapies.

The next logical step for the field of molecular medicine was to ask whether non-mutated versions of disease-causing genes could be used for therapy. The concept of treating life-threatening diseases with genes remains compelling in its simplicity, but implementing this idea has proven highly challenging. The problems hindering realization of the promise offered by gene therapy techniques include technical difficulties in gene delivery and control, clinical failures, and over-hyped expectations, the latter of which is shared by other areas of genetic research. However, despite these problems, there are few who doubt that one day the technology to deliver successful gene therapy will be sufficiently mature and robust to achieve widespread clinical acceptance. For many genetic disorders, there are no satisfactory pharmacologic or cell-based therapies, and the persuasive idea of treating the root cause of such diseases has never lost its appeal. This book addresses a question that will arise once the technical hurdles of somatic cell gene transfer (SCGT) are overcome: whether genetic modification of the human germ line and other types of inheritable genetic modification (IGM) will ever be ethically and socially justifiable.

Genes cannot function outside the context of a cell, and thus any potential gene therapy must use specific target cells as vehicles. Since stem cells are long-lived and capable of massive expansion in number, they offer an obvious, if not straightforward, cellular target for gene therapies. Assuming that medical therapy using genes is a worthwhile goal, what would be the "minimum therapeutic unit" to transfer the genetic payload, so to speak? In one sense, whole organ transplantation is a "macroscopic" version of gene therapy, insofar as organ transplantation uses tissues that contain cells, whose genes deliver a therapeutic function. These therapies have been used successfully for decades to treat particular diseases, and include transplantation of kidney, liver, lung, and/or heart tissue. For those proponents of stem cell therapy (whether involving therapeutic cloning or, less controversially, adult stem cells), a "minimum therapeutic unit" involves the transplantation of whole cells such as skin, bone marrow, or peripheral blood hematopoietic stem cells, which are commonly used to treat malignant disorders of blood cells such as leukemia. The problem confronting each of the above cellular and tissue-based therapies is immune rejection and the consequent commitment to long-term immune suppression of the recipients, which in turn makes them vulnerable to infection.

Downscaling in terms of size, those wishing to use therapies based on chromosomes or genes adopt a more reductionist approach with the aim of modifying the existing genome of the recipient's cells. Although the genetic engineering of cells could be achieved on organ-, tissue-, or cell-based levels, parsimony dictates that, all other things being equal, the smallest intervention required for success should be preferred. Of central importance to this book is the important distinction between those gene transfer procedures that could lead to inheritable changes and those that do not. Interventions that could lead to IGM consist of ooplasmic transfer, gene transfer to reproductive cells and their precursor cells, and embryonic stem (ES) cell manipulations including reproductive cloning. Current therapeutic interventions that might never be expected to lead to IGM include the whole organ transplantation procedures described above and adult stem cell therapies such as hematopoietic stem cell transplantation.

This chapter does not examine the development of, and procedures involved in, human gene transfer in detail. A number of excellent books detail technical aspects of gene transfer and stem cell technology,[3] which also are summarized in essays in this book by John E.J. Rasko and Douglas J. Jolly, and Rudolph Jaenisch.[4] However, certain highly-publicized tragedies, failures, and mistakes have taken place in the brief history of gene therapy research that provide the historical and experimental context out of which some of the more controversial aspects of gene transfer have emerged.

Once the recombinant DNA revolution became well-established in the 1970s, early experiments in mice suggested that gene therapy might work.[5] In 1980, Martin Cline at the University of California at Los Angeles (UCLA) sought to transfect bone marrow cells from an Italian patient and an Israeli patient with a gene in order to treat their thalassemia. As has been documented, the trial was not approved (as was required) by the UCLA Institutional Review Board; there was an intention to hide the true nature of the experiment; there was no clinical or scientific follow-up of the two patients; and there were scientific reasons at the time that argued against the likelihood of success of such an experiment.[6] Hence, Cline received severe academic punishment and ceased research in this field. This first non-viral human gene therapy trial led to substantial scientific and public furor that eventually forced the United States federal government to expand the responsibilities of the Recombinant DNA Advisory Committee (RAC) to include human gene therapy. Eventually, approved clinical trials were initiated in 1990. The first involved a 4-year-old child, Ashanti de Silva – who suffered from severe combined immunodeficiency (SCID) – being re-infused with her own gene-modified cells; and the second involved the use of gene-modified tumor-infiltrating blood cells aimed at treating cancers. Since then, over 1000 clinical trials have been undertaken worldwide involving thousands of individuals.[7] To date, no gene transfer procedure has been approved by the Food and Drug Administration (FDA) for use in the U.S.A. However, in 2004 China approved production of an anti-cancer gene therapeutic.[8] The biotechnology investment market does not tolerate delays and failures well, and the peak of over 100 biotechnology companies with a focus on gene therapy has dwindled to about one-fifth of these original numbers.

Cline's ethically- and scientifically-suspect gene transfer experiments provided an inauspicious start for the field, but worse was to come when the first fatality directly attributable to a gene therapy trial was reported. In 1999, 18-year-old Jesse Gelsinger, who suffered from a rare enzyme disorder affecting the liver, but who had been relatively healthy before participating in the trial, died soon after receiving a high dose of experimental adenovirus designed to provide gene therapy. His death shocked the gene therapy field and led to the suspension of all gene therapy trials being conducted at the time. However it was not the death of a human volunteer *per se* that caused the storm, but subsequent revelations regarding problems with trial design, informed consent, and the lack of medical caution exercised at the time of gene delivery, as well as the compromise of the chief investigator who had significant financial incentives if the trial was successful. Six years after this death, a settlement was reached between the U.S. Justice Department and the chief investigator of the trial.[9]

The final example highlights the greatest clinical achievement in gene transfer to date, which was tempered by profound disappointment and was described by a leader in the field as "The Best of Times, The Worst of Times."[10] In a trial initiated in France, over 10 young children suffering from SCID have been treated with their own gene-modified hematopoietic stem cells because they were not able to receive a potentially-curative bone marrow transplant from a matched donor. Within a short time, it was clear that the clinical and cellular response to this gene therapy was close to miraculous, leading to the successful restoration of the immune system in recipients.[11] After a period of re-invigoration and rekindled optimism fueled by this result, the field was struck a serious blow when it was revealed that leukemia had developed in a minority of the experimental gene transfer trial participants.[12] Not only was it shown that the gene transfer itself had led to the leukemias (due to induced mutations caused by the viral gene transfer technology), but that this technical problem might affect other promising forms of experimental gene transfer. Similar trials were put on hold owing to these safety concerns until a review of the technology indicated that the unexpectedly high occurrence of leukemia was likely to be unique to this specific trial.[13] After 15 years of clinical trials, this seeming "triumph" of gene therapy has become another example of the difficulties that this novel technology has continued to experience. Despite the serious side effects, however, the French SCID trial was the first example where not only was the specific root genetic cause of a disease diagnosed, but a gene therapeutic was successfully used to treat it.

1.2   Are there "natural" precedents for IGM?

Scientific discussions about the future of gene therapy often focus on the technologic problems that have occurred in these early trials, as reviewed above. But most ethical and social critiques of gene therapy have focused on the problematic nature of IGM, and objections to it often stem from ideas about what is "natural" and arguments against intentionally causing genetic changes in future generations. However in recent years there has been what might be considered to be a provocative "precedent" for IGM in the demonstration that there are now human babies who have three biologic parents as a result of medical intervention.

In 2001, a reproductive medicine group in the U.S.A. reported the existence of two 1-year-old children who inherited genetic material from three unrelated genetic "parents".[14] In a follow-up letter, the researchers noted that 16 babies had been conceived by the same ooplasmic transplantation method.[15] In 2002, an FDA Advisory Committee reported at least two dozen births using this method that have been supervised by three fertility clinics since 1998.[16] This experimental method of ooplasmic transfer is designed to improve successful pregnancy rates for couples who are infertile due to recurrent implantation failure. The proponents of ooplasmic transfer argue that unknown factors are defective in the cytoplasm of some oocytes, leading to loss of viability of the pregnancy. The "therapy" involves the introduction of cytoplasmic material from a healthy donor oocyte, which is intended to provide beneficial factors and sub-cellular components, including mitochondria. However, mitochondria carry their own unique DNA, which encode almost 40 known genes not found in the nuclear DNA. The mitochondrial DNA (mtDNA) represents only one-tenth of a percent of the known genes present in cells, but abnormalities in it can transmit approximately 50 genetic diseases (e.g., Leber's Hereditary Optic Neuropathy).

What is often neglected in descriptions of classical Mendelian inheritance is that mtDNA is almost completely (about 99.99%) inherited from one's mother.[17] Because mitochondria must self-replicate independent of somatic nuclear division, and because they do not participate in the careful segregation that occurs when nuclear chromosomes replicate, they are apparently randomly allocated to daughter cells during mitosis. Thus children produced as a result of ooplasmic transfer followed by *in vitro* fertilization have one set of nuclear DNA each from the mother and the father, as well as a mixture of mtDNA from the mother and the woman who donated the cytoplasm, a phenomenon known as heteroplasmy. The female descendents of children conceived by ooplasmic transfer would receive the genetic inheritance of three parents. Such a reproductive intervention produces a situation that is scientifically akin to the ultimate aim of IGM, namely to provide therapy for, or prevent, genetic disease by the addition of new genetic material from a third source. In late 2004, an application was submitted to the U.K. Human Fertilization and Embryology Authority to perform a variant of ooplasmic transfer in which the nucleus from a fertilized egg from a woman with a genetic disease carried by her mitochondria would be transplanted into an enucleated donor egg. Thus inheritance of the woman's faulty mitochondria might be avoided, but such nuclear transfer would intentionally lead to children with three genetic parents.

Perhaps even more shocking for those who hold dear one's "right" to a "relatively fixed" genome (i.e., one inherited from two parents) is the fact that heteroplasmy occurs naturally in most animals, including humans.[18] Although the mechanism for heteroplasmy is far from clear, its existence has famously been used to resolve a genetic discrepancy in descendents of the Tsar Nicholas II who was slaughtered along with his Tsarina and their five children during the Bolshevik uprising in 1917.[19]

The simple fact is that, through ooplasmic transfer, new genetic information has been purposefully introduced into the germ line of humans, and at very least a scientific precedent has been set for intentional transfer of genes under some circumstances. Since mtDNA represents only a tiny percentage of the total genome, some have dismissed the precedent set by ooplasmic transfer as a "red herring" in terms of the ethical and social issues raised by other types of IGM. But such arguments neglect the overwhelming attention paid by some regulators and ethicists to the problematic nature of the inadvertent addition of even one gene to the genome, let alone IGM intended as therapy. Indeed, the FDA has called ooplasmic transfer a "*de facto* germ-line gene transfer" technique and, along with the governments of China and the U.K., has effectively banned it.[20] Without doubt this technology remains experimental and the possibility that its use may predispose children to an increased risk of genetic abnormalities needs to be carefully tested using preclinical models and monitoring of the health of children already conceived in this manner.

The facts that heteroplasmy occurs naturally in human populations and may be experimentally introduced by ooplasmic transfer highlights a question, and a theme, of this book: is IGM really a dividing line that should not be crossed or even considered? The question considered in various ways by the authors of the essays in this book is whether IGM is intrinsically morally objectionable, and what limits (if any) should be placed on it.

1.3   Why focus on "IGM"?

Early in this project, we decided to define the types of genetic interventions to be examined in terms of their intended and potentially-realizable effects (i.e., IGM), rather than in terms of the biologic materials or means used in their application (e.g., germ-line gene modification). This distinction arose because we consider intentional inheritability to be the essential characteristic of the interventions in question, which distinguishes them from other types of interventions that have been argued to be less ethically problematic (e.g., SCGT), and that the tissues and means of mediating them are secondary aspects of the process.

The term "IGM" hence indicates those procedures where the material and means used have the capacity to facilitate the intended transmission of particular genetic alterations to future generations. If our primary focus was on the secondary aspects of the interventions (i.e., the tissues targeted for modification), our considerations could have been confounded by the definitional problems that have characterized discussions about intentional IGM of humans for the last 20 years, namely, the blurring of the boundaries between somatic and germ-line tissues, and between intentional and inadvertent effects. For example, we might have argued about whether ooplasm does or does not constitute part of the germ line, and we might have concluded that it does not, probably on the basis that its genetic content is too small to contribute significantly to the total genetic make-up of an individual. But, as discussed above, the recent history of assisted reproductive technology makes this question difficult to answer, as it is not clear that the answer to it lies in quantitative estimates of genetic contribution.

In choosing to use the term "IGM" instead of "germ-line gene modification," we are not rejecting the idea of the "germ line" in any sense. The germ line has a definite existence and is a clearly definable biologic tissue (despite its various other interpretations). It constitutes the reproductive cells of an organism (i.e., the germ cells, including their products, and gametes) that can transmit genetic information from one generation to the next. The germ line has the major role to play in inheritable genetic interventions and is essential to discussions about them.[21]

In rejecting the term "germ-line gene modification" for general use in this book, we hope to prevent confusion between the aims of IGM and of germ-line engineering, which are often quite distinct. For example, one could aim to engineer the germ line for the sole purpose of introducing a genetic change into every cell of an individual (while controlling tissue-specific expression) without wishing for the change to be inherited by his or her progeny. In this situation, one would have to figure out how auxiliary chromosomes could be blocked "from passing through the sexual cycle to the next generation."[22] The rationale behind this aim is that rapid development of the science means that each new generation will want to have more up-to-date versions of the change and not be tied to a fixed version embedded within it.

Alternatively one might aim to engineer the germ line for the purposes of introducing a genetic change into every cell of an individual (while controlling tissue-specific expression) and *want* the change to be inherited by his or her progeny. In this situation, one would have to determine how auxiliary chromosomes could be consistently passed through the sexual cycle to the next generation. The rationale behind this aim is that each new generation would not have to undergo modification (i.e., the disease phenotype in question would be removed from future generations). These two situations show how useful the term "germ line" is, and at the same time how confusing the term "germ-line gene modification" can be (at least as it has been used in the literature to date), and how IGM more precisely describes the subject of this book.

Based on our criterion of intentional heritability, IGM is a biomedical intervention (molecular, genetic, or cellular) that alters the set of genes that a subject has available to transmit to his or her offspring. It includes all interventions performed at an early enough stage in an organism's development to have inheritable effects on its germ cells (gametes and gamete-forming tissues). Audrey Chapman and Mark Frankel, among others, have relied on this definition when discussing these types of interventions.[23] Thus this book focuses on intentional IGM by the application of techniques such as the use of artificial chromosomes, viral vectors, oligonucleotides, cell fusion, and sub-cellular component transplantation (e.g., mitochondria). Other potentially powerful mediators of IGM such as social and cultural practices, alteration of the environment (e.g., by nuclear radiation), and side effects of non-genetic treatments for infertility or other diseases (e.g., by chemotherapeutic agents) are not considered. Germ cell and ES cell modification constitute the major IGM subtypes.

1.4   What about the "dividing line"?

Discussions about the potential for biotechnologic alteration of human germ cells and whole human beings reflect concerns about benefits, risks, safety, and consent among other ethical, biomedical, and social issues. They also reflect a deep concern about the destiny of "human freedom, equality, and dignity,"[24] as well as human identity and where the limits of human intervention should be drawn. They are a sign of deep fears that hitherto natural attributes will be brought "within the sphere of social control, and thereby within the domain of justice."[25] Hence commentators have traditionally focused on constructing dividing lines between what should and should not be permissible, and on determining the conditions that must be satisfied before these lines might be crossed, if ever.

All discussions are partly shaped by the language used in them, and debates about intentional inheritable genetic interventions are no exception, as overt "dividing line" language has been used for over 20 years.[26] Dividing lines have been constructed, and then invariably deconstructed, between the natural and the social or technologically-engineered; the somatic cell and the germ line; enhancement and therapy; the intentional and the inadvertent; and humans and other species. The language of the "dividing line" is often accompanied by that of the "slippery slope" – the idea that once a technology has begun to be implemented, its application cannot be controlled, and some dividing line will inevitably be crossed between what is moral and what is immoral. The dividing line was further blurred by the appeal of some commentators to the "principle of double effect," whereby ethical difficulties are not associated with crossing moral lines, so long as the "crossing" is unintentional, or a sort of side effect of another, morally just action.[27]

Science has also blurred these lines, sometimes by crossing them in unexpected ways. The somatic cell/germ line divide has been crossed by somatic cell nuclear transfer (SCNT) in animals;[28] the enhancement/therapy divide is becoming untenable as enhancement and therapy are becoming less distinguishable as disease is being constantly redefined;[29] the intentional/inadvertent divide is not sustainable in terms of moral consequences;[30] and there does not appear to be a unified definition of species.[31] The problem with "dividing line" language is that it polarizes debate and competing, diametrically opposed, positions are compared with one another, often in isolation from other possible combinations of diverse positions.

It is our hope that while use of the term "IGM" is unlikely to fully dissolve the barriers to constructive discussion, it will invoke a different type of dividing line that facilitates social, ethical, and biologic assessment of intentional inheritable gene interventions by allowing clear distinctions between targets, and tissues, means, intentions, effects, and consequences, and their inter-comparison, without attempting to "solve the moral questions by artful redefinition or by denying to some morally crucial element a name that makes clear that there is a moral question to be faced."[32] In using the term "IGM," and even in grounding this book at the outset with technical and scientific explorations of these and related technologies,[33] we have no desire to create a new barrier to discussion by "subordinating social and ethical issues to technical and scientific debate in the regulatory arena."[34] At the same time, we support Katherine

High's wise counsel that we must "stay grounded in science and the realities of drug development if we wish to develop novel therapeutics."[35]

The term "IGM" conveys a change in focus within the field of gene transfer research from the question of "can we find a disease in which we can justify attempting [IGM]?", to the question of "can we use the new tools to identify a safe basis from which to proceed?"[36] It also emphasizes the need to move towards using the more ethically and technically appropriate language associated with experimental trials rather than "therapy" language, particularly given the nascent status of this field. We generally avoid using the term "germ-line gene therapy" (except where used in its strictest meaning to indicate something that is actually intended to be therapeutic) in part because human IGM, at this stage, is experimental. But in addition, if IGM were to be implemented on a widespread basis, in many cases its primary aim would be to prevent a genetic condition in a potential, future individual, rather than to treat a disease condition in the individual receiving the transferred gene(s).[37]

1.5   IGM as a tool for ethical debate

Against this background, the essays in this book are designed to examine ethical and policy issues associated with IGM and related technologies using a range of disciplinary approaches. Rather than viewing ethical debate as narrowly grounded in science, the biomedical/clinical context, or moral philosophy, the contributors to this book explore ethical issues within their wider scientific, political, social, cultural, and legal contexts. There is considerable confusion amongst members of the public (and even many expert commentators) as to the connections between technical/biologic and ethical issues in this domain, and many essays in this book attempt to disentangle this new Gordian knot.

Several essays take the form of thought experiments, imagining a range of potential futures and how we might react to them, or perhaps prevent them from occurring. For instance, Peter Singer introduces the volume using Robert Nozick's metaphor of the "genetic supermarket" to lay out a framework that can be used to examine moral questions related to genetic technologies for enhancement.[38] Singer also questions what counts as therapy and as disability, in order to project for us a picture of a future where IGM and other genetic technologies might become more widely available, for those who can afford them. The crucial questions then become not whether or not we should permit enhancement, or what counts as therapy, but instead whether these technologies should be privately or publicly controlled, and by what mechanisms. The themes of public policy and control in a not-so-distant future are echoed in Roberta Berry's essay, which claims that "bioethics can speak helpfully to politics about gene transfer by explicating both the past and an imagined future."[39] To reflect in a useful manner on any potential future for IGM requires a solid grounding in our past

history of uses and abuses of genetic medicine, eugenics, and genetic counselling, as well as clear reflection on what our societal norms have been, and
what norms should be furthered in public policy.

Françoise Baylis and Jason Scott Robert imagine a different future, one
where intentional IGM has become widespread, in order to consider how some
fundamental boundaries, or perhaps dividing lines, might be crossed.[40] They
use the concept of "radical rupture" as a heuristic device to explore the ways in
which volitional IGM could cause major disruptions to our concepts and ideas
associated with genetic inheritance, genetic legacy, and species. Eric T. Juengst,
in contrast, examines a future that is already here: one of strange alliances
forged on the basis of shared commitment to prohibiting IGM.[41] He argues
that although talk of "preserving the species" (such as that used in draft legislation promoted to the United Nations) may initially seem attractive, it smuggles
in dangerous, essentializing assumptions not only about the human species and
genetics, but about how we assign moral rights. As he argues, "The human gene
pool, unlike the sea, has no top, bottom, or shores: it cannot be 'preserved.' The
reservoir of human mutual respect, good will, and tolerance for difference,
however, seems perennially in danger of running dry. *That* is the truly fragile
heritage that we should work to preserve in monitoring genetic research on
behalf of the future." Denis Kenny undermines a different set of dangerous
assumptions, namely those that envision our universe as static and nature as
given, with human beings having no right to intervene in this order in any significant ways.[42] Instead, he advocates a notion of a "creative universe" with an
alternative cosmology, one that might lead us to conclude that in fact IGM is
part of our responsibilities to ourselves and this universe.

The fragility of various concepts – notably disease, normality, and human
identity – is taken up in several essays, most notably by Jackie Leach Scully in her
examination of IGM in relation to disability.[43] She argues that we must look at
the ethical and social issues about these technologies from a disability perspective, not only because disabled and chronically ill people are likely to be those for
whom IGM and related technologies will have the greatest and most pressing
impacts, but also because disabled people have novel perspectives particularly
with regard to identity and other fundamental aspects of human life. Isabel
Karpin and Roxanne Mykitiuk[44] take a feminist legal approach to investigate legislative controls on reproductive technologies and particularly those associated
with genetic modifications which provide limits on scientific innovation in order
to ensure safe and ethical research, but also reveal how such legislation and its
language is attempting to dictate what is to count as "normal" reproduction.
Thus as also argued by Rosemarie Tong,[45] rather than rehearsing the usual
bioethical debates, disability and feminist perspectives should lead us to recast
the very questions that we ask, and to whom we address those questions.

Indeed, rather than addressing our questions about genetic technologies,
IGM, and other bioethical dilemmas solely to bioethical experts or policy

makers, Joan A. Scott contends that we must listen to those most affected by these technologic developments, and attempt to determine what they want and how they conceptualize the main issues, in order to provide them appropriate guidance in any current or future clinical setting.[46] Christoph Rehmann-Sutter also draws on typically ignored voices of those suffering from or at risk for genetic illness, as well as the "voices" implicit in our popular cultural narratives that touch on issues associated with IGM.[47] From the Frankenstein monster story to H.G. Wells' *The Island of Dr Moreau*, we have been fascinated and terrified about scientific power and creation; IGM is a further step along a technologic path whose wonders and risks have been long recognized, if we look beyond our usual source materials. Gabrielle M. O'Sullivan draws our attention to IGM that is already widespread, namely non-human animal genetic modification, and introduces the debates that surround its use as a mirror through which we could usefully consider the parallel ethical issues likely to be raised when these technologies are applied to humans, notably concerns about animal welfare and risks to human health and the environment.[48]

In the ever-more complicated social and political context within which science and medicine operate today, bioethics must be accountable to the broader public and cultivate its participation in decision-making about key issues, such as those associated with IGM. Accordingly, this book has been designed to provide alternative viewpoints in an accessible format for a wide scientific, academic, and general audience by developing a dialogue between authors located around the globe and across different disciplinary and institutional perspectives. Although we seem to be entering a troubling political period where controls are increasingly being placed not only on what is allowed but also even on what can be discussed,[49] it is crucial to actively foster debate. In this sense, we endorse the so-called "navigational approach" advocated by Berry. This approach "acknowledges that there is no authoritative source of all the practical principles that should guide our conduct as we encounter novel problems over time, but a collection of practical reasoners who develop these principles through engagement with experience and one another. The approach is risky for those who know resolutions to the questions of gene transfer in advance, but hopeful for those who do not know but want to."[50] We do not claim to know the answers or to provide any resolutions, but we hope this book can help you to begin to ask the right questions not only about IGM, but more generally about bioethics and our shared, yet fragile, human future.

NOTES

1   J.A. Wolff and Joshua Lederberg, An early history of gene transfer and therapy, *Human Gene Therapy* 5 (1994), 469–80.

2 Colin F. Macilwain, World leaders heap praise on human genome landmark, *Nature* 405 (2000), 983–6.

3 Theodore Friedmann, *The Development of Human Gene Therapy*. Cold Spring Harbor, NY: Cold Spring Harbor Laboratory Press (1999); Angel Cid-Arregui and Alejandro Garcia Carranca, *Viral Vectors: Basic Science and Gene Therapy*. Natick, MA: Eaton Publishing (2000); Thomas F. Kresina, *An Introduction to Molecular Medicine and Gene Therapy*. New York: Wiley-Liss (2001).

4 John E.J. Rasko and Douglas J. Jolly, The science of inheritable genetic modification (Chapter 2, this volume); Rudolf Jaenisch, Nuclear cloning, embryonic stem cells, and gene transfer (Chapter 3, this volume).

5 K.E. Mercola and M.J. Cline, Sounding boards: the potentials of inserting new genetic information, *New England Journal of Medicine* 303 (1980), 1297–300.

6 See National Reference Center for Bioethics Literature, Scope note 24 – Gene therapy, The Joseph and Rose Kennedy Institute of Ethics, Georgetown University http://www.georgetown.edu/research/nrcbl/publications/scopenotes/sn24.htm (last accessed 4 April 2005).

7 M. Edelstein, *The Journal of Gene Medicine* Clinical Trial Site, www.wiley.co.uk/genmed/clinical/ (last accessed 31 March 2005).

8 Sue Pearson, Hepeng Jia and Keiko Kandachi, China approves first gene therapy, *Nature Biotechnology* 22 (2004), 3–4.

9 Erika Check, Sanctions agreed over teenager's gene-therapy death, *Nature* 433 (2005), 674.

10 W. French Anderson, Gene therapy: the best of times, the worst of times, *Science* 288 (2000), 627–9.

11 Marina Cavazzana-Calvo, Salima Hacein-Bey, Geneviève de Saint Basile, *et al.*, Gene therapy of human severe combined immunodeficiency (SCID)-X1 disease, *Science* 288 (2000), 669–72.

12 S. Hacein-Bey-Abina, C. Von Kalle, M. Schmidt, *et al.*, LMO2-associated clonal T cell proliferation in two patients after gene therapy for SCID-X1, *Science* 302 (2003), 415–9.

13 Donald B. Kohn, Michael Sadelain and Joseph C. Glorioso, Occurrence of leukaemia following gene therapy of X-linked SCID, *Nature Reviews Cancer* 3 (2003), 477–88.

14 Jason A. Barritt, Carol A. Brenner, Henry E. Malter, *et al.*, Mitochondria in human off-spring derived from ooplasmic transplantation, *Human Reproduction* 16 (2001), 513–6. "Parents" has been placed in scare quotes here by us to draw attention to the unusual nature of the genetic relation in these cases but also to remain neutral as how parentage should be defined in such cases. For a related discussion on the power of terminology and our biases with regard to "normal reproduction," see Isabel Karpin and Roxanne Mykitiuk, Regulating inheritable genetic modification, or policing the fertile scientific imagination? A feminist legal response (Chapter 11, this volume).

15 Jason A. Barritt, Carol A. Brenner, Henry E. Malter, *et al.*, Rebuttal: interooplasmic transfers in humans, *Reproductive Biomedicine Online* 3 (2001), 47–8.

16 U.S. Food and Drug Administration (FDA), Biological Response Modifiers Advisory Committee (BRMAC), Briefing Document for Day 1, Ooplasm transfer as method

to treat female infertility, 9 May 2002, http://www.fda.gov/OHRMS/DOCKETS/ac/02/briefing/3855B1_01.pdf (last accessed 29 March 2005).

17 Friderun Ankel-Simons and Jim M. Cummins, Misconceptions about mitochondria and mammalian fertilization: implications for theories on human evolution, *Proceedings of the National Academy of Sciences USA* 93 (1996), 13859–63.

18 Paul D. Olivo, Michael J. Van de Walle, Philip J. Laipis, *et al.*, Nucleotide sequence evidence for rapid genotypic shifts in the bovine mitochondrial DNA D-loop, *Nature* 306 (1983), 400–2.

19 Pavel L. Ivanov, Mark J. Wadhams, Rhonda K. Roby, *et al.*, Mitochondrial DNA sequence heteroplasmy in the Grand Duke of Russia Georgij Romanov establishes the authenticity of the remains of Tsar Nicholas II, *Nature Genetics* 12 (1996), 417–20.

20 U.S. FDA, BRMAC, Ooplasm transfer as method to treat female infertility.

21 It is interesting to note that ooplasmic transfer techniques point us to parallels between ooplasm and germ plasm. The term "germ plasm" (as currently used) refers to complex (sometimes undefined) components in the germ cells that contribute to their function, such as the protoplasm, which consists of the nucleus and the cytoplasm with which it interacts. Thus viewed in this way, ooplasm could be claimed to be a "form" of germ plasm.

22 John Campbell and Gregory Stock, A vision for practical human germ-line engineering. In: Gregory Stock and John Campbell (eds.), *Engineering the Human Germline: An Exploration of the Science and Ethics of Altering the Genes We Pass to Our Children.* Oxford: Oxford University Press (2000), p. 11.

23 Audrey R. Chapman and Mark S. Frankel, Framing the issues. In: Audrey R. Chapman and Mark S. Frankel (eds.), *Designing Our Descendents: The Promises and Perils of Genetic Modification.* Baltimore, MD: John Hopkins University Press (2003), pp. 5–6. Note that the term "heritable genetic modification" is synonymous with IGM, whereas the term "germ-line gene modification" is not always interchangeable with IGM, although it is sometimes used as such.

24 The President's Enquiry on Bioethics, *Human Cloning and Human Dignity: An Ethical Enquiry.* Washington, DC (July 2002), p. xviii.

25 Allen Buchanan, Dan W. Brock, Norman Daniels, *et al.*, *From Chance to Choice: Genetics and Justice.* Cambridge: Cambridge University Press (2000), p. 83.

26 President's Commission for the Study of Ethical Problems in Medicine and Biology and Behavioral Research, *Splicing Life: A Report on the Social and Ethical Issues of Genetic Engineering with Human Beings.* Washington, D.C.: The Commission (1982).

27 Ray Moseley, Commentary: maintaining the somatic/germ-line distinction: some ethical drawbacks, *Journal of Medicine and Philosophy* 16 (1991), 641–7.

28 See Jaenisch, Nuclear cloning, embryonic stem cells and gene transfer.

29 Sheldon Krimsky, Human gene therapy: must we know where to stop before we start? *Human Gene Therapy* 1 (1990), 171–3.

30 Ray Mosley, Commentary.

31 Jason S. Robert and Françoise Baylis, Crossing species boundaries, *The American Journal of Bioethics* 3 (2003), 1–13.

32 The President's Enquiry on Bioethics, *Human Cloning and Human Dignity,* p. xviii.

33 See Rasko and Jolly, The science of inheritable genetic modification; Jaenisch, Nuclear cloning, embryonic stem cells, and gene transfer.

34 Emily Marden and Dorothy Nelkin, Displaced agendas: current regulatory strategies for germ-line gene therapy, *McGill Law Journal* 45 (2000), 461–81, 461.

35 Katherine A. High, The risks of germ-line gene transfer, *Hastings Center Report* 33 (2003), 3.

36 Kenneth W. Culver, Gene repair, genomics and human germ-line modification. In: Audrey R. Chapman and Mark S. Frankel (eds.), *Designing Our Descendents: The Promises and Perils of Genetic Modification.* Baltimore, MD: Johns Hopkins University Press (2003), p. 86; and note that the Recombinant DNA Advisory Committee (RAC) will not *at present* entertain proposals for germ-line alterations but will consider proposals involving somatic cell gene transfer as long as the proposals meet the established criteria. See RAC, Guidelines for research involving recombinant DNA molecules, Appendix M; National Institutes of Health (NIH), Points to consider in the design and submission of protocols for the transfer of recombinant DNA into the genome of human subjects, in Regulatory issues: the revised "Points to consider" document, *Human Gene Therapy* 1 (1990), 93–103.

37 We do acknowledge that correction of a genetic "fault" in an individual's germ cells may be interpreted as not just a form of preventive health for future individuals, but in some sense as being "therapeutic" for the present individual because his/her reproductive cells are being "treated." Under this view, Starr (Esther) Rose Kaplan interprets the patient "as the parents of the embryo, the embryo itself, or the embryo's future offspring"; see her "Germ-line genetic engineering revisited," *The Pharos* (Fall 1997), 21–5.

38 Shopping at the genetic supermarket (Foreword, this volume).

39 Can bioethics speak to politics about the prospect of inheritable genetic modification? If so, what might it say? (Chapter 13, this volume).

40 Radical rupture: exploring biological sequelae of volitional inheritable genetic modification (Chapter 7, this volume).

41 "Alter-ing" the human species? Misplaced essentialism in science policy (Chapter 8, this volume).

42 Inheritable genetic modification as moral responsibility in a creative universe (Chapter 5, this volume).

43 Inheritable genetic modification and disability: normality and identity (Chapter 10, this volume).

44 Regulating inheritable genetic modification, or policing the fertile scientific imagination?

45 Traditional and feminist bioethical perspectives on gene transfer: is inheritable genetic modification really the problem? (Chapter 9, this volume).

46 Inheritable genetic modification: clinical applications and genetic counseling considerations (Chapter 12, this volume).

47 Controlling bodies and creating monsters: popular perceptions of genetic modifications (Chapter 4, this volume).
48 Ethics and welfare issues in animal genetic modification (Chapter 6, this volume).
49 On politics and bioethics, see for instance Eric M. Meslin, The President's Council:
   fair and balanced? *The Hastings Center Report* 34 (2004), 6–8.
50 Can bioethics speak to politics about the prospect of inheritable genetic modification?

The science of inheritable genetic modification

John E.J. Rasko and Douglas J. Jolly

2.1 The scope of inheritable genetic modification

Inheritable genetic modification (IGM) can be defined as the modification of the inheritable genetic information of an animal or person so that the alteration or added trait(s) corresponding to the transferred gene(s) are passed on to descendants. However, IGM has also been used to describe early intervention in the developing embryo that results in large-scale modification of the cells of the eventual person or animal that is not aimed at being inheritably transmitted. This methodology has been proposed to treat genetic diseases that result in perinatal death, so-called *in utero* gene therapy.[1] Although the two procedures are quite different in their goals, they overlap both in terms of their technology and in the heightened possibility that somatic embryo modification might lead to an inadvertent germ-line change compared to other types of somatic cell gene transfer (SCGT). This is simply due to the small size of the embryo and the rapid turnover of cells, circumstances that favor transduction of a large number of cells in the embryo, but also make it seem more likely that inadvertent germ-line alterations will be made. Indeed any gene when delivered to the systemic circulation may cause the unintended consequence of the modification of germ cells. The consequences presumably would be unintentional because in most jurisdictions including the U.S.A., the U.K., and Australia, any intentional modification of the germ line is, for practical purposes, forbidden.[2] The systemic delivery of a gene vector and possible IGM may result from direct injection into the circulation or through indirect means, such as might occur when it is injected into the muscle and escapes into local blood vessels.

Another related technology which overlaps with IGM is the use of modified stem cells including genetically-modified embryonic stem (ES) cells. Although therapeutic cloning to reconstitute or augment tissue in an animal or person[3] would not *per se* be a form of IGM, if the therapeutic tissue included germ cells in order to treat a disorder of reproduction, then IGM would be a potential consequence. Conversely, purely reproductive cloning also would not be defined as IGM because modification of the germ line would not have taken place. The example of ooplasmic transfer discussed in a previous chapter[4] sets a scientific precedent for IGM, as it involves a modification of the germ line that has already been performed in humans.

Germ-line genetic interventions, even for the purpose of therapy, are highly controversial.[5] While there appears to be justification for considering the embryo therapy discussed above, there is almost universal condemnation of intentional modification of the germ line.[6] Most of these criticisms are ethically and morally driven, but there are also technical limitations, which will be discussed in this chapter, that make the dispute a hypothetical one, at least for the time being. Therefore it is unclear whether there will ever be acceptance of germ-line genetic interventions for therapeutic goals. A further step beyond this, in terms of a decreased probability of general acceptance, is the use of germ-line modification for improvement in athletic performance.

There are two major sets of issues to be investigated with regard to IGM: first, how would a society be organized and motivated to engage in pursuing these sorts of procedures? Second, are they actually possible? The majority of this chapter will be devoted to the second question, but of course its answer has implications for the first. The following sections primarily examine the science and technology surrounding intentional IGM. Further discussion concerns embryo gene therapy and the use of modified stem cells for somatic tissue replacement. A detailed analysis of the technology of nuclear transfer (NT) is provided in a separate chapter.[7]

2.2   Methods of creating transgenic animals

It is now commonplace to create rodents and lower-order model organisms such as fruit flies and worms using recombinant DNA technology. In considering the science of IGM as it pertains to human animals, much can be learnt from the many years of experience with transgenic non-human animals.[8]

Current methods for making transgenic animals are cumbersome, have inherently high levels of unpredictability, and require a dedicated breeding program. Germ-line transfer of genes has been achieved in a number of animals in various ways as described below. These include the micro-injection of fertilized eggs, the manipulation of ES cells, the delivery of somatic nuclei to enucleated eggs, and the mixing of DNA with sperm, as well as the delivery of genes into the male germ line in potential fathers.

In general there have been three reasons to create animals using recombinant DNA technology: the first was to investigate the basic biologic and physiologic processes of differentiation, gene expression, and disease; the second was to create animals that produce useful proteins (generally for therapeutic purposes); and the third was to more easily select strains of domesticated animals that have some advantage. Examples of the first type of use of recombinant DNA technology abound in the scientific literature: from creating hemophilic mice as models for the human disease to investigating gene function in general.[9] There are several examples of the second type of use, one of which is the production of human growth hormone in the milk of lactating rabbits.[10] Despite a number of attempts to achieve the third aim, there are no current examples of improved domesticated breeds that are actually used in agriculture or elsewhere for commercial purposes. If the technology is ever applied to humans, obviously it will follow on the technical advances made in animals.

2.2.1 Micro-injection of fertilized eggs

Transgenic methods first appeared in 1980,[11] 2–3 years after the cloning of the first human gene. The animals in question were inbred laboratory mice and the steps in the technology were as follows: female mice were induced to super-ovulate (produce many eggs), then mated with males; the resulting fertilized eggs then were collected from the female mice. The male pro-nucleus of each egg was micro-injected with purified DNA (the transgene), and the eggs were re-implanted into the oviducts of pseudo-pregnant female mice (i.e., those that had previously been placed with vasectomized males). In this first experiment, the success rate for obtaining mice showing retention of the introduced transgene was about 2.5%. Gene expression levels were not measured in the first experiment, but these tests are now routinely performed to demonstrate that the gene is functional in its new host. This method has been standardized and the equipment used has become more sophisticated so it is now the most frequent method of creating transgenic mice used today in research laboratories. Hundreds, if not thousands, of strains of transgenic mice have been generated in academic and commercial laboratories.[12] In addition, methods based on this technology have been used to create other transgenic animals including chickens, rabbits, pigs, sheep, goats, and primates.[13,14] However, the frequency of success has rarely been better than 10% of implantations (and often much lower). The use of viral gene transfer technology using a vector based on the human immunodeficiency virus (lentiviral vector) has greatly improved transgenic rates in rodents.[15]

In addition to unacceptably low success rates, there are a number of further technical drawbacks to micro-injection methods, if one were to contemplate creating transgenic humans. The first drawback is that insertion into the genome is random, leading to unpredictable expression levels and possible inactivation or inappropriate activation of endogenous genes. This in turn can lead to cancer induction, or non-viable or enfeebled animals. The second drawback is mosaicism, where the gene is expressed in some but not all appropriate cells/tissues; a third is the lack of understanding of how to control gene expression appropriately (see below for further discussion). Driven in part by these deficiencies, there has been considerable interest in developing other methods of creating transgenic

Table 2.1. Methods for creating transgenic animals

Method	Gene delivery method	Transgenic animals	Efficiency	Mosaic offspring	Comments
Injection of fertilized eggs or blastocyst	DNA with micro-needle or viral vector	Mice, rats, rabbits, sheep, pigs, cattle	1–10%, lower in farm animals	Yes	Most transgenic animals are produced this way. Lentiviral vectors are promising
ES cells plus DNA vector	ES cells modified in culture, then injected into embryo	Mice only (so far)	Varied, <10%	Yes	Competent ES cells only in mice. Allows homologous recombination
Enucleated egg plus gene-modified somatic nucleus	Transfer of nucleus from gene-modified cell to enucleated oocytes and implanted	Mice, sheep, chicken	0.1–1%	No	First generation animals have abnormalities that require further breeding to eliminate
Sperm plus DNA	DNA is mixed with sperm, used for fertilization	Mice, pigs	Varied, up to 60%	Yes, but reduced	Insufficient experience
Modification of male germ-line germ cells	DNA introduced *in vitro* and the cells then reimplanted	Mice	~5%	Probably not	Insufficient experience; may require pretreatment of host

animals; the most prominent of these are listed in Table 2.1. As can be seen, there is a wide variety of methods that have had some success.

2.2.2   ES cells

The use of ES cells is well-studied as the cells can be grown and manipulated *in vitro* for extended periods of time and then be implanted in pseudo-pregnant female animals.[16] Genes can be introduced by almost any technique available for cells maintained in tissue culture and the best evidence available confirms that rodents develop normally.[17] However, only mouse ES cells have been shown to be fully competent for creating transgenic mammals, so the technique is used solely for research. Generating ES cells for other mammalian species (with the exception of non-human primate and man) has not been successful and the true totipotency of current human "ES" cell lines is unknown.[18] The only convincing test of totipotency would be to reproduce the steps outlined for the mouse cells, that is, produce an animal descended from a cell line. This would require the generation of mosaic non-human animals or humans as a first step followed by the need for successive second and third generations to validate germ-line transmission and guarantee 100% derivation of all cells in the body from the original gene-modified injected ES cell. Such genetic/cellular engineering in humans is considered to be medically unsafe and unethical by most regulatory bodies.

2.2.3   Delivery of somatic nuclei to enucleated eggs

The delivery of a nucleus from a somatic cell to an enucleated oocyte is the technique that is usually used to generate cloned animals, the famous first example being Dolly the sheep.[19] It has now been possible to add genes to the somatic cell before nuclear transplantation (NT) and subsequently generate viable animals; thus this is one way to generate transgenic animals.[20] One major drawback is that, to date, all the cloned animals are abnormal.[21] This is primarily the result of a lack of "reprogramming" of the transferred genetic material that normally occurs at meiosis and initial embryogenesis.[22] However, if the cloned animal is reproductively competent, the next generation of animals produced by normal breeding will have been successfully reprogrammed and will be likely to be relatively robust. Demonstration of this possibility in animals with long gestation periods and lengthy maturation timelines presents some difficulties. Use of this technique in humans would similarly be limited by all of these factors, in addition to the profound ethical questions discussed in many other chapters in this volume.

2.2.4   Mixing DNA with sperm

It is now generally accepted that creation of transgenic animals may be achieved by simply mixing DNA with sperm or semen and then fertilizing ovulating females.[23,24] Originally this technique proved very difficult to perform reliably and therefore was not adopted. With further experience, however, it has begun to appear that this simple technology can be applied more widely, allowing easier generation of transgenic animals. However, the animals produced are still mosaic and a further round of breeding is required to eliminate mosaicism. This technology has not been explored fully as yet, and would require more basic and translational research before contemplating its use in humans.

2.2.5   Delivery of genes to the male germ line in the father

Some laboratories have had technical success in delivering genes to male germline germ cells or the descendants of these cells before spermatogenesis.[25] Such target cells may be harvested from testes, transduced with the desired gene, and re-implanted into the testes of recipient animals. The animals with the re-implanted, transduced germ-line germ cells yield transgenic sperm and hence transgenic offspring on mating. So far this technique seems to work well only in animals (mice) that have some "space" in the testes and do not have a competing endogenous germ cell development process.

2.2.6 Summary

Table 2.1 lists the techniques in terms of these broad categories outlined above, and also outlines some of the issues surrounding each of the technologies with regard to reproducibility, ease of use, and risks of unwanted side effects. Each of these IGM techniques creates a risk of insertional mutagenesis unless the transgene is introduced by homologous recombination. Of all of the transgenic techniques described above, sperm-mediated transgenesis seems to have promise as a relatively undemanding technology with good rates of success. However, this technology is very much in its infancy.

In summary, it appears that the current predominant IGM method using micro-injection of fertilized eggs is sufficient for research purposes. This method can be used reliably to make transgenic mice or strains of animals as research tools and as bioreactors for protein production. It has not yet been possible to produce improved livestock in a meaningful way and generate animals that are useful for farming.[26] If any research is directed towards creating transgenic humans, the experience gained from studies into pronuclear injection of fertilized eggs would provide important guidance.

2.3 Gene delivery systems

The term "somatic gene therapy" refers to the addition of genes to non-germ-line tissues such as muscle or liver for a therapeutic purpose. In this context, there has been broad clinical testing of potential gene therapeutics for many diseases including cardiovascular,[27] hematologic,[28] and pulmonary diseases,[29] as well as cancer.[30] These approaches have a reasonable likelihood of wide applicability in the future. Somatic gene therapies are generally agreed to resemble conventional drugs in terms of their acceptability, the trials through which they would be tested, and the indications for their use as legitimate "medicines."

In contrast to somatic gene therapy, IGM refers to genetic modification of the genes that a subject has available to transmit to his or her offspring. Genes have been delivered to germ-line cells for IGM using various approaches. In this section, the gene transfer methods that are commonly applied or most likely to succeed are discussed. There are several types of vectors that have been used clinically to deliver genes to non-germ-line tissues for somatic gene therapy.[31] With the exception of live viral vaccines such as the Sabin polio vaccine, smallpox vaccines, and the recent chickenpox vaccine,[32] none of these products had been approved for sale until recently. The exception is the acceptance by the Chinese government of an anti-cancer gene therapeutic.[33] The vectors that have been used in the clinic are listed in Table 2.2, along with some of their relevant

Table 2.2. Methods of transferring genes and construction of transgenic animals

Vector	Genome size	Insert size	RNA or DNA?	Integrates into cell genome?	Clinical use?	Produced transgenic animals?	References
DNA	NA	~ 50–100 kb	DNA	Yes, low efficiency	Yes, 15%	Yes	58
DNA plus carrier	NA	~ 50–100 kb	DNA	Yes, low efficiency	Yes, 8.5%	No	59
Retrovirus	10 kb	<8 kb	RNA/DNA	Yes	Yes, 27%	Yes	62
Lentivirus	10 kb	<8 kb	RNA/DNA	Yes	Yes, 0.3%	Yes	61
Adenovirus	36 kb	8–30 kb	DNA	Low efficiency	Yes, 26%	No	63
Adeno-associated virus	4.5 kb	<4.1 kb	DNA	Usually low efficiency	Yes, 2.5%	No	64
Herpes virus	160 kb	>20 kb	DNA	No	Yes, 3%	No	65
Vaccinia virus	180 kb	2–20 kb	DNA	No	Yes, 7%		57
Hybrids (e.g., transposons in adenovirus)	Herpes or adenovirus sizes	8 kb	RNA/DNA	Yes	No	No	66
Micro-cell fusion	Chromosome	≥200 kb	DNA	Persists as a mini-chromosome	No	Yes	67

The percentage of the approximately 1000 gene therapy clinical trials to date that have used the specific vector is shown[57] (NA: not applicable).

properties, as far as these are understood. Also included are two methods that have not been used in the clinic but that may be useful for making transgenic animals. The key factor for utility is the stability of the added gene(s), which usually means that the genes integrate into the host cell genome or persist alongside it. This is necessary to ensure that the genes persist in all cells in the body, as well as in the germ cells. Consequently many of the vectors on the list are unsuitable as a means of achieving IGM because they do not lead to stable modification of the genome.

Traditionally, gene delivery methods have been divided into viral and non-viral systems because they depend on disparate technologies and exhibit distinct features. In general, the viral systems have been much more efficient and consequently have been used in about three-quarters of all human clinical trials. All of the viral systems take advantage of nature's evolved solution to the problem of gene transfer, since naturally-occurring viruses are masters of introducing their own genetic payload to specific target cells. Viral vectors designed to transfer genes as therapeutics for genetic disorders typically have been rendered incapable of self-replication. They are usually designed to introduce a corrected or functional version of the existing disease-causing gene anywhere in the genetic complement of the cell, but they do not *replace* or *correct* the existing gene that remains. However, the very idea of using viruses (which of course remain a widespread cause of human disease) as therapeutics makes their non-viral counterparts seemingly more attractive. Non-viral systems depend on plasmids (autonomously replicating minichromosomes in bacteria) or chemically-synthesized nucleic acids. The most promising gene transfer vectors for IGM, apart from routine DNA micro-injection, are retroviruses,[34] lentiviruses,[35] hybrids with transposons,[36] and minichromosomes.[37] The next criterion for ranking these methods is appropriate expression, and it is possible that the minichromosome method has some inherent advantage in this respect because the gene of interest is transferred in a much larger piece of the immediately surrounding DNA and may be more likely to respond and act in a natural or physiologic way. The problems associated with this method are that it may be difficult to control precisely what is transferred with the larger DNA segment, and also that gene delivery has, to date, been cumbersome. These systems are summarized in Table 2.2 along with references to reviews in the scientific literature.

2.4   Limitations of current gene delivery systems

As noted above, a further set of questions with respect to the generation of transgenic animals concern gene expression. This includes the risks of mosaicism, activating or inactivating an important existing gene, and transgene expression levels in animals receiving IGM.

2.4.1   Risk of inactivating a useful gene and directed integration

The risk of inactivating a useful gene results from the random nature of integration of gene transfer vectors throughout the target genome. Since the random integration can cause mutations in genes due to interruption in their continuity or due to activation of nearby genes resulting from powerful gene control elements incorporated into vector design, this side effect of vector integration is called "insertional mutagenesis." In the case of IGM, such factors could lead to decreased fitness due to non-lethal insertional mutagenesis; the potential for contributing events that promote tumor formation; and variable gene expression due to positional effects. Although the risk of insertional mutagenesis has always been recognized, it has taken on a greater significance for hemopoietic stem cells (and by implication other stem cells) owing to its unexpectedly high occurrence in the otherwise-successful gene therapy trial of children with severe combined immune deficiency (SCID).[38] To address these issues, methods have been developed in animals for inserting genes by homologous recombination into targeted chromosomal segments. These methods can work quite well but reduce further (by about 10- to 100-fold) the odds of creating the desired IGM animal in the first place. This technology has been used with ES cell genetic modification,[39] and is also employed in NT. A further targeting method that is well-suited to answering research questions is the insertion of a specific short target site in the genome, then directing genes to this site by use of enzymes.[40] However, this approach presupposes insertion of the specific target site which itself would integrate randomly. Other methods of achieving control over the site of integration such as the "sleeping beauty" transposon system and targeted gene repair methods with RNA/DNA or triplex-forming oligonucleotides are in their infancies.[41]

2.4.2   Mosaicism and chimerism

Mosaicism and chimerism as strictly defined refer to different phenomena, inasmuch as the former situation arises from a single fertilized egg whereas the latter arises from more than one. Both situations refer to the presence of cell populations from distinct genetic lineages. Thus in the case of IGM, a true transgenic with all of its tissues carrying the same transgene integrated in the same place in the genome can only be achieved by a further round of breeding, identification, and selection *after* the original gene transfer procedure has been performed. At this stage the animal is heterozygotic for the transgene and must go through a further round of breeding to generate homozygotic transgenic animals, if such an animal is actually viable. While such rounds of breeding are tedious in mice, they greatly attenuate the advantages that transgenic cattle, pigs, and sheep should have over conventional breeding techniques. Avoiding mosaicism would create presumably insurmountable barriers for the creation of transgenic humans.

2.4.3   Control of gene expression

The third major issue limiting gene transfer for IGM is the lack of understanding of how to control transgene expression appropriately. Although some strains of mice have been created that express genes in a specific location (e.g., in breast milk) and with various local control regions, most often this is not the case.[42] Expression in every tissue and at all times is rarely desirable. If controlled or appropriate gene expression is needed, this can only be achieved in a limited number of cases, and so the numbers of transgenic animals to be screened for a desired phenotype increases further, thereby lowering the current efficiency of 1–10%. One situation in which IGM animals might have an advantage over those receiving standard gene transfer methods is the ability to use drug-controlled induction of gene expression. Control is achieved with compounds such as antibiotics or small molecules to modulate expression of the particular introduced gene by interacting with a protein encoded by a second introduced gene that controls expression of the first gene.[43] In this system, animals are administered a non-toxic drug to induce gene expression. This system could be very useful, as transgenic animals appear to be immunologically tolerant of the regulatory protein since in this case it becomes endogenously produced.

2.5   Difficulty in programming complex traits by adding genes

Even if we simply assume that eventually there will be sufficient knowledge to create transgenic humans in a reliable fashion which does not have an unacceptable level of failure or side effects, it is unclear how it will be possible to improve complex traits in animals or in humans by single or multiple gene additions. For instance, there are clearly genetic differences predisposing one athlete to perform better than another for a particular competitive sport.[44] Probably the most common example is the proportion of fast twitch to slow twitch muscle in an athlete.[45] These have definably different metabolism, are determined largely by genetic make-up, and predispose individuals to have natural ability in sprint and endurance athletic events, respectively. How this is programmed during pre- and post-natal development is completely unclear, although it can be possibly influenced in a number of ways by gene and cell manipulation in mature animals. Whereas for somatic tissue gene delivery it seems possible to at least identify a few genes, such as erythropoietin and growth hormone, which are potentially deliverable and could improve performance, this seems extremely unlikely to be feasible in the context of IGM.

An example of the unpredictability of IGM by DNA micro-injection is the use of the growth hormone gene. The growth hormone protein is used to treat children who have very small stature and has been shown to increase strength in aging individuals. While mice transgenic for growth hormone grew bigger than normal litter mates and otherwise seemed more or less normal, the corresponding transgenic pigs were only slightly larger and had slightly reduced fat levels while suffering from a number of deleterious effects.[46] These included movement difficulties and heart enlargement due to being "muscle-bound," reduced fertility, and increased susceptibility to stress. Therefore, until experiments could be performed in humans, if ever, we cannot predict *a priori* what the effects of introducing a single gene into the germ line would be.

2.6   Technologies related to IGM

In this section we consider two methods which, although not strictly designed for IGM, demand inclusion in this review due to their relevance.

2.6.1   *In utero* gene transfer

This method has been proposed because many genetic diseases start to cause clinical impairment before or soon after birth.[47] Examples of diseases that might be treated with *in utero* gene transfer include neurologic disorders (such as many lysosomal storage diseases); immunologic deficiencies (such as the SCID syndromes); hematologic disorders (such as thalassemia); and metabolic diseases (such as Lesch Nyhan syndrome or osteopetrosis).[48] The technology involves directly injecting genes into the developing embryo *in utero* as has been performed using animal models.[49] In principle this is a variant of the common research method for constructing transgenic mice (injection of fertilized eggs or blastocyst), with the difference that the embryos are at later stage, and perhaps much later. The gene transfer systems that would be expected to be useful are those that permanently modify target cells (e.g., retroviral and lentiviral vectors), but others have been used in animal models. Attractive features of this approach for "somatic" therapy include that a large proportion of the cells of the whole organism can be gene-modified and the possibility of providing immunologic tolerance (i.e., not provoking an immune reaction) to the transgene product. Drawbacks include those previously discussed, such as the potential for insertional mutagenesis; mosaicism; issues with the control of gene expression; and difficulties in programming complex traits by adding genes. In addition, there appears to be increased potential for genuine germ-line modification. On the other hand, it is worth noting that this "twilight zone" between somatic and germ-line gene interventions is one that could conceivably be applied to individual humans, if these technical hurdles can be overcome.

2.6.2   Transplantation of transduced ES cells into somatic tissue

Several types of stem cells, including ES cells, have been shown in animal models to have the potential to differentiate into tissue resembling the specific host target tissue following injection.[50] This idea relates to the stem cell concepts of tissue plasticity and transdifferentiation.[51] Attempts to genetically modify stem cells and eventually re-implant them in certain organs have had limited success.[52] Strictly such interventions are forms of somatic tissue gene transfer, but much of the expertise involved overlaps with that required for efficient IGM. As such, the study of gene-modified transplanted ES cells provides a legitimate scientific space to develop such technologies which have potential for application to IGM technology.

2.7   Summary of known technical limitations and consequences for attempts at IGM in humans

The hurdles obstructing the reliable generation of transgenic humans are daunting, even if it was to be actively pursued. These include the following:

1. It takes 15–20 years for humans to mature to a reproductive age.
2. There appears to be a universal need to passage the transgene through a further generation to either remove mosaicism or reset the epigenetic imprint on the genome. Consequently humans would require about a 30-year lead time to achieve stable IGM.
3. Current methods are difficult to control in terms of appropriate gene expression, and the desired outcome or phenotype is selected from a group of transgenic animals.
4. The current methods appear very inefficient in terms of the failure-to-success ratio.
5. In many situations, there is a considerable risk of negative alterations to the genome that can have devastating consequences on the individual.
6. Without a clear understanding of genetic reprogramming of nuclear-transferred material, cloning will never be safe for humans.[53]

2.8   Difficulties in predicting future technical advances

It has always been difficult to predict the speed and scope of technologic and intellectual advances in biomedicine. For example, a review of germ-line gene transfer (GLGT) and SCGT in 1990 concluded that both of these were so difficult and unpredictable that it was not really worth worrying about either possibility.[54] This can no longer be said of SCGT methods. It is possible that in another 15 years that the same evolution will occur with IGM. As noted above the technology has yet to produce strains of commercially useful "improved" livestock, but efforts are continuing in this area, so the technology is likely to develop further. In addition, as noted before, the use of modified stem cells for somatic transfer may provide enhanced understanding as well as techniques that could be used to achieve IGM in humans. Such developments might be pursued underground and not publicized if bans are universally adopted, driven perhaps by intended illicit use of such technology, which suggests regulation without prohibition would be most appropriate.

Two other ongoing scientific efforts could contribute to IGM methods becoming technically feasible. These are the sequencing and annotation of the human genome,[55] and the current "systems biology" efforts which try to explain and predict outcomes from multifactorial interactions in cells and animals.[56] Both efforts are directed towards a general understanding of the underlying causes of disease and other complex phenotypes. Such approaches could ultimately provide an understanding of how complex traits are genetically determined and offer insights into facilitating IGM more efficiently. Even if it is theoretically possible, it seems unlikely that the hurdle of human maturation time could ever be overcome for the implementation of true IGM, so this is likely to remain an unbreakable technical barrier. There exists an unsettling "halfway house" where mosaic individuals could be produced by embryo injection. Although there are many technical barriers, it is possible to imagine some groups that might devote 15–20 years (after the technology is developed) to produce such a mosaic adult, even if such procedures were to be prohibited.

2.9   Conclusions

As noted above, SCGT for clinical use is widely accepted as non-controversial, as long as the risk/benefit profile is acceptable. On the other hand, IGM, even as a therapeutic method, is highly controversial. The current technology is not suited to creation of transgenic humans, although it is possible that this will change over the next 20 years. Although the technology to achieve IGM safely in humans still appears to be many years in the future, it is clear that success in non-human animal models has identified potentially fruitful avenues for study. It remains uncertain whether scientific and technical impasses will render the idea of human IGM entirely theoretical, or whether social and ethical objections will ultimately prevent its realization. An examination of the latter question is the concern of most of the other chapters in this volume.

NOTES

1 John J. Rossi, Primate *in utero* gene transfer comes of age, *Molecular Therapy* 3 (2001), 274–5.
2 National Institutes of Health (NIH), Points to consider in the design and submission of protocols for the transfer of recombinant DNA molecules into one or more

human research participants, Appendix M, *Guidelines for Research Involving Recombinant DNA Molecules* (2002).

3 Megan J. Munsie, Anna E. Michalska, Carmel M. O'Brien, *et al.*, Isolation of pluripotent embryonic stem cells from reprogrammed adult mouse somatic cell nuclei, *Current Biology* 10 (2000), 989–92.

4 See John E.J. Rasko, Gabrielle M. O'Sullivan and Rachel A. Ankeny, Is inheritable genetic modification the new dividing line? (Chapter 1, this volume).

5 Nancy M.P. King, Accident and desire: inadvertent germ-line effects in clinical research, *Hastings Center Report* 33 (2003), 23–30.

6 Ezmail D. Zanjani and W. French Anderson, Prospects for *in utero* human gene therapy, *Science* 285 (1999), 2084–8.

7 See Rudolf Jaensich, Nuclear cloning, embryonic stem cells, and gene transfer (Chapter 3, this volume).

8 See Gabrielle M. O'Sullivan, Ethics and welfare issues in animal genetic modification (Chapter 6, this volume).

9 L. Bi, R. Sarkar, T. Naas, *et al.*, Further characterization of factor VIII-deficient mice created by gene targeting: RNA and protein studies, *Blood* 88 (1996), 3446–50.

10 D. Lipinski, J. Jura, R. Kalak, *et al.*, Transgenic rabbit producing human growth hormone in milk, *Journal of Applied Genetics* 44 (2003), 165–74.

11 John W. Gordon, George A. Scangos, Diane J. Plotkin, *et al.*, Genetic transformation of mouse embryos by microinjection of purified DNA, *Proceedings of the National Academy of Sciences USA* 77 (1980), 7380–4.

12 C.C. Linder, Mouse nomenclature and maintenance of genetically engineered mice, *Comparative Medicine* 53 (2003), 119–25.

13 Masumi Hirabayashi, Ri-itchi Takahashi, Kazumi Ito, *et al.*, A comparative study on the integration of exogenous DNA into mouse, rat, rabbit, and pig genomes, *Experimental Animals* 50 (2001), 125–31.

14 A.W. Chan, K.Y. Chong, C. Martinovich, *et al.*, Transgenic monkeys produced by retroviral gene transfer into mature oocytes, *Science* 291 (2001), 309–12.

15 Carlos Lois, Elizabeth J. Hong, Shirley Pease, *et al.*, Germ-line transmission and tissue-specific expression of transgenes delivered by lentiviral vectors, *Science* 295 (2002), 868–72.

16 Achim Gossler, Thomas Doetschman, Reinhard Korn, *et al.*, Transgenesis by means of blastocyst-derived embryonic stem cell lines, *Proceedings of the National Academy of Sciences USA* 83 (1986), 9065–9.

17 D.A. Williams, Embryonic stem cells as targets for gene transfer: a new approach to molecular manipulation of the murine hematopoietic system, *Bone Marrow Transplantation* 5 (1990), 141–4.

18 Woo Suk Hwang, Young June Ryu, Jong Hyuk Park, *et al.*, Evidence of a pluripotent human embryonic stem cell line derived from a cloned blastocyst, *Science* 33 (2004), 1669–74.

19 K.H. Campbell, J. McWhir, W.A. Ritchie, *et al.*, Sheep cloned by nuclear transfer from a cultured cell line, *Nature* 380 (1996), 64–6.

20 Yoshimi Kuroiwa, Poothappillai Kasinathan, Yoon J. Choi, *et al.*, Cloned transchromosomic calves producing human immunoglobulin, *Nature Biotechnology* 20 (2002), 889–94; K.J. McCreath, J. Howcroft, K.H. Campbell, *et al.*, Production of gene-targeted sheep by nuclear transfer from cultured somatic cells, *Nature* 405 (2000), 1066–9.

21 Ian Wilmut, Are there any normal cloned mammals? *Nature Medicine* 8 (2002), 215–6.

22 For more details, see Jaenisch, Nuclear cloning, embryonic stem cells, and gene transfer.

23 Kijong Chang, Jin Qian, Meisheng Jiang, *et al.*, Effective generation of transgenic pigs and mice by linker based sperm-mediated gene transfer, *BMC Biotechnology* 2 (2002), 5.

24 Marialuisa Lavitrano, Maria L. Bacci, Monica Forni, *et al.*, Efficient production by sperm-mediated gene transfer of human decay accelerating factor (hDAF) transgenic pigs for xenotransplantation, *Proceedings of the National Academy of Sciences USA* 99 (2002), 14230–5.

25 Makoto Nagano, Clayton J. Brinster, Kyle E. Orwig, *et al.*, Transgenic mice produced by retroviral transduction of male germ-line stem cells, *Proceedings of the National Academy of Sciences USA* 98 (2001), 13090–5.

26 John Clarke and Bruce Whitelaw, A future for transgenic livestock, *Nature Reviews Genetics* 4 (2003), 825–32.

27 John E. Rasko and David S. Celermajer, Gene therapy for vascular diseases: closer to delivering the goods? In: Roger T. Dean and David T. Kelly (eds.), *Atherosclerosis: Gene Expression, Cell Interactions and Oxidation*. Oxford: Oxford University Press (2000), 112–36.

28 K.A. High, Gene transfer as an approach to treating hemophilia, *Seminars in Thrombosis and Hemostasis* 29 (2003), 107–20.

29 J.A. Wagner, I.B. Nepomuceno, A.H. Messner, *et al.*, A phase II, double-blind, randomized, placebo-controlled clinical trial of tgAAVCF using maxillary sinus delivery in patients with cystic fibrosis with antrostomies, *Human Gene Therapy* 13 (2002), 1349–59.

30 K. Brand, Gene therapy for cancer. In: Nancy Smyth Templeton (ed.), *Gene and Cell Therapy: Therapeutic Mechanisms and Strategies*. New York: Marcel Dekker (2004), 531–84.

31 Templeton (ed.), *Gene and Cell Therapy: Therapeutic Mechanisms and Strategies*.

32 U.S. Food and Drug Administration, Center for Biologics Evaluation and Research. Vaccines licensed for immunization and distributed in the U.S. (2003).

33 Sue Pearson, Hepeng Jia and Keiko Kandachi, China approves first gene therapy, *Nature Biotechnology* 22 (2004), 3–4.

34 P.M. Cannon and W. French Anderson, Retroviral vectors for gene therapy In: Templeton (ed.), *Cell and Gene Therapy*, 1–16.

35 Douglas J. Jolly, Lentiviral vectors. In: Templeton (ed.), *Gene and Cell Therapy: Therapeutic Mechanisms and Strategies*, 131–46.

36 Zsuzsanna Izsvák and Zoltán Ivics, Sleeping beauty transposition: biology and applications for molecular therapy, *Molecular Therapy: The Journal of the American Society of Gene Therapy* 9 (2004), 147–56.

37 Kuroiwa, Kasinathan, Choi, *et al.*, Cloned transchromosomic calves producing human immunoglobulin; Richard Saffery and K.H. Andy Choo, Strategies for engineering human chromosomes with therapeutic potential, *Journal of Gene Medicine* 4 (2002), 5–13.

38 S. Hacein-Bey-Abina, C. Von Kalle, M. Schmidt, *et al.*, LMO2-associated clonal T cell proliferation in two patients after gene therapy for SCID-X1, *Science* 302 (2003), 415–9; Donald B. Kohn, Michael Sadelain and Joseph C. Glorioso, Occurrence of leukaemia following gene therapy of X-linked SCID, *Nature Reviews Cancer* 3 (2003), 477–88.

39 Mario R. Capecchi, Altering the genome by homologous recombination, *Science* 244 (1989), 1288–92.

40 Mark Lewandoski and Gail R. Martin, Cre-mediated chromosome loss in mice, *Nature Reviews Genetics* 17 (1997), 223–5.

41 Aron M. Geurts, Ying Yang, Karl J. Clark, *et al.*, Gene transfer into genomes of human cells by the sleeping beauty transposon system, *Molecular Therapy: The Journal of the American Society of Gene Therapy* 8 (2003), 108–17.

42 Christoph W. Pittius, Lothar Hennighausen, Eric Lee, *et al.*, A milk protein gene promoter directs the expression of human tissue plasminogen activator cDNA to the mammary gland in transgenic mice, *Proceedings of the National Academy of Sciences USA* 85 (1988), 5874–8; Patrick A. Navas, Kenneth R. Peterson, Qiliang Li, *et al.*, Developmental specificity of the interaction between the locus control region and embryonic or fetal globin genes in transgenic mice with an HS3 core deletion, *Molecular and Cellular Biology* 18 (1998), 4188–96.

43 Manfred Gossen and Hermann Bujard, Studying gene function in eukaryotes by conditional gene inactivation, *Annual Review of Genetics* 36 (2002), 153–73; C. Toniatti, H. Bujard, R. Cortese, *et al.*, Gene therapy progress and prospects: transcription regulatory systems, *Gene Therapy* 11 (2004), 649–57.

44 H.E. Montgomery, R. Marshall, H. Hemingway, *et al.*, Human gene for physical performance, *Nature* 393 (1998), 221–2.

45 Gregory J. Crowthers, Sharon A. Jubrias, Rodney K. Gronka, *et al.*, A "functional biopsy" of muscle properties in sprinters and distance runners, *Medicine and Science in Sports and Exercise* 34 (2002), 1719–24.

46 Vernon G. Pursel, Carl A. Pinkert, Kurt F. Miller, *et al.*, Genetic engineering of livestock, *Science* 244 (1989), 1281–8.

47 Charles R. Scriver, William S. Sly, Belinda Childs, *et al.* (eds.), *The Metabolic and Molecular Bases of Inherited Disease*. New York: McGraw-Hill Professional (2000).

48 Zanjani and Anderson, Prospects for *in utero* human gene therapy.

49 Nam D. Tran, Christopher D. Porada, Yi Zhao, *et al.*, *In utero* transfer and expression of exogenous genes in sheep, *Experimental Hematology* 28 (2000), 17–30; Janet E. Larson, Susan L. Morrow, Joseph B. Delcarpio, *et al.*, Gene transfer into the fetal

primate: evidence for the secretion of transgene product, *Molecular Therapy: The Journal of the American Society of Gene Therapy* 2 (2000), 631–9.

50 R. McKay, Stem cells: hype and hope, *Nature* 406 (2000), 361–4; Antonio Musaro, Christina Giacinti, Giovanna Borsellino, *et al.*, Stem cell-mediated muscle regeneration is enhanced by local isoform of insulin-like growth factor 1, *Proceedings of the National Academy of Sciences USA* 101 (2004), 1206–10.

51 Marc H. Dahlke, Felix C. Popp, Stephen Larsen, *et al.*, Stem cell therapy of the liver – fusion or fiction? *Liver Transplantation* 10 (2004), 471–9.

52 Yutaka Hanazono, Takayuki Asano, Yasuji Ueda, *et al.*, Genetic manipulation of primate embryonic and hematopoietic stem cells with simian lentivirus vectors, *Trends in Cardiovascular Medicine* 13 (2003), 106–10.

53 See Jaenisch, Nuclear cloning, embryonic stem cells, and gene transfer.

54 B.D. Davis, Limits to genetic intervention in humans: somatic and germline, *Ciba Foundation Symposium* 149 (1990), 81–6.

55 Francis S. Collins, Michael Morgan and Aristides Patrinos, The Human Genome Project: lessons from large-scale biology, *Science* 300 (2003), 286–90.

56 Eric H. Davidson, Jonathan P. Rast, Paola Oliveri, *et al.*, A genomic regulatory network for development, *Science* 295 (2002), 1669–78.

57 Z.S. Guo and D.L. Bartlett, Vaccinia as a vector for gene delivery, *Expert Opinion on Biological Therapy* 4 (2004), 901–17.

58 M. Edelstein, *The Journal of Gene Medicine* Clinical Trial Site, www.wiley.co.uk/genmed/clinical/ (last accessed 31 March 2005).

59 Templeton, *Gene and Cell Therapy*.

60 Ann Boyd, Exogenous DNA expression in eukaryotic cells following microinjection, *Methods in Cell Science* 24 (2002), 115–22.

61 Lois, Hong, Pease, *et al.*, Germ-line transmission and tissue-specific expression.

62 A. Dusty Miller, Daniel G. Miller, J. Victor Garcia, *et al.*, Use of retroviral vectors for gene transfer and expression, *Methods in Enzymology* 217 (1993), 581–99.

63 X. Danthinne and M.J. Imperiale, Production of first generation adenovirus vectors: a review, *Gene Therapy* 7 (2000), 1707–14.

64 Hildegard Büning, Markus Braun-Falco and Michael Hallek, Progress in the use of adeno-associated viral vectors for gene therapy, *Cells Tissues Organs* 177 (2004), 139–50.

65 D. Wolfe, W.F. Goins, D.J. Fink, *et al.*, Engineering herpes simplex viral vectors for therapeutic gene transfer. In: Templeton (ed.), *Gene and Cell Therapy: Therapeutic Mechanisms and Strategies,* 103–30.

66 Izsvak and Ivics, Sleeping beauty transposition.

67 Kuroiwa, Kasinathan, Choi, *et al.*, Cloned transchromosomic calves producing human immunoglobulin.

Nuclear cloning, embryonic stem cells, and gene transfer

Rudolf Jaenisch

An emerging consensus is that somatic cell nuclear transfer (SCNT) for the purpose of creating a child (also called "reproductive cloning") is not acceptable for both moral and scientific reasons. In contrast, SCNT with the goal of generating an embryonic stem (ES) cell line (so-called "therapeutic cloning") remains a controversial issue. Although therapeutic cloning holds the promise of yielding new ways of treating a number of degenerative diseases, it is not acceptable to many because the derivation of an ES cell line from the cloned embryo (an essential step in this process) necessarily involves the loss of an embryo and hence the destruction of potential human life.

In this chapter, I develop two main arguments that are based on the available scientific evidence. First, in contrast to an embryo derived by *in vitro* fertilization (IVF), a cloned embryo has little, if any, potential to ever develop into a normal human being. By circumventing the normal processes of gametogenesis and fertilization, nuclear cloning prevents the proper reprogramming of the clone's genome, which is a prerequisite for development of an embryo to a normal individual. It is unlikely that these biologic barriers to normal development can be solved in the foreseeable future. Therefore, from a biologist's point of view, the cloned human embryo which is to be used for the derivation of an ES cell and the subsequent transfer into a patient in need has little if any potential to create a normal human life. Second, ES cells developed from a cloned embryo are functionally indistinguishable from those that have been generated from embryos derived by IVF. Both types of ES cells have an identical potential to serve as a source for therapeutically useful cells.

ES cells can be used to correct inherited gene defects by gene targeting. This approach is not complicated by serious side effects as have been seen recently in gene therapy trials using retroviral vectors to introduce genes into hematopoietic stem cells. The goal of this chapter is to summarize the biology of stem cell-based therapy and to contribute further more informed discussion of therapeutic cloning founded on scientific evidence rather than on misconceptions or misrepresentations of the available scientific data.

3.1   Promise and problems of gene transfer

Gene transfer is a therapeutic approach that involves the insertion of genetic material into some cells of a patient with the goal to correct an inborn error of metabolism or to provide the cells with a new function.[1] Genes can be either transferred into germ cells (germ-line genetic transfer, GLGT) or into somatic cells (somatic cell genetic transfer, SCGT). In addition to serious scientific issues, GLGT and other forms of inheritable genetic modification (IGM) face considerable ethical concerns not examined in this chapter.

In SCGT, a "therapeutic" gene (i.e., a functional copy of the mutated or dysfunctional gene of a patient), is introduced into the patient's cells. For example, severe combined immune deficiency (SCID) is an inherited disorder that is caused by the deficiency of an enzyme which is crucial for normal immune cell function. The transfer of a normal copy of this gene into bone marrow stem cells would fully restore enzymatic activity resulting in an effective cure of the disease. As gene transfer is inefficient at best, most gene therapy trials to date have used viral vectors to transfer the functional gene into hematopoietic stem cells (i.e., those cells that are able to generate the full range of red and white cells in the blood). Indeed, SCID was cured in 10 diseased infants by retrovirus mediated interleukin receptor gene transfer into blood progenitors. However, the therapy trials were abruptly halted when 2 of the 10 treated patients developed leukemia.[2] This unanticipated and serious complication was caused by the accidental insertion of the retroviral vector into an oncogene leading to its activation and to leukemic transformation.

Gene repair by homologous recombination (gene targeting) represents a safer approach, as it would exclude the chance activation of an endogenous gene by random insertion of a gene vector into the genome. However, gene targeting cannot be done in hematopoietic stem cells (or in other adult stem cells) because somatic stem cells are rare and difficult to propagate in culture. In contrast, gene targeting can routinely be accomplished in permanently growing ES cells. This chapter does not discuss the scientific issues surrounding gene transfer technology, which can be found in recent literature reviews.[3] Instead I focus on ES cells and the promise and problems of "therapeutic cloning" approaches as a basis for tissue repair and gene therapy.

3.2   Nuclear cloning and ES cells

For nuclear cloning it is important to distinguish between "reproductive cloning" and "nuclear transplantation therapy" (also referred to as SCNT or therapeutic cloning). In reproductive cloning, a cloned embryo is generated by transfer of a somatic nucleus into an enucleated egg with the goal to create a cloned individual. In contrast, the purpose of nuclear transplantation therapy is to generate an ES cell line (referred to as ntES cells) that is "tailored" to the needs of a patient who served as the nuclear donor. The ntES cells could be used as a source of functional cells that would be suitable for treating an underlying disease by transplantation.

There is now experience from cloning of seven different mammalian species that is relevant for three main questions that are of general, public interest: first, would cloned human embryos be "normal"? Second, could the problems currently seen with cloning be solved in the foreseeable future? Three, could ES cells derived from cloned human embryos be "normal" and useful for cell therapy? The arguments advanced in this chapter are strictly based on molecular and biologic evidence that has been obtained largely in the mouse.[4]

3.2.1 Most cloned animals die or are born with abnormalities

The majority of cloned mammals derived by nuclear transfer (NT) die during gestation, and those that survive to birth frequently display "large offspring syndrome," a neonatal phenotype characterized by respiratory and metabolic abnormalities, and enlarged and dysfunctional placentas.[5] In order for a donor nucleus to support development into a clone, it must be reprogrammed to a state compatible with embryonic development. The transferred nucleus must properly activate genes important for early embryonic development and also suppress differentiation-associated genes that had been transcribed in the original donor cell. Inadequate "reprogramming" of the donor nucleus is most likely the principal reason for developmental failure of clones.[6] Since few clones survive to birth, the question remains whether survivors are fully normal or merely the least affected animals who carry through to adulthood despite harboring subtle abnormalities that originate in faulty reprogramming but that are not severe enough to interfere with survival to birth or beyond.

3.2.2 Reprogramming of the genome during normal development and after nuclear transfer

The fundamental difference between nuclear cloning and normal fertilization is that the nucleus used in nuclear cloning comes from a somatic cell that has not undergone the developmental events required to produce the egg and sperm. Nuclear cloning involves the transplantation of a somatic nucleus into the oocyte from which the nucleus has been removed. However, the genes in the somatic nucleus are not in the same state as those in the fertilized egg because nuclear transplantation short-cuts the complex process of egg and sperm maturation which involves extensive "reprogramming" of the genome, a process that shuts some genes off and leaves others on. Reprogramming during gametogenesis prepares the genome of the two mature gametes with the ability to activate faithfully the genetic program that ensures normal embryonic development when they combine at fertilization. This reprogramming of the genome begins at gastrulation,

when primordial germ cells (PGCs) are formed, and continues during differentiation into mature gametes resulting, in a radically different chromatin configuration of sperm and oocyte.[7]

Experiments have shown that uniparental embryos (embryos whose genomes
are derived solely from either the maternal or paternal parent) do not develop
normally. Uniparental embryos at first seem normal; they direct cleavage (early
development to the blastocyst stage) despite profound differences in their epigenetic organization.[8] However, uniparental embryos fail soon after the implantation of the embryo into the wall of the uterus, indicating that both parental
genomes are needed and functionally complement each other beginning at this
later step of embryogenesis. Presumably, the different epigenetic organization of
the two genomes is crucial for achieving normal development. Moreover, it has
been well established that the imbalance of imprinted gene expression represents an important cause of embryonic failure.[9]

In order for cloned embryos to complete development, genes normally
expressed during embryogenesis but silent in the somatic donor cell must be reactivated. This complex process of epigenetic remodeling (i.e., the reconfiguration of
the genome by turning on and off specific genes) that occurs during gametogenesis in normal development ensures that the genome of the zygote can faithfully
activate early embryonic gene expression.[10] In a cloned embryo, reprogramming,
which in normal gametogenesis requires months to years to complete, must occur
in a cellular context radically different from gametogenesis and within the short
interval (probably within hours) between transfer of the donor nucleus into
the egg and the time when zygotic transcription becomes necessary for further
development. Given these radically different conditions, one can envisage a spectrum of different outcomes to the reprogramming process ranging from (i) no
reprogramming of the genome, resulting in immediate death of the NT embryo;
through (ii) partial reprogramming, allowing initial survival of the clones, but
resulting in an abnormal phenotype and/or lethality at various stages of development; to (iii) faithful reprogramming producing fully normal animals. The phenotypes observed over the past 5 years in cloned embryos and newborns suggest
that complete reprogramming is the exception, if it occurs at all.

3.2.3   Development of clones depends on the differentiation-state of the donor nucleus

The majority of cloned embryos fail at an early step of embryonic development,
soon after implantation in the wall of the uterus, an early step of embryonic
development.[11] Those that live to birth often display common abnormalities
irrespective of the donor cell type (see Table 3.1). In addition to symptoms
referred to as "large offspring syndrome," neonate clones often suffer from respiratory distress and kidney, liver, heart, or brain defects.[12] However, the abnormalities characteristic of cloned animals are not inherited by their offspring,[13]

Table 3.1. Development of normal embryos and embryos cloned from ES cell and somatic donor nuclei. Note that normal and ES-cell-derived blastocysts have a similar potency to develop to term if calculated from the fraction of transplanted blastocysts

Donor nucleus	Mice (% of blastocysts)	Phenotype
Fertilized zygote	30–50%	Normal
NT from		Most (if not all) clones are
ES cell	15–30%[14]	abnormal
Cumulus cell, fibroblast	1–3%[15]	
B and T cells	<1/3000[16]	

indicating that epigenetic aberrations (i.e., failure of genome reprogramming) rather than genetic aberrations (changes in the sequences within the DNA) are the cause.

The efficiency of creating cloned animals is strongly influenced by the differentiation-state of the donor nucleus (Table 3.1). In the mouse, for example, only 1–3% of cloned blastocysts derived from somatic donor nuclei (e.g., those prepared from fibroblasts or cumulus cells) will develop to adult cloned animals.[17] In certain cases, such as those using terminally differentiated B or T cell donor nuclei, the efficiency of cloning is so low as to preclude the direct derivation of cloned animals. In stark contrast to these examples, cloning using donor nuclei prepared from ES cells is significantly more efficient (between 15% and 30%, see Table 3.1). This correlation with differentiation-state suggests that embryonic nuclei require less reprogramming of their genome, ostensibly because the genes essential for embryonic development are already active and need not be reprogrammed. In fact, the nucleus of an embryonic cell such as an ES cell may well have the same high efficiency to generate postnatal mice after NT as the nucleus prepared from a recently fertilized egg (see Table 3.1; and *cf.* Fig. 3.3). Nonetheless, most if not all mice that have been cloned from ES cell donor nuclei, in contrast to mice derived through natural fertilization from the zygote, are abnormal, indicating that the processes of gametogenesis and fertilization endows the zygote nucleus with the ability to direct normal development. In summary, these data indicate that the potential of a nucleus to generate a normal embryo is lost progressively with development.

3.2.4   Adult cloned animals: how normal are they?

The observation that apparently healthy adult cloned animals have been produced in seven mammalian species (albeit at low efficiency) is being used by some as a justification for attempting to clone humans. In fact, even those that survive to adulthood, such as Dolly, may succumb relatively early in adulthood because of numerous health problems. Insights into the mechanisms responsible for clone failure before and after birth have come from molecular and biologic analyses of mouse clones that have reached the blastocyst stage, the perinatal period, and adulthood, respectively.

3.2.4.1   Most clones fail early

As stated above in order for clones to develop, the genes that are normally expressed during embryogenesis, but are silent in the somatic donor cell, must be reactivated.[18] It is the failure to activate key "embryonic" genes that are required for early development that leads to the demise of most clones just after implantation. Recently, a set of about 70 key embryonic genes termed "Oct-4 like" genes have been identified that are active in early embryos but not in somatic donor cells. Importantly, the failure to faithfully activate this set of genes can be correlated with the frequent death of cloned animals during the immediate postimplantation period.[19] These results define "faulty reprogramming" as the cause of early demise of cloned embryos through the failure to reactivate key embryonic genes that are silent in the donor cell.

3.2.4.2   Newborn clones misexpress hundreds of genes

Clones that survive to birth suffer from serious problems, many of which appear to be due to an abnormal placenta. The most common phenotypes observed in animals cloned from either somatic or ES cell nuclei are fetal growth abnormalities such as increased placental and birth weight. This has suggested that surviving clones had accurately reprogrammed the "Oct-4 like" genes that are essential for the earliest stages of development (i.e., those immediately following implantation of the embryo into the uterus). The abnormal phenotype of those clones that do survive through these early stages and develop to birth indicates that other genes that are important for later stages of development but are not essential for early survival are not correctly reprogrammed. To assess the extent of abnormal expression of various genes in the cells of clones, global gene expression has been assessed by microarray analysis of RNA prepared from the placentas and livers of neonatal cloned mice (i.e., clones that survived development and were viable at birth); these clones had been derived by NT of nuclei prepared either from cultured ES cells or from freshly isolated cumulus cells (somatic cells that surround the egg).[20] Direct comparison of gene expression profiles of over 10,000 genes (of the 30,000 or so in the mammalian genome) showed that for both classes of cloned neonatal mice, approximately 4% of the expressed genes in their placentas differed dramatically in expression levels from those in controls, and that the majority of abnormally expressed genes were common to both types of clones. When imprinted genes, a class of genes that express only one allele (either from maternal or paternal origin), were analyzed, between 30% and 50% were not correctly activated. These data represent strong molecular evidence that cloned animals, even those that survive to birth, suffer from serious gene expression abnormalities.

3.2.4.3   Cloned animals develop serious problems with age

The generation of adult and seemingly healthy adult cloned animals has been taken as evidence that normal cloned animals can be generated by NT, albeit with low efficiency. Indeed, a routine physical and clinical laboratory examination of 24 cloned cows of 1–4 years of age failed to reveal major abnormalities.[21] Cloned mice whose ages correspond to those of the cloned cows (2–6 months in mice versus 1–4 years in cows) also appear "normal" by superficial inspection. However, when cloned mice aged, serious problems, not apparent at younger ages, became manifest. One study found that the great majority of cloned mice died significantly earlier than normal mice, succumbing with immune deficiency and serious pathologic alterations in multiple organs.[22] Another study found that aged cloned mice became overweight with major metabolic disturbances.[23] Thus, serious abnormalities in cloned animals may often become manifest only when the animals age.

Firm evidence about aging and "normalcy" of cloned farm animals is incomplete or anecdotal because cloned animals of these species are still comparatively young (relative to their respective normal life span). For example, the premature death of Dolly[24] is entirely consistent with serious abnormalities in cloned sheep that become manifest only at later ages. Also, 2 of the analyzed cloned cows developed disease soon after the study on "healthy and normal cattle"[25] had appeared: 1 animal developed an ovarian tumor and another one suffered brain seizures.[26] While it cannot be ruled out that these are "spontaneous" maladies unconnected with the cloning procedure, a more likely alternative is that these problems were direct consequences of the NT procedure.

3.2.4.4   Are there any "normal" clones?

It is a key question in the public debate whether it is ever possible to produce a normal individual by nuclear cloning, even if only with low efficiency. The available evidence suggests that it may be difficult if not impossible to produce normal clones for the following reasons. First, as summarized above, all analyzed clones at birth showed dysregulation of hundreds of genes. The development of clones to birth and beyond despite widespread epigenetic abnormalities suggests that mammalian development can tolerate dysregulation of many genes. Second, some clones survive to adulthood by compensating for gene dysregulation. Though this "compensation" assures survival, it may not prevent the manifestation of maladies at later ages. Therefore, most if not all clones are expected to have at least subtle abnormalities that may not be so severe as to result in an obvious phenotype at birth but will cause serious problems later as seen in aged mice. Clones may just differ in the extent of abnormal gene expression: if the key

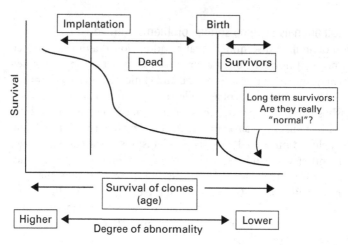

Degree of abnormalities in clones
A continuum without defined stages

Figure 3.1. The phenotypes are distributed over a wide range of abnormalities. Most clones fail at two defined developmental stages: implantation and birth. More subtle gene expression abnormalities result in disease and death at later ages.

"Oct-4 like" genes are not activated, clones die immediately after implantation. If those genes are activated, the clone may survive to birth and beyond.

The two stages when the majority of clones fail are immediately after implantation and at birth (see Fig. 3.1). These are two critical stages of development that may be particularly vulnerable to faulty gene expression. Once cloned newborns have progressed through the critical perinatal period, various compensatory mechanisms may counterbalance abnormal expression of other genes that are not essential for the subsequent postnatal survival. However, the stochastic occurrence of disease and other defects at later age in many or most adult clones implies that such compensatory mechanisms do not guarantee "normalcy" of cloned animals. Rather, the phenotypes of surviving cloned animals may be distributed over a wide spectrum from abnormalities causing sudden demise at later postnatal age or more subtle abnormalities allowing survival to advanced age. These considerations illustrate the complexity of defining subtle gene expression defects and emphasize the need for more sophisticated test criteria such as environmental stress or behavior tests. However, the available evidence suggests that truly normal clones may be the exception.

It should be emphasized that "abnormality" or "normalcy" are defined here by molecular and biologic criteria that distinguish cloned embryos or animals from control animals produced by sexual reproduction. The most informative data for the arguments presented above come from the mouse. There is, however, every reason to believe that these difficulties associated with producing mice and a variety of other mammalian embryos by nuclear transplantation will also afflict the process of human reproductive cloning.[27]

3.2.4.5 Is it possible to overcome the problems inherent in reproductive cloning?

It is often argued that the "technical" problems in producing normal cloned mammals will be solved by scientific progress that will be made in the foreseeable future. The following considerations argue that this may not be so.

A principal biologic barrier that prevents clones from being normal is the "epigenetic" difference (such as distinct patterns of DNA methylation[28]) between the chromosomes inherited from mother and father (i.e., the difference between the "maternal" and the "paternal" genome of an individual). Methylation of specific DNA sequences is known to be responsible for shutting down the expression of nearby genes. Parent-specific methylation marks are responsible for the expression of imprinted genes and cause only one copy of an imprinted gene, derived either from sperm or egg, to be active while the other allele is inactive.[29] When sperm and oocyte genomes are combined at fertilization, the parent-specific marks established during oogenesis and spermatogenesis persist in the genome of the zygote. Of interest for this discussion is that within hours after fertilization, most of the global methylation marks (with the exception of those on imprinted genes) are stripped from the sperm genome whereas the genome of the oocyte is resistant to this active demethylation process.[30] This is because the oocyte genome is already in an "oocyte-appropriate" epigenetic state whereas the incoming sperm genome has to alter its epigenetic state to become "oocyte-appropriate." The oocyte genome becomes only partially demethylated within the next few days by a passive demethylation process. The result of these postfertilization changes is that the two parental genomes are epigenetically different (as defined by the patterns of DNA methylation) in the later stage embryo and remain so in the adult in imprinted as well as non-imprinted sequences.

In cloning, the epigenetic differences that are established during gametogenesis may be erased because both parental genomes of the somatic donor cell are introduced into the egg from the outside and are thus exposed equally to the demethylation activity present in the egg cytoplasm.

This predicts that imprinted genes may be particularly vulnerable to inappropriate methylation and associated dysregulation in cloned animals. The results summarized earlier are consistent with this prediction. For cloning to be made safe, the two parental genomes of a somatic donor cell would need to be physically separated and separately treated in an "oocyte-appropriate" and a "sperm-appropriate" way, respectively. At present, it seems that this is the only rational approach to guarantee the creation of the epigenetic differences that are normally established during gametogenesis. Such an approach is beyond our present abilities. These considerations imply that serious biologic barriers exist that interfere with faithful reprogramming after NT. It is a safe conclusion that these biologic barriers represent major stumbling blocks to efforts aimed at making nuclear cloning a safe reproductive procedure for the foreseeable future.

It has been argued that the problems in mammalian cloning are similar to those encountered 30 years ago with IVF. Thus, following this argument, the methods of culture and embryo manipulations merely would need to be improved to develop reproductive cloning into a safe reproductive technology that is as acceptable as IVF. This argument appears to be fundamentally flawed. It is certainly correct that merely "technical" problems needed to be solved to make IVF efficient and safe. But it is important to distinguish between the perfection of technical skills to imitate a biologic event and the development of wholly new science to overcome the blocks to events that have severe biologic restrictions. Nuclear cloning faces serious biologic barriers that cannot be addressed by mere adjustments in experimental technique. Indeed, since the birth of Dolly, no progress has been made in solving any of the underlying biologic issues of faulty gene reprogramming and resulting defective development.

3.3   Therapeutic applications of SCNT

3.3.1   Reproductive cloning versus therapeutic cloning

In spite of the biologic and ethical barriers associated with reproductive cloning, NT technology has significant therapeutic potential that is within our grasp. There is an enormous distinction between the goals and the end product of these two technologies. The purpose of reproductive cloning is to generate a cloned embryo that is then implanted in the uterus of a female to give rise to a cloned individual. In contrast, the purpose of nuclear transplantation therapy is to generate an ES cell line (ntES cells) that is derived from a patient and can be used subsequently for tissue replacement.

Many scientists recognize the potential of ntES cells for organ transplantation. Nearly all organ transplants undertaken at present involve the use of donor organs that are recognized as foreign by the immune systems of the recipient and thus are targeted for destruction by these immune systems. To treat this "host versus graft" disease, immunosuppressive drugs are routinely given to transplant recipients in order to suppress this organ rejection. Such immunosuppressive treatment has serious side effects, including increased risks of infections and malignancies. In principle, ES cells can be created from a patient's nuclei using NT. As ntES cells will be genetically identical to the patient's cells, the risks of immune rejection and the requirement for immunosuppression will be eliminated. Moreover, ES cells provide a renewable source of replacement tissue allowing for repeated therapy whenever needed. Finally, if ES cells are derived from a patient carrying a known genetic defect, the mutation in question can be corrected in the ntES cells using standard gene targeting methods before introducing these ES cells (or derived tissue-specific stem cells) back into the patient's body.

3.3.2 Combining nuclear cloning with gene and cell therapy

In a "proof of principle" experiment, nuclear cloning in combination with gene and cell therapy has been used to treat a mouse genetic disorder that has a human counterpart (Fig. 3.2). To do so, the well-characterized Rag2 mutant mouse was used as the "patient."[31] This mutation causes SCID, because the enzyme that catalyzes immune receptor rearrangements in lymphocytes is non-functional. Consequently, these mice are devoid of mature B and T cells, a disease resembling human Omenn syndrome.[32]

In a first step, somatic (fibroblast) donor cells were isolated from the tails of Rag2-deficient mice and their nuclei were injected into enucleated eggs. The resultant embryos were cultured to the blastocyst stage and isogenic ES cells were isolated. Subsequently, one of the mutant Rag2 alleles was targeted for repair by homologous recombination in ES cells to restore normal Rag2 gene structure and function. In order to obtain somatic cells for treatment, these genetically-repaired ES cells were differentiated into embryoid bodies and further into hematopoietic precursors by expressing HoxB4, a transcription factor that is responsible for programming the behavior of the hematopoietic stem cells. Resulting hematopoietic precursors were transplanted into irradiated Rag2-deficient animals in order to treat the disease caused by their Rag2 mutation. Initial attempts to engraft these cells were, however, unsuccessful because of an increased level of natural killer (NK) cells in the Rag mutant host. ES-cell-derived hematopoietic cells express low levels of the MHC antigens and thus are a preferred target for NK mediated destruction. Elimination of NK cells by antibody depletion or genetic ablation allowed the ntES cells to efficiently populate the myeloid and to a lesser degree the lymphoid lineages of these mice. Functional B and T cells that had undergone proper rearrangements of their immunoglobulin and T cell receptor alleles as well as serum immunoglobulins were detected in the transplanted mutants. Hence, important cellular components of the immune system were restored in mice that previously were unable to produce these cells.

This experiment demonstrated that ES cells derived by NT from somatic cells of a genetically-afflicted individual can be combined with gene transfer to treat the underlying genetic disorder. As Rag2 deficiency causes an increase in NK activity and necessitated the elimination of NK cells prior to transplantation in the above-described experiments, some have concluded that "the experiment failed to show success with therapeutic cloning"[33] and that "this indicates that the only successful therapy using cloned embryos would be through 'reproductive' cloning, to produce born clones who can serve as tissue donors for patients."[34] This is a troublesome, indeed willful misrepresentation of the data. First, it has been shown that

Correction of a genetic defect by combination of therapeutic cloning and gene therapy

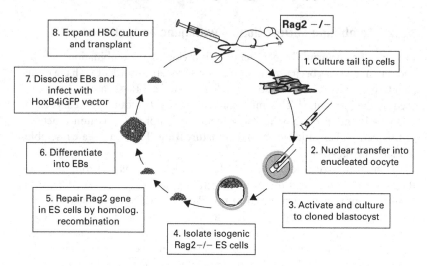

Figure 3.2. Scheme for therapeutic cloning combined with gene and cell therapy. A piece of tail from a mouse homozygous for the recombination activating gene 2 (Rag2) mutation was removed and cultured. After fibroblast-like cells grew out, they were used as donors for NT by direct injection into enucleated MII oocytes using a Piezoelectric driven microma-nipulator. ES cells isolated from the NT-derived blastocysts were genetically repaired by homologous recombination. After repair, the ntES cells were differentiated *in vitro* into embryoid bodies (EBs), infected with the HoxB4iGFP retrovirus, expanded, and injected into the tail vein of irradiated, Rag2-deficient mice.

ES-cell-derived hematopoietic cells can successfully engraft and rescue lethally irradiated mice indicating that increased NK activity is a peculiarity of Rag2-deficiency.[35] Therefore, it would seem that for most diseases no anti-NK treatment would be required to assure engraftment of ES-cell-derived somatic cells. Second, it is correct that treatment of a human patient with Omenn syndrome, which is equivalent to Rag2 deficiency, by SCNT may also require anti-NK treatment to transiently reduce NK activity. This would allow the transplanted cells to engraft as in the mouse experiment. Once these cells are successfully engrafted, there is every reason to believe that such anti-NK treatment would no longer be necessary.

In conclusion, the mouse experiment indicates that, unlike the situation with reproductive cloning, no biologic barriers exist that in principle prevent the use of SCNT to treat human diseases. The technical issues in using SCNT and human stem cells for therapeutic purposes need, however, to be solved, but there are no indications at present that these represent formidable problems that will resist relatively rapid solution.

3.4   Faulty reprogramming after nuclear transfer: does it interfere with the therapeutic potential of embryonic stem cells?

As summarized above, most if not all cloned animals are abnormal because of faulty reprogramming after NT. Does this epigenetic dysregulation affect the potential of ntES cells to generate functional somatic cells that can be used for cell therapy? To address this question, I first compare the *in vivo* development of embryos with the *in vitro* process of ES cell derivation from explanted embryos, and then discuss the epigenetic state of the ES cell genome. Finally, I contrast the phenotype of cloned mice derived from ES cell donor nuclei with that of chimeric mice generated by injection of ES cells into blastocysts.

3.4.1   The phenotype of an embryo is determined by its donor nucleus

As mentioned repeatedly above, embryos can be derived from the fertilized egg or from a somatic nucleus by SCNT. The potential of the resulting blastocyst, when implanted into the womb, to develop into a fetus and a postnatal animal depends strictly on the nature of the donor nucleus (Fig. 3.3).

First, when derived from the zygote, most embryos develop to birth and generate a normal animal. Second, similarly, most blastocysts cloned from an ES cell donor nucleus develop to birth but, in contrast to the normally fertilized embryo, the great majority of the cloned animals will be abnormal ("large offspring syndrome").[36] Third, the great majority of cloned blastocysts derived from somatic donor nuclei such as fibroblasts or cumulus cells will die soon after implantation and only a few clones will survive to birth and these too will be abnormal, suffering once again from the large offspring syndrome.[37] Finally, the likelihood of cloned blastocysts derived from another type of somatic donor nucleus – present in terminally differentiated lymphoid cells – to generate a cloned animal is extremely low and has not been achieved except by using a two-step procedure involving the intermediate generation of ES cells.[38] These observations suggest that a blastocyst retains an "epigenetic memory" of its donor nucleus. This memory determines its potential for fetal development: while a fertilized embryo develops normally, any embryo derived by SCNT will be abnormal though the efficiency of a given clone to develop to birth is strongly influenced by the differentiation-state of the donor cell (see Table 3.1). In other words, the cloned embryo after implantation into the womb will be abnormal because the cloned blastocyst retained an epigenetic memory of its donor nucleus and this causes faulty fetal development. This epigenetic memory is erased when a blastocyst, either derived by nuclear cloning or from the fertilized egg, is explanted into tissue culture and grown into an ES cell. Erasure of the epigenetic memory has major consequences for the "normalcy" of ES cells.

**Epigenetic memory of blastocyst
nuclear donor determines phenotype of embryo**

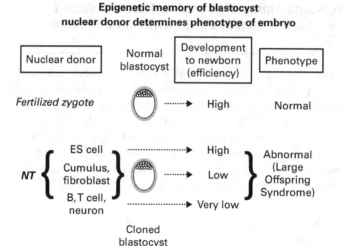

Figure 3.3. Blastocysts retain epigenetic memory of donor nucleus. Blastocysts can be derived from the fertilized egg or by NT. After implantation development of the embryo strictly depends on the donor nucleus: blastocysts derived from a fertilized egg will develop with high efficiency to *normal* animals; blastocysts derived by NT from an ES cell donor will develop with high efficiency to *abnormal* animals; blastocysts derived by NT from a fibroblast or cumulus cell donor will develop with low efficiency to *abnormal* animals; blastocysts derived by NT from B or T donor cells will not develop to newborns by direct transfer into the womb (but only by a two-step procedure).

3.4.2   The derivation of embryonic stem cells is a highly selective process

ES cells, regardless of whether they have been generated from a fertilized egg or by SCNT, are derived from the cells of a blastocyst that have been explanted and propagated in tissue culture (Fig. 3.2). Of the blastocyst cells that are explanted in this way, those that derive from the portion of the blastocyst termed the inner cell mass (ICM) initially express "key" embryonic genes such as Oct-4. However, soon after explantation, most ICM cells extinguish Oct-4 expression and cease proliferating.[39] Only one or a few of the ICM-derived cells will eventually re-express Oct-4 and these few Oct-4-positive cells are those that resume rapid proliferation, yielding the cell populations that we designate as "ES" cells. These cells represent a cell population that has no equivalent in the normal embryo and may be considered a tissue culture artifact, though a useful one.

The important point for this discussion is that the propagation of blastocyst cells *in vitro* results in a rare population of surviving cells that have erased the "epigenetic memory" of the donor nucleus. This process results ultimately in ES cells that have, regardless of donor nuclear origin, an identical developmental potential. In other words, ES cells derived from embryos produced by normal fertilization and those produced from cloned embryos are functionally indistinguishable.[40] As the ES cells that derive from normally fertilized embryos are able to participate in the generation of all normal embryonic tissues, we can conclude that the ES cells derived from cloned embryos have a similar potential to generate the full range of normal tissues.

3.4.3   Embryonic stem cells, epigenetic instability, and therapeutic potential

Epigenetic instability appears to be a consistent characteristic of ES cells, regardless of whether they are derived from NT or a fertilized egg. This was shown when individual ES cells were analyzed for expression of imprinted genes: even cells in a recently subcloned ES cell line differed strongly in the expression of genes such as H19 or Igf2. The variable expression was correlated with the DNA methylation status of the genes, which switched from an unmethylated to a methylated state between sister cells.[41] This was a surprising result in view of the known potential of ES cells to generate terminally differentiated cells that function normally after transplantation into an animal. Possible explanations include:

1. that epigenetic instability in ES cells is a consequence of propagation of cells in tissue culture, or
2. that epigenetic instability is a prerequisite for cells to be pluripotent (i.e., this instability may be a manifestation of a plasticity in the gene expression program that is required to enable the ES cells to generate a wide variety of differentiated cell lineages).

Whatever the explanation for the observed epigenetic instability of ES cells may be, it supports the view that the process of generating ES cells erases all epigenetic memory of the donor nucleus and, as a consequence of the selection process, generates epigenetic instability in the selected cells. In other words, epigenetic instability appears to be an intrinsic characteristic of ES cells regardless of whether derived by SCNT or from a fertilized egg. This is consistent with the conclusion that both types of ES cells have an equivalent potency to generate functional cells in culture and, in the longer term, fully normal differentiated tissues upon implantation of these cells *in vivo*.

3.4.4   Embryonic stem cells form normal chimeras but abnormal nuclear clones

As outlined above, faulty reprogramming leads to abnormal phenotypes of cloned mice derived from ES cell donor nuclei. Why is faulty reprogramming and epigenetic instability a problem for reproductive cloning but not for therapeutic applications? The main reason for this seeming paradox is that, in contrast to reproductive cloning, the therapeutic application of NT does not require the formation of a fetus. Therapeutic applications involve the ability of cloned ES cells to form a single tissue or organ, not to recapitulate all of fetal development. For example, normal fetal development requires faithful expression of the imprinted genes. As outlined above, nuclear cloning causes between 30% to 50% of imprinted genes to be dysregulated consistent with the notion that disturbed imprinting is a major contributing factor to clone failure. As most imprinted genes have no known function in the postnatal animal, the dysregulation of imprinting would not be expected to impede functionality of *in vitro* differentiated ES cells because this process does not require the formation of a fetus. Therefore, the functionality of mature cells derived in culture from ES cells would not depend on the faithful reprogramming of the imprinted genes. Dysregulation of some imprinted genes such as Igf2 are known, however, to cause disease in the adult. Thus, it will be important to test whether dysregulation of such genes has adverse effects on the function of somatic cells derived from ES cells.

When injected into a blastocyst, ES cells form normal chimeras. It appears that the presence of surrounding "normal" cells (i.e., cells that are derived from a fertilized embryo) prevents an abnormal phenotype of the chimera such as the "large offspring syndrome" that is typical for cloned animals. Any therapeutic application creates, of course, a chimeric tissue where cells derived from ntES cells are introduced into a diseased adult individual and interact with surrounding "normal" host cells. Therefore, no phenotypic abnormalities, such as those seen in cloned animals, would be expected in patients transplanted with cells derived from ntES cells.

3.5 SCNT for cell therapy: destruction of potential human life?

A key concern raised against the application of the nuclear transplantation technology for tissue therapy in humans is the argument that the procedure involves the destruction of potential human life. From a biologic point of view, life begins with fertilization when the two gametes are combined to generate a new embryo that has a unique combination of genes and has a high potential to develop into a normal baby when implanted into the womb. A critical question for the public debate on SCNT is this one: is the cloned embryo equivalent to the fertilized embryo?

In cloning, the genetic contribution is derived from one individual and not from two. Obviously, the cloned embryo is the product of laboratory-assisted technology, not the product of a natural event. From a biologic point of view, nuclear cloning does not constitute the creation of new life, but rather the propagation of existing life because no meiosis, genetic exchange, and conception are involved. Perhaps more important is, however, the overwhelming evidence obtained from the cloning of seven different mammalian species that a cloned human embryo would have little if any potential to develop into a normal human being. As summarized above, the small fraction of cloned animals that survive beyond birth are likely to be abnormal, even if they appear "normal" upon superficial inspection. In other words, a cloned human embryo will lack the essential attributes that characterize the beginning of normal human life.

Taking into account the potency of fertilized and cloned embryos, the following scenarios regarding their possible fates can be envisaged (Fig. 3.4). Fertilized embryos that are "left over" from IVF have three potential fates: disposal, generation of normal ES cells, or implantation into the womb in hopes of production of a normal baby. Similarly, the cloned embryo has three potential fates: it can be destroyed or could be used to generate a normal ntES cell line that has the same potential for therapy as an ES cell derived from a fertilized embryo. In contrast to the fertilized embryo, the cloned embryo has little, if any, potential to ever generate a normal baby. An ES cell line derived by NT may, however, help sustain existing life when used as a source for cell therapy that is "tailored" to the need of the patient who served as its nuclear donor.

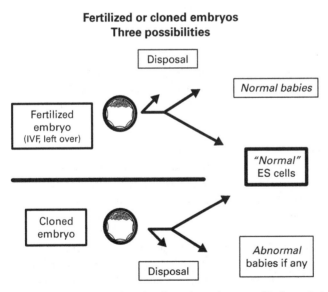

Figure 3.4. Normal and cloned embryos have three possible fates. Embryos derived by IVF ("left over embryos") have three fates: they can be disposed, create *normal* babies if implanted or can generate ES cells if explanted into tissue culture. Cloned embryos have also three fates: they can be disposed, can generate *abnormal* babies if any when implanted or can generate ES cells when explanted. The ES cells derived from an IVF embryo or a cloned embryo are indistinguishable.

If SCNT were accepted as a valid therapeutic option, a major concern of its implementation as medical procedure would be the problem of how to obtain sufficient numbers of human eggs that could be used as recipients. Commercial interests may pressure women into an unwanted role as egg donors. The demonstration that ES cells can be coaxed into a differentiation pathway that yields oocyte-like cells[42] may offer a solution to this dilemma. If indeed functional oocytes could be generated from a generic human ES cell line, sufficient eggs could be generated in culture and serve as recipients for NT without the need of a human egg donor. It seems that technical issues, not fundamental biologic barriers, need to be overcome so that transplantation therapy can be carried out without the use of human oocytes.

Acknowledgements

I thank my colleagues Bob Weinberg, Gerry Fink, George Daley, and Andy Chess for critical and constructive comments on this manuscript. The content of this chapter is largely based upon a review commissioned by the U.S. President's Council on Bioethics.[43]

NOTES

1 Alexander Pfeifer and Inder M. Verma, Gene therapy: promises and problems, *Annual Review of Genomics and Human Genetics* 2 (2001), 177–211; Neeltje A. Kootstra and Inder M. Verma, Gene therapy with viral vectors, *Annual Review of Pharmacology and Toxicology* 43 (2003), 413–39.

2 S. Hacein-Bey-Abina, C. Von Kalle, M. Schmidt, *et al.*, LMO2-associated clonal T cell proliferation in two patients after gene therapy for SCID-X1, *Science* 302 (2003), 415–20; D.B. Kohn, M. Sadelain and J.C. Glorioso, Occurrence of leukaemia following gene therapy of X-linked SCID, *Nature Reviews Cancer* 3 (2003), 477–88.

3 See also John Rasko and Douglas Jolly, The science of inheritable genetic modification (Chapter 2, this volume).

4 I do not attempt to review the cloning literature comprehensively, but only refer to selected papers on cloned mice. The relevant literature on cloning of mammals can be found in recent reviews such as L.E. Young, K.D. Sinclair and I. Wilmut, Large offspring syndrome in cattle and sheep, *Reviews in Reproduction* 3 (1998), 155–63; J.B. Gurdon, Genetic reprogramming following nuclear transplantation in Amphibia, *Seminars in Cell and Developmental Biology* 10 (1999), 239–43; W.M. Rideout, K. Eggan and R. Jaenisch, Nuclear cloning and epigenetic reprogramming of the genome, *Science* 293 (2001), 1093–8; Ian Wilmut, How safe is cloning? *Cloning* 3 (2001), 39–40; J.A. Byrne and J.B. Gurdon, Commentary on human cloning, *Differentiation* 69 (2002), 154–7; Konrad Hochedlinger and Rudolf Jaenisch, Nuclear transplantation: lessons from frogs

and mice, *Current Opinion in Cell Biology* 14 (2002), 741–8; B. Oback and D. Wells, Donor cells for cloning: many are called but few are chosen, *Cloning Stem Cells* 4 (2002), 147–68.

5 Young, Sinclair and Wilmut, Large offspring syndrome in cattle and sheep; Rideout, Eggan and Jaenisch, Nuclear cloning and epigenetic reprogramming of the genome.

6 The genome of a somatic cell is in an epigenetic state that is appropriate for the respective tissue from which it derives and assures the expression of the tissue-specific genes (in mammary gland cells, for example, those genes important for mammary gland function such as milk production). In contrast, the genes that are normally expressed in early development are in a "silent" epigenetic state (see Note 9 below). In cloning, the somatic nucleus must activate those genes that are needed for embryonic development but which are silent in the donor cell in order for the cloned embryo to survive. The egg cytoplasm contains "reprogramming factors" that can convert the epigenetic state characteristic of the somatic donor nucleus to one that is appropriate for an embryonic cell so it can activate the genes that are needed for embryonic development to proceed. This process is very inefficient leading to inappropriate expression of many genes and causes most clones to fail early.

7 Rideout, Eggan and Jaenisch, Nuclear cloning and epigenetic reprogramming of the genome.

8 Wolf Reik, Wendy Dean and Jörn Walter, Epigenetic reprogramming in mammalian development, *Science* 293 (2001), 1089–93.

9 For most genes, both copies, the one inherited from father and the one inherited from mother, are expressed. In contrast, only one of the two copies of an imprinted gene, either the maternal one or the paternal one, is active. The two copies are distinguished by methylation marks (see Note 28 below) that are imposed on imprinted genes either during oogenesis (maternally-imprinted genes) or during spermatogenesis (paternally-imprinted genes). Thus, the two copies of imprinted genes are epigenetically different in the zygote and remain so in all somatic cells. These epigenetic marks distinguish the two copies and cause only one copy to be expressed whereas the other copy remains silent. It is estimated that between 100 and 200 genes (of the total of 30,000 genes) are imprinted. Disturbances of normal imprinted gene expression lead to growth abnormalities during fetal life and can be the cause of major diseases such as Beckwith–Wiedeman and Prader–Willi syndromes.

10 Cells of a multicellular organism are genetically identical but express different sets of genes ("tissue-specific genes") depending on the particular cell type. These differences in gene expression arise during development and must be retained through mitosis. Stable alterations of this kind are said to be "epigenetic," as they are heritable in the short term (during cell divisions) but do not involve mutations of the DNA itself.

11 Rideout, Eggan and Jaenisch, Nuclear cloning and epigenetic reprogramming of the genome; Hochedlinger and Jaenisch, Nuclear transplantation; Oback and Wells, Donor cells for cloning.

12 Jose B. Cibelli, Keith H. Campbell, George E. Seidel, *et al.*, The health profile of cloned animals, *Nature Biotechnology* 20 (2002), 13–14.

13 Kellie L. Tamashiro, Teruhiko Wakayama, Hidenori Akutsu, *et al.*, Cloned mice have an obese phenotype not transmitted to their offspring, *Nature Medicine* 8 (2002), 262–7.

14 William M. Rideout, Teruhiko Wakayama, Anton Wutz, *et al.*, Generation of mice from wild-type and targeted ES cells by nuclear cloning, *Nature Genetics* 24 (2000), 109–10; Kevin Eggan, Hidenori Akutsu, Janet Loring, *et al.*, Hybrid vigor, fetal overgrowth, and viability of mice derived by nuclear cloning and tetraploid embryo complementation, *Proceedings of the National Academy of Science USA* 98 (2001), 6209–14; Kevin Eggan, Anja Rode, Isabell Jentsch, *et al.*, Male and female mice derived from the same embryonic stem cell clone by tetraploid embryo complementation, *Nature Biotechnology* 20 (2002), 455–9.

15 Teruhiko Wakayama, D.G. Whittingham and Ryuzo Yanagimachi, Production of normal offspring from mouse oocytes injected with spermatozoa cryopreserved with or without cryoprotection, *Journal of Reproduction and Fertility* 112 (1998), 11–7; Teruhiko Wakayama and Ryuzo Yanagimachi, Cloning of male mice from adult tail-tip cells, *Nature Genetics* 22 (1999), 127–8.

16 Konrad Hochedlinger and Rudolf Jaenisch, Monoclonal mice generated by nuclear transfer from mature B and T donor cells, *Nature* 415 (2002), 1035–8.

17 Hochedlinger and Jaenisch, Nuclear transplantation.

18 Rideout, Eggan and Jaenisch, Nuclear cloning and epigenetic reprogramming of the genome; Hochedlinger and Jaenisch, Nuclear transplantation.

19 Alex Bortvin, Kevin Eggan, Helen Skaletsky, *et al.*, Incomplete reactivation of Oct4-related genes in mouse embryos cloned from somatic nuclei, *Development* 130 (2003), 1673–80.

20 David Humpherys, Kevin Eggan, Hidenori Akutsu, *et al.*, Abnormal gene expression in cloned mice derived from ES cell and cumulus cell nuclei, *Proceedings of the National Academy of Science USA* 99 (2002), 12 889–94.

21 Humpherys, Eggan, Akutsu, *et al.*, Abnormal gene expression in cloned mice derived from ES cell and cumulus cell nuclei.

22 Narumi Ogonuki, Kimiko Inoue, Yoshie Yamamoto, *et al.*, Early death of mice cloned from somatic cells, *Nature Genetics* 30 (2002), 253–4.

23 Tamashiro, Wakayama, Akutsu, *et al.*, Cloned mice have an obese phenotype not transmitted to their offspring.

24 Jim Giles and Jonathan Knight, Dolly's death leaves researchers woolly on clone ageing issue, *Nature* 421 (2003), 776.

25 Robert P. Lanza, Jose B. Cibelli, David Faber, *et al.*, Cloned cattle can be healthy and normal, *Science* 294 (2001), 1893–4.

26 Jose B. Cibelli, personal communication.

27 Rudolf Jaenisch and Ian Wilmut, Developmental biology: don't clone humans! *Science* 291 (2001), 2552.

28 "DNA methylation" is defined as reversible modification of DNA (methylation of the base cytosine) that affects the "readability" of genes: usually, methylated genes are silent and unmethylated genes are expressed. DNA methylation represents an important determinant of the "epigenetic state" of genes and affects the state of the

chromatin: methylated regions of the genome are in a "silent" state and unmethylated regions are in an "open" configuration that causes genes to be active.

29 Wolf Reik and Jörn Walter, Genomic imprinting: parental influence on the genome, *Nature Reviews Genetics* 2 (2001), 21–32.

30 Wolfgang Mayer, Alain Niveleau, Jörn Walter, *et al.*, Demethylation of the zygotic paternal genome, *Nature* 403 (2000), 501–2.

31 William M. Rideout, Konrad Hochedlinger, Michael Kyba, *et al.*, Correction of a genetic defect by nuclear transplantation and combined cell and gene therapy, *Cell* 109 (2002), 17–27.

32 Rideout, Hochedlinger, Kyba, *et al.*, Correction of a genetic defect by nuclear transplantation and combined cell and gene therapy.

33 Coalition of Americans for Research Ethics, Do no harm–reality check: proof of "therapeutic cloning?" www.stemcellresearch.org/pr/pr_2003-03-10.htm, 2003 (last accessed 30 March 2005).

34 David Prentice, Why the "successful" mouse "therapeutic" cloning really didn't work, www.cloninginformation.org/info/unsuccessful_mouse_therapy.htm, 2002 (last accessed 30 March 2005).

35 Michael Kyba, Rita C. Perlingeiro and George Q. Daley, HoxB4 confers definitive lymphoid-myeloid engraftment potential on embryonic stem cell and yolk sac hematopoietic progenitors, *Cell* 109 (2002), 29–37.

36 David Humpherys, Kevin Eggan, Hidenori Akutsu, *et al.*, Epigenetic instability in ES cells and cloned mice, *Science* 293 (2001), 95–7; Eggan, Akutsu, Loring, *et al.*, Hybrid vigor, fetal overgrowth, and viability of mice derived by nuclear cloning and tetraploid embryo complementation.

37 Teruhiko Wakayama and Ryuzo Yanagimachi, Mouse cloning with nucleus donor cells of different age and type, *Molecular Reproduction and Development* 58 (2001), 376–83.

38 Hochedlinger and Jaenisch, Monoclonal mice generated by nuclear transfer from mature B and T donor cells.

39 M. Buehr, J. Nichols, F. Stenhouse, *et al.*, Rapid loss of oct-4 and pluripotency in cultured rodent blastocysts and derivative cell lines, *Biology of Reproduction* 68 (2003), 222–9.

40 Teruhiko Wakayama, Viviane Tabar, Ivan Rodriguez, *et al.*, Differentiation of embryonic stem cell lines generated from adult somatic cells by nuclear transfer, *Science* 292 (2001), 740–3; Hochedlinger and Jaenisch, Nuclear transplantation; Rideout, Eggan and Jaenisch, Nuclear cloning and epigenetic reprogramming of the genome.

41 Humpherys, Eggan, Akutsu, *et al.*, Epigenetic instability in ES cells and cloned mice.

42 Karin Hubner, Guy Fuhrmann, Lane K. Christenson, *et al.*, Derivation of oocytes from mouse embryonic stem cells, *Science* 300 (2003), 1251–6.

43 Rudolf Jaenisch, *The Biology of Nuclear Cloning and the Potential of Embryonic Stem Cells for Transplantation Therapy* (2003), http://www.bioethics.gov/background/jaenisch.html (last accessed 30 March 2005).

Controlling bodies and creating monsters: popular perceptions of genetic modifications

Christoph Rehmann-Sutter

4.1 Introduction

The idea of modulating the human genome to fit human plans and desires is stuff for fertile imagination and intellectual creativity. Ingenuous creators of popular culture (writers, film makers, cartoonists, and others) exceed the genetic engineers in their inventiveness. Even though their monsters might still be enclosed in the plastic test tubes of imagination, and even if not all of their content is meant to be taken as a serious forecast of a future technology or a future society, it is still meant to be seen as a contribution to the assessment of the powers and dangers of genetic manipulation of human and non-human bodies and to the decisions to be undertaken in the present. Pop culture is part of an enlarged bioethical discourse. The monsters of fiction sometimes demonstrate an imminent monstrosity, not primarily of those affected by gene transfer, but of the geneticists who perform it, and of the powers that influence and control them.

Genetic fantasies depend on how the genome is intellectualized. Images and phobias of genetic modifications presuppose – or reveal – an implicit understanding of what genes mean for human existence. A story about genetic change must seize in some terms on what it is that should be changed and the consequences that an intervention will have for the lives of those affected. The manipulators and also the authors of the imagination need a causal account of the genome. They need to have at least a rough idea of the mechanism connecting the effects of a possible intervention (e.g., a particular position in the DNA sequence), with an intended effect (e.g., the enhancement of a desired capacity). Otherwise they would not be able to plan (imagine) efficient intervention strategies.

Their account of the genome happens also to have ontologic implications. DNA is thought to contain in its sequence something like the "instruction book" of the human organism, a "program" to be executed or the like. This double-edged physical/metaphysical account cannot be developed by a strict application of scientific methods alone, because scientific results primarily give only answers to one aspect of the question: the causal. Their ontology remains implicit. The metaphysics of narratives may be, by contrast, debated more explicitly. There is no methodologic need to abstain from a certain kind of proposition in art and literature. It is an arena of free construction and decon-struction of ideas, identities, and life plans, and of metaphysics. Answers to questions about the meaning of genes for the existence and identity of humans and other species are given, repeated, ritualized, and sometimes also modified.[1] Through this process, the life science and biotechnology complex is engaged in an ongoing, indissoluble joint venture with cultural discourses. The double-edged causal and ontologic account of the genome will be its joint achievement.

The topic of this chapter is the popular narrative imagery of genetic alter-ations. It is a fascinating co-production of knowledge by scientists, pop culture producers, and average people through their everyday conversations. By its nature this topic is too large to be grasped in these few pages; this chapter there-fore is restricted to a few rather accidental examples which are interpreted in a qualitative way. The abundance of examples is impressive, and my sampling is the result of unsystematic participant-observation within contemporary high-tech culture.[2]

The overarching goal of interpreting the examples presented in this chapter is to learn more about the mechanisms of joint production of narratives in metaphysico-moral matters. Its mixture of skeptical questions and fascinating attractions is sometimes explosive. The questions these narrations deal with include: who wants to engage in genetic modification? For what purpose? What will be the collateral damage? Will our species be split between "Naturals" and "Rectifieds"? Or between "Normals" and genetic "Perverts," or between those in power, in part through their genetic superpowers, and those who will be genet-ically prevented from revolting against them? The narratives can be seen as contributions to moral reflections. This is the first role of pop culture: con-tributing to ethical discourse. Film is a medium that can contribute to ethical discourse in a much more direct way than theoretical texts can. Pictures touch the heart; a film's narrative can argue by constructing a case and getting the viewers involved.

But apart from that, the study of science fiction also reveals how our ways of dealing with the practices, changes, and risks of human biotechnologies, our ethical questions we pose are formed by those texts. People only infrequently refer directly to the scientific discourse but use well-known stories and myths from (mostly occidental) cultural traditions to endow the unknown with familiar meanings.[3] The unknown is transformed to a *fascinosum* that is both terrifying and attractive, a transformation that would not be possible without extensively drawing from our culture's meaning resources. Based upon this sec-ond role of science fiction in the process of cultural reproduction,[4] we can learn about the ontogeny of the perspective patterns and the frameworks of mean-ings that precede the issues which we discuss.

4.2   Explicit metaphysics

Some of the narratives about genetics may appear in popular culture and elsewhere merely as fragments or in an abbreviated form. An example of this is the "genetic program." It is a narrative presented in the nutshell of two words, a narrative with tremendous significance, as I will discuss below.[5] Others appear in larger packages, comprising the length of a novel or motion picture. But many of them are intertwined with each other. They form a narrative network in which the self is entangled, in which we find meanings, make our life plans, and in which we participate by finding our identities: answers to the question of what specifies ourselves, what makes what we are and what we want to realize.

Let us start with a simple three-panel cartoon by Nicole Hollander[6] showing two women speaking but not listening to each other. The woman on the left mentions her blind Saturday night date; on the right, the other says: "Scientists are genetically altering pigs to produce more muscle than fat." The woman on the left continues her own line of thought: "I know it's shallow, but I'd like to know what he looks like." The right, obviously concerned with her make-up, adds: "Soon humans will be genetically altered to conform to a single standard of beauty…" In the final panel, the first woman tries to interrupt her friend: "Could I have a little attention?" to which the other says, "But not by this weekend."

Superimposed on this story of casual non-communication is an account of what it might be desirable to do, once scientists are capable of modifying the genes: they could at least try to make love matters easier. But it also contains the suggestion that the alteration of genes could confer the power to do that: the power to make people conform to a single standard of beauty to decide what it means to treat humans similarly than pigs and so forth. The underlying story, however, is about the power biotechnology learns to utilize: the power of our genes over human appearance. This might also draw attention to the complementary gene technologic strategy which could be directed to the other part of an aesthetic relationship. The characteristics of *desire*, what people *see* as beautiful, might also be subject to genetic control and an object of intervention.

The power of our genes over human identity is sometimes predicted by lay participants to be enormous. A particularly striking example is available from a recent research study. In a qualitative interview when asked how she imagines the genes, B, an 18-year-old woman with severe cystic fibrosis (CF), said: "Basically, I have no idea of how a gene looks … Probably we could not see it with the naked eye … Humans consist of genes. They determine, for instance, the color of the hair or whether somebody will get ill with CF or not. You can inherit a gene … I do not know, perhaps a gene is small and round?"[7] "Humans consist of genes" – this is an awkward phrase. But it contains a very direct personal answer to the metaphysical question of what it is that *makes* a human being. It is information about her personal metaphysics. B says also that she knows that her disease has a genetic cause. When she said that she consists of genes and that CF is caused by one of them, she also said something about the relationship between herself and the condition CF. She obviously believes that her identity also includes the disease from which she is suffering. Her attitude towards gene therapy for CF is not negative but cautious. She imagines somebody who is offered a gene correction: "Perhaps this person does not want those other genes."[8] This may be a surprise for those who are used to identifying humanity with a healthy body, and disease with some dysfunction. But it is less a surprise for people who are suffering from chronic illnesses and disability.[9]

B and other lay people are not alone in drawing a connection between identity and the genes, in other terms between Aristotle's question about the *ti en einai* (what it means to be this) and DNA. Max Delbrück, one of the founders of molecular biology, claimed (rhetorically) that "this wonderful man [Aristotle] discovered DNA."[10] Why did he claim this? In his account of procreation, Aristotle insisted that, as Delbrück put it, "the male contributes, in the semen, a *form principle*, not a mini-man."[11] DNA has not only been an organizing principle for twentieth-century life sciences, it has also been one of the twentieth-century answers to the questions of metaphysics, and clearly not only in pop culture. Delbrück was not a professionally trained philosopher. If he had been, he probably would not have accepted the kind of answer that he proposes, for a number of good reasons. He would have thought that identifying this substance DNA (in this case via the semen) with the *eidos* is not a correct interpretation of Aristotle's ontology which identified essence with form (not matter), but rather a crude materialistic naturalism. It is hard to think that the form principle, the ontological "essence," sticks to a molecule. But nonetheless, in everyday life, the gene has indeed provided this kind of answer.[12]

In 2000, at the occasion of the public presentation of the "working draft" of the human genome, there was a need to explain the significance of the genome and its sequence. A problem had to be solved. Why should this sequence of one copy of human DNA, nothing but a boring list of ATCG letters produced by an industry of automatic sequencers, a huge load of mechanical work, be a milestone for humanity? U.S. President Bill Clinton fulfilled this task brilliantly by playing on the keyboard of the great narratives of western culture. An excerpt of his White House address on June 26, 2000 reads: "After all, when Galileo discovered he could use the tools of mathematics and mechanics to understand the motion of celestial bodies, he felt, in the words of one eminent researcher, that he had learned the language in which God created the universe ... Today we are learning the language in which God created life."[13] Galileo, the icon of Renaissance science and a symbol for modernity, understood the mathematical language in which the Book of Nature is written. God wrote it; humans learn to read it. God made the universe; humans learn to use his skills which come within their reach if they understand the basic natural laws. The genome has a parallel meaning to this. God wrote the Book of Life; humans learn to read it.[14] It is written in DNA letters, and the language is not yet known, except a few words. But here too humans have a lesson to learn. They are supposed to learn a new set of skills to understand and use DNA.

This metaphysics is obviously religious. The story, here only partially told, but mostly implicit, presents an image of God as the creator of the universe and life. God is an omniscient eternal being who guarantees that all parts of nature, all characters of life, have their meanings. But with this turn of the narration, the human scientific endeavor has also been glorified. Science is not merely the pragmatic activity of our species driven by natural selection, admittedly lacking in formal truth value but perhaps necessary for our survival. Science, particularly genomics, is rather the insight into eternal truths, like an intellectual private audience *(privatissimum)* with the Lord and Creator himself.

The occasion for communicating this to the public, mostly over their TV screens, itself contained an ambivalent message. It was not the scientists who announced it somewhere in a university hall, but their respective politicians: the President of the U.S.A., together with the British Prime Minister, speaking over video.[15] The human genome was also their business. This brings me to the double-sidedness of the story, in which there is only a one-handed humility. The other hand contributes to the glory of the storyteller himself. DNA, through this religious symbolism of the "language of creation," has not been made sacred and therefore immunized against manipulative changes or other kinds of technical exploitation. Nobody would have invested billions of dollars into the sequencing projects unless they had possible future utility value. Science on this scale of financing is not undertaken for pure intellectual satisfaction. There will be gene tests, there will be genetic modification, and there will also be rich fruits for all kinds of research in the life sciences and biotechnologies. All this investment will pay off. But is this all there is to consider? What about the genetic manipulation of the human constitution itself? What about inheritable genetic modification (IGM)?

This narrative, of course, has a direct consequence for the issue of IGM: it is tampering with God's ideas. Or, if we put more weight on the other half of the story, the side that glorifies the human intellect which is now capable of reading the Book of Life, IGM would be imitating the Creator *(imitatio Dei)*. Even if we allow room for those participating to be morally ambivalent and keep a critical distance from hubris, engaging in these interventions is still *playing* God. We are forced to admit that the Book of Life narrative definitely has a certain pay-off for the sanctification of IGM. BBC Radio explained the significance of the completion of the Human Genome Project as follows: "It is a complete manual for building and running the human body. We will be the only species who knows how to build ourselves [sic], to know who we are and where we came from."[16]

But there is still a gap between understanding the role of DNA in one organism and understanding the significance of the germ line. The germ line is what physically connects one generation to the next. August Weismann, who discovered the germ line, identified a lineage of cells within multicellular organisms which differentiates into the germ cells. They contain the germ plasm and carry in the chromosomes what he called *ids*, that is, elements of the architectural plan of the body. Germ cells bring those ids into the process of fertilization.[17] The gene's eye view of twentieth-century molecular biology has transformed this picture of cellular interactions and differentiation into a molecular variant; it is no longer the cell but the genes within them that produce the (somatic) body, which then dies off. Within a life time, the somatic body can replicate its genes such that they can enter a new process of procreation. This is "molecular Weismannism."[18] What is its metaphysical side?

The metaphysics underlying this view are related to the reality of the unifying principle of humanity. The germ line is sometimes seen as a physical representative of the universality of the species. In this view each individual is a particular instance, or a physical representation, of that universal humankind. According to the late thirteenth-century theologian William Ockham, the worst error of philosophy was precisely this: to believe that universals are real things rather than names or concepts.[19] He argued that everything real is just individual and particular, while universality is a property pertaining only to mental concepts (like names) due to their signification relations. In contrast to the metaphysical realism of universals, this nominalistic view has been a prerequisite for the development of the experimental methodology of modern science. Humankind, therefore, strictly scientifically speaking exists only in our minds. What *is* real are the individuals, each probably different from other individuals in some respects, in other respects similar.[20] All of them are related via family pedigrees. The germ line, in the nominalistic view, has no ontologic significance beyond physically representing those pedigrees. The germ line is not the representative of "the species."[21] But, as we have seen, the popularized understanding of the genes typically is far from strictly scientific.

If we take seriously the metaphysical overemphasis which has been placed on the genome, the germ line becomes more burdened as well. Because the germ cells transport the genes, they also confer the essential principle to a new organism. The germ line becomes a "metaphysical string" that not only connects individuals of different generations but also is the foundation for their possibilities of existing. This metaphysical overload makes IGM appear to be taboo; touching the germ line would mean doing the unthinkable: touching that universal principle upon which the character and individuality of every human being depends. It would change the species. It would change the origins.

4.3   Monsters

One key example of a species manipulator is Moreau in the John Frankenheimer film, *The Island of Dr Moreau*.[22] A biologist with a Nobel Prize for "gene manipulation," Moreau (played by Marlon Brando) was driven out of the U.S.A. by animal rights activists because of his experiments. He moved to an island in the middle of the ocean and established his laboratories there. For 17 years, he studied the fusion of animal and human genes and created a whole island full of monstrous, hideous half-humans. They had brutal instincts and had to be controlled strictly: Moreau used small electronic implants that caused terrible pain in the body of the creatures whenever they were switched on by a remote control device which always remained in his possession. Suffering from hypersensitivity to the sun, he always had to wear white clothes over his enormous body, put white make-up on his face, and protect himself with a veil, traveling around mounted on a huge all-terrain car that gave him a truly papal appearance. And he was indeed called "Father" by the creatures.

He both represented and enforced the law. "The Law is not to kill for any reason," said one of the creatures, in a court-like scene in front of Moreau. This scene occurs just before one of his own sons, the evil one of his four children (all partly animals) with the most brutal instincts ("to hunt, to kill"), shoots one of the other creatures without any motivating reasons. Its mourning parent discovers his child's implant among the ashes of the body, and realizes that these devices must be causing the pain and subduing them to Moreau. He rips his own implant out of his body and became immune to Moreau's remote control. A violent revolt breaks out, in the course of which Moreau and his family are killed, and the most monstrous islanders and the laboratories destroyed. Only a few of the creatures survive, among them a sort of primitive priest. The remaining inhabitants keep the wisdom they have acquired: "No more scientists! No more laboratories! We have to be what we are."

The story is told in retrospect by Douglas, the only survivor of an airplane accident over the ocean, who by chance was rescued by Moreau's assistant. He became an unintentional witness of the horrible events on the island. After he narrowly escaped the riot he fled from the island on a small ship and carried home the message from Moreau's island, which was a moral lesson. The last words of Douglas at the end of the film serve "…as a warning to all who want to follow Dr Moreau's footsteps. And I go in fear."

A key scene of the film is the conversation at a festive family dinner table in Moreau's house. After playing a moving Chopin composition on a grand piano, accompanied by a goblin on a tiny piano, Moreau explains his plans and ideas: "Well, permit me, Mr. Douglas, to tell you something of the devil … The devil is that element in human nature that impels us to destroy and debase." Douglas asks what Moreau has done other than debase, for instance in giving his progeny such dreadful monstrous appearances. Moreau responds:

The 17 years I have been striving to create some measure of refinement in the human species … And it is here, on this very island that I, sir, have found the very essence of the devil. I have seen him. I have seen the devil in my microscope and I have changed him … I have cut him into pieces. The devil I have found is nothing more than a tiresome collection of genes. And it is with great assurance that I can tell you that Lucifer is no more.

Douglas asks: "How does this justify these monstrous disfigurements?" "Very simply," states Moreau, "They represent a stage in the process of eradication of destructive elements found in the human psyche. And I have almost achieved perfection of a divine picture. It is pure, harmonious, absolutely incapable of malice."

This film is a very typical example of a moralistic tradition of narration which tells the story that tinkering with genes is dangerous because monsters will emerge and they will turn against their creators. We are in the vast story world of the Frankenstein myth. Frankenstein-story novels, plays, and films typically share three central themes: the transgression of a taboo, the figure of the mad scientist, and the loss of control over his monstrous creatures.[23] Remarkably enough, the taboo transgressed in *The Island of Dr Moreau* is animal experimentation, not gene modification. Moreau has been "thrown out of the States" by animal rights activists because of his inhumane experiments, but for genetic engineering he has been rewarded by a Nobel Prize. The madness of Moreau consists in his obsession, his *idée fixe* of eradicating the evil from human nature. He wanted to make humans ideal and absolutely incapable of malice, but ended up debasing them. Not even Aissa, his beautiful daughter ("a pussycat" as Montgomery, the assistant, calls her) was able to maintain her seeming perfection. She was slowly deteriorating; cat teeth were growing in her mouth. "I am changing," she cries in despair, "The syrup Montgomery gives me in the lab will stop my regression." Moreau's creatures could not even regain their dignity by removing their implants and revolting against their ruler; too much had already been destroyed in their natures.

One is forced to take the morals of this film seriously. It is not one of those light concoctions of the science fiction industry that you can put out of your mind after viewing it. The film gives a warning not to jeopardize the respect of the nature of the species. Human nature certainly has some elements of imperfection built into it. The film does not focus on the human imperfections of disease, the shortness of our lifespan, or our mortality, but malice, that "devil" inside ourselves which can lead us to be destructive, mean, and bad. Moreau compares the reality of human nature with an image of *moral* perfection, purity, and harmony. As a naïve moralist he believes that the difference between the ideal and the reality of human nature can, or even should, be exterminated for the better. As this goal is so highly esteemed, all means necessary to attain it seem to him to be justifiable.

This sort of moral caution against a blinding ideal that makes us inattentive to the means is not irrational and could also be seen to apply to other circumstances where we compare the reality with an ideal and try to eradicate the difference by gene technology. Max More, the founder of "extropianism," a movement to reverse the trend to increase entropy, for example sees an ideal in the absence of disease and aging ("we will no longer tolerate the tyranny of aging and death") and calls for all sorts of technologic interventions (including IGM) which he sees legitimized alone by the sadness of the actual *conditio humana*: "We will … take charge over our genetic programming and achieve mastery over our biologic and neurologic processes."[24] In all of these types of cases of technoeuphoristic naivety, we are likely to forget first that what we discern as a negative element distancing us from the ideal might have *positive* aspects; second that the result of the technologic procedure of making humans perfect might prove different than imagined, and not prove to be a direct realization of our mental image of the ideal; and third that the trail leading towards the goal of perfection is littered with debasement of those beings who will be used as mere "stages in the process." These types of arguments make a contribution to the ethical discourse on genetics, worth to be considered.

The Moreau story also is reminiscent of Mephisto in Goethe's *Faust*, who describes himself as part of the force that always wants evil but does good.[25] In *The Island*, Moreau as the prototype of the gene-manipulating scientist, is a mirror image of this force. He is part of the force which always wants good and does not care that in reality he produces evil. He wrestles the devil out of human genes but proves to be the devilish figure himself. It is not the genes that are Lucifer; Moreau does not really cut Lucifer "into pieces," but instead makes himself into a devilish figure who does not care about the reality of the effects of his deeds. He is enclosed by his own mind and sees only his ideals, not the real living creatures as other living beings. Even his own sons and his only and beloved daughter are mere "steps in the process," representing deviations from the ideal. But his creatures see in him their "father," even a God. As a means for self-protection and for guaranteeing his control over the brutes, he contributes to constructing and maintaining that picture of himself as a God-like figure.

There is another interesting element in *The Island*. Douglas, the inadvertent witness, identifies the spectators of the film as well as the island's creatures, as *monsters*. He complains of their "monstrous disfigurements." But what is a monster? An element of any monstrosity is certainly its abnormality, its misshapenness. But there are two other arguably more essential elements to the idea of a monster. First, not all abnormal and misshapen animals, plants, or persons are seen as monsters. The monster is frightening; it causes horror. If we think of a creature as a monster, we put this creature into a certain *position* in relation to ourselves. We construct or change a distinct relationship with the creature. The term "monster" only makes sense in a perceptive relationship; in fact, it *defines* a perceptive relationship. The perceptive relationship itself has normative and practical implications: the monster is not something you are supposed to help, support, or love. Quite the contrary, a monster is something to be feared and controlled, because it might possibly be dangerous. A monster is an outcast from all moral relationships. It may be fatal for a creature if others see it as a monster.

Second, monsters are imaginary creatures. This is obviously true for Moreau's monsters or Frankenstein's monster. But it also would be the case for real monsters, because monstrosity is merely an image projected onto a being. The real monster would be a combination of the reality of the perceived other being and of the mental image projected upon it. And in being imaginary creatures, monsters make sense only within a context of meanings, within a narrative. The crucial point of this meaning is hidden in the lingual root of the word "monster" – from the Latin verb *monstrare* – to show, to lead a way, to point to something. *Monstrum* also has stood for a sign of wonder.[26] Monster stories want to show something to us. As narrative elements they have a message. The appearance of a monster, if we were to encounter one, would reveal that something unusual is going on in our relationship with this being. In *The Island of Dr Moreau*, the monsters show their status as outcasts of moral relationships. They demonstrate the risk accompanying each project involving the modification of human nature (via genes), the risk that the creations will be outcasts of society and of moral relationships, because they are in some respect still (or accidentally even more) imperfect, and because their characters now can be attributed to human manufacture.

The simple fact of construction and interference will change moral relationships. At the beginning of the riot, one of the creatures asks Moreau: "Tell me why you made the pain?" Pain is no longer a natural phenomenon, but is due to the planning of a human being, which changes the meaning of pain considerably. It turns from being a misfortune to an injustice. Judith Shklar has argued that the defining element of injustice in comparison to misfortune is its dependence on decisions and therefore its avoidability.[27] On the island, the pain to which the creature refers was caused by the implants and the remote control. But the same is evidently true for all other sources of pain and suffering that trace back to genetic interventions.

IGM could cause harms as side effects. These harms, from the perspective of the person affected, will be the fault of his or her parents and doctors who have been involved in the decisions. It will no longer be attributable to fate or nature, but instead to other humans. This change also would alter the moral meaning of the suffering which would be connected with such side effects. But in principle this understanding will be equally valid for all other pains, diseases, and disabilities *not* changed by genetic intervention, because the element of change brings in arbitrariness. Such negative elements of the human body will be elements that have *not been* changed. Therefore, the moral meaning of all negative elements of the human constitution will be transformed from misfortune to injustice, as soon as the project of IGM begins. This is an important change in the moral universe that affects the perception of nearly everything of our bodies, every aspect that might be seen as undesirable. The anticipation of this change may be at the core of a powerful argument against the whole project of IGM.

Mary Wollstonecraft Shelley, in her original *Frankenstein* novel, borrowed three verses from John Milton's *Paradise Lost* to serve as a motto on the title page: "Did I request thee, Maker, from my clay / To mould Me man? Did I solicit thee / From darkness to promote me?"[28] In quite similar words in a reproach against Victor Frankenstein, his creator, the creature exclaims: "Cursed creator! Why did you form a monster so hideous that even you turned from me in disgust? God in pity made man beautiful and alluring, after his own image; but my form is a filthy type of yours, more horrid from its very resemblance."[29] Shelley's *Frankenstein* may be dissimilar to Frankenheimer's depiction of *The Island* in many respects, but both stories make an issue of the transformation of moral relationships occurring when the characters, the shape, and the construction of human descendants can be attributed to human responsibilities. Shelley's creature is a key figure. He makes biotechnologically-altered human procreation – a radically new type of interhuman relationship – morally translucent from the point of view of the progeny.

Closely connected to this theme is the issue of identity. At a gathering resembling a divine service, the creatures on *The Island* ask insecurely, "We are men, are we not?" Aissa, Moreau's daughter, sobbing because of her growing cat teeth, whispers to her father: "I want to be like you." Frankenstein's creature declares: "And what was I? ... Was I then a monster, a blot upon the earth, from which all men fled, and whom all men disowned?"[30] Both the film and the novel pose this question of identity for the products (or victims) of genetic manipulation. They are different from natural humans. Will the natural humans always have the generosity to accept every genetically-caused difference from the normal human constitution? Will genetic discrimination acquire another, even more forceful, dynamic when genetic features leading to discrimination are not natural, but the product of the gene technologic interventions of other people? How will genetically-altered human beings find their identities? Identity is not something we just invent. We do not have it simply in hand as a given, because identity is a joint production and accomplishment by many people interconnected in moral relationships. It depends on being loved by others, on trust, on being accepted as an equal.[31]

Another important detail from the film is the image of the island itself. Moreau, the mad scientist, has found a loophole in the international legal network by moving to the island. There, nobody can keep him from doing what he wants. Science is uncontrollable, because our legal systems are based on the institution of the states. This theme corresponds to a widespread fear that "rogue" scientists (like the supposed cloners in the media of our time) may exploit those differences and find a spot on the earth where nobody can control them.

Comparing *The Island of Dr Moreau* with Shelley's novel *Frankenstein* and a prototypic film version *Frankenstein* made in 1931,[32] two features of *The Island* warrant further attention. First, women have almost no active roles. They are shown only as the objects of sexual desire among the creatures. Aissa, Moreau's daughter who is the incomplete image of perfection and beauty, is desired by Douglas. Second, the inspiring moral model for *The Island* is an ethic of control, not an ethic of care. Shelley, an advocate of an ethic of care, showed *why* Frankenstein's creature became dangerous and monstrous: because of unrealized parental responsibility and a lack of relationships. But on the island, some of the creatures just are good, and others are mean, both as a result of their instincts. Consequently, ethical issues are grouped around the motives of risk and control.

Finally, there is also a strong dose of DNA mythology in the film *The Island*. There is a scene toward the end where Douglas discovers in the remnants of the laboratory that Montgomery had kept blood samples from Douglas in the refrigerator. Reading the corresponding lab manuals, he comes to understand that Moreau had tried to use Douglas's DNA to stop the regression in Aissa, his creation who came closest to perfection. Douglas, astonished, declares to Aissa that: "He saved my life. But all the time he intended to take it … to abuse it, to take my DNA to stop your regression." Douglas obviously identifies his life with his DNA, taken from a blood sample. And he equates taking DNA from the blood sample with the taking of his life. This is a rational argument only within the framework of a gene myth whose underlying principle is that genetic information contains not only the ontologic essence of what it means to be human, but the very substance of human life. When someone takes DNA from another, he takes away life. From a strictly scientific point of view, this view is quite odd. It seems to be a sort of magical DNA voodoo, reflecting the belief that what is done to our DNA, extracted from a drop of blood in vials outside our bodies, affects our lives.

4.4 Clones

When I was preparing the materials for this chapter, I explained my project in a few words to our younger daughter Judith, who was then 9 years old. She brought me one of her Mickey Mouse cartoons which was about copying, cloning, and modifying. The cartoon depicts a new 3-D doubling machine. It copies an apple (together with the worm in the apple), and it copies Goofy. The copy of Goofy gets a green shawl for identification. At first, the two Goofys have fun together, but then they begin to fight until they decide that one of them has to leave. But this does not work for emotional reasons: they love each other too much, they hug – and hugging merge into one Goofy as he was before.[33] This simple story is reminiscent of Harold Ramis's hilarious 1995 film comedy *Multiplicity*,[34] where Doug Kinney (Michael Keaton), the handsome but chronically overworked family father, accepts an offer to be cloned. From a blood probe, an accurate copy of Doug is produced. Soon there are three of them, then four and five. The last one is slightly off, a little mad. He is a copy of a copy – and thus cannot be as sharp as the original. This degenerative logic of the reproductive process is applied to the multiplication of Dougs.

What again is striking in this example is the role of DNA. The film does not give many details of the process, but DNA alone is presented as being sufficient to make the whole person again together with his education, skills, memories, and habits, even his haircut. Nobody would be able to identify which is the copy of which, not even his wife or their little daughter. DNA is seen as the carrier not only of species identity but of personal, social, and psychic identity – the whole Doug Kinney from hair to toes, and nobody else. If this DNA were to be modified, then Doug Kinney, the person, the social self, and the psyche would also be modified. The idea of reproductive cloning as "photocopying" nourishes the misunderstanding that nuclear transfer means a transfer of the identity and of the soul.

This is the reason why a discussion of genome modification fictions should also take into consideration stories about cloning. Not only those novels and films that deal with IGM explicitly are relevant.[35] By providing the (germ-line) genome with the role of making the person in all aspects, narratives about nuclear transfer powerfully shape also the expectations and fears about IGM. As we have strong scientific reasons to believe that in reality the genome does *not* provide personal identity, paradoxically those clone stories are perhaps less a contribution to the ethics of cloning itself than to the popular perception of the genes and their modification.

The 2000 film *The 6th Day*[36] is a bit more complex – and less funny. Cloning is shown as a procedure for remaking the body out of a DNA sample within a few hours. But the DNA does not carry memories and thoughts. All conscious and unconscious records have to be downloaded and stored on a computer disk. When the body is finished, a machine transfers the data from the disk to the brain. Only after this double transfer of two types of personal information, genetic and mental, can the cloned person be the same as the original. Here, the powers of DNA are reduced to the construction of the body and the infrastructure for consciousness: they make the hardware and the inbuilt programs, so to speak. The data are provided separately. But nonetheless the DNA makes the full person except for the sum of his or her experiences.

The story of *The 6th Day* is located in a thoroughly high-tech world. The head of the cloning company, a ruthless capitalist exploiting the restrictive law against reproductive cloning of humans, protects his business by all means available. The legal ban on human cloning includes draconic detentions, and, inadvertently is the breeding ground for a thriving black market. Therefore, those who want to clone themselves must do so secretly. The cloning company takes advantage of this situation, reducing the lifespan of the clones by adding a disease gene, for instance a gene for CF or cancer. This intervention allows them more control over the situation in the black market, and, as a welcome side-effect, keeps the clients dependent on the services of the company: they need to have a periodic re-cloning.

Adam Gibson (Arnold Schwarzenegger), the main character, comes home on his birthday and discovers by looking through the window of his house that another Adam Gibson, who looks exactly like him, is merrily celebrating together with his wife Natalie, their daughter, and friends. Two brutal killers from the clone company attack him, telling him that he has been cloned and that they have an order to kill one of them. The criminal act of cloning would otherwise be detected. Of course Adam would not be played by Schwarzenegger if the plot were for him not to escape. In the course of the story, our hero discovers that he himself is the clone without knowing it, and the other Adam is the original Adam. There is a sign of this: each cloning procedure produces a small mark under the lid of the eye. The killers have several marks already; each time one of them is killed in the course of their work they are remade and can continue their jobs.

It is in this narrative context that the moral side of IGM is quite sensibly examined in one case. Dr Griffin Weir (Robert Duvall), the chief scientist of the cloning company, is about to lose his beloved wife, who is suffering from CF. He offers to help her in his clinic, but she refuses, saying that her time to die has come. Weir loves his wife and understands that respecting her will is a necessary element of his love. Then he finds out that the gene associated with CF was inserted intentionally by his own company, without telling him. He quits his job, seeing that this procedure of genetic weakening was evil.

The figure of Dr Weir in *The 6th Day* is different from the typical mad scientist. He is not shown as inconsiderate of the feelings of his patients. Rather, he is a stereotype of the "good doctor," who believes that cloning is a real help and can save lives. He shows respect and does not want to impose his treatment on the patients. But he is deceived. The company he is working for exploits his skills ruthlessly. The moral qualities of the scientists or physicians are of no use in a world of faceless power interests. The institutional context of medicine turns it into an evil means for securing the power of those controlling it. This warning, that a procedure that is ethically defensible in principle might look very different when realized within the power networks of our real world, is clear and might even be well-justified. In professional bioethics discourse about genetics, however, these contextual aspects of the implementation of genetic technologies are rarely discussed.

In *The 6th Day*, DNA modification is used as an overtly destructive technology serving the interests of the evil powers. It is used to shorten lifespans. Perhaps this could also prove a cynically realistic scenario. As long as gene transfer is difficult and not particularly successful, at the same time as increasingly large numbers of genes are being identified as associated with a high risk of severe disease, it would indeed be easier technically to use this knowledge for damaging a person's health rather than for improving it. Knocking out a function of the body is easier than repairing it, but destruction is not a medical goal. Atomic power also had its first application in bombs, not in controlled civil use. The film is a story about power relations, and about the contextual effects of power relations on biomedical technology. Power relations change the role of technology within a society. Cloning technology confers control over the germ line to the powerful; gene modification technology, it could be argued, in turn confers them the power over the course of our lives.

4.5   Eugenics

But not everything is in the genes and not all pop culture acts as another ally for genetic determinism. Andrew Niccol wrote and directed *GATTACA* (1997),[37] a piece of narrative bioethics of IGM. The title, composed of letters from the DNA alphabet, is the name of a prestigious company of space engineering. There, only engineers are allowed whose genes have been enhanced before pregnancy. It is irrelevant whether the technology applied includes only preimplantation genetic diagnosis (PGD) and rigorous embryo selection or also interventions to cause enhancement. The focus of the film is on the potential consequences of all these technologies within a society that accepts a genetic-determinist ideology.

In the future world that *GATTACA* depicts, parents are encouraged to decide the genetic makeup of their children before birth. But not everybody has access to the technology. Those who underwent the procedure are considered as "valid," the others as "invalid," and they encounter severe discrimination. Vincent, the hero of the film, is an invalid, but his dream is to become a space engineer nonetheless. With the help of Eugene, a valid, who after an accident is bound to a wheelchair and no more able to pursue an active role otherwise, Vincent fakes a valid genetic profile. He uses Eugene's blood samples in false fingertips, Eugene's urine in little plastic bags, and so forth. Because everybody believes that he has Eugene's profile, he is able to obtain a job at Gattaca and prepares for off-world expeditions. But he can keep up this deceit only by devoting much of his energies in the avoidance of any stray skin cell or body hair. A lost eyelash finally provides DNA evidence and makes Vincent (falsely) the prime suspect of a murder. Vincent's battle is to show that also the genetically unenhanced is actually a superior human being and capable of being an astronaut.

There are a series of striking issues raised by this film. I can only highlight a few. Perhaps the most important is the question which criteria are to be used to select the "valid" traits and to discriminate the "invalids." In the film, it is not something that would make a person extravagant in any respect, like doubling brain volume, multiplying lifespan, or changing the construction pattern of the body. It is rather assumed that the traits modified and selected through genetic technologies will be exactly those that are broadly seen as desirable and confer obvious social advantages, like a full head of hair (no premature baldness), tall stature, health, perfect vision, or low body weight. This modifies the standard bioethical concern about IGM that the definition of the range of diseases is subject to selections that may be influenced by what human geneticists or medicine in general at a certain time see as desirable and undesirable.[38] The definition of disease is not value-free. In the film those decisions are made with reference to what will improve the life chances within the existing society ("You want to give your child the best possible start"). Genetics is in a service position to those who want to integrate into the culturally and politically pre-established value systems. And the brute fact is that when the technology is introduced and becomes accessible for the elite class, it will change the structures of this very society. What makes discrimination on the basis of genetics obviously unjust is the impermeability of the glass barriers that separate the classes.

4.6   Desires

Science fiction has the job of experimentally contextualizing a new technology before it becomes reality. Science fiction stories can be read as moral tales experimenting with possible worlds. Model worlds are often based on accurate observations of selected parts of our real world. They highlight some of its elements and tell us what the effects of human biotechnology on the social reality are likely to be. Above all they give lessons in the mechanisms of the social construction of desires. Consider the desire for genetic modification as portrayed in *The 6th Day*. Reducing the lifespan is not a normal human desire. But it can be generated within a particular perspective at a discrete moment and place in a world of tense power relations.

A cartoon by Jimmy Margulies published in 2000 shows industrial buildings with signs on them: "Biotechnology Research," "DNA EXPRESS – That 10-min gene therapy place. Drive thru."[39] And from behind one of the buildings appears the speech balloon of an unseen person with the words: "I wonder how the HMO [health maintenance organization] industry will adapt to the human genome findings?" Indeed, a good question. We must also face this kind of questions in our ethical deliberations. The effects of these real world mechanisms of desire production need to be scrutinized before they take over medical genetics. How can we do this? Theoretical speculation about possible moral dilemmas is certainly still important. But in order to get an imagination of the many different angles of potential involvement, the medium of the narrative (novels, plays, films, and so on) has the advantage of being open to be entered from many different sides. They are "models of possible worlds" inhabited by characters that guide our imagination to a variety of perspectives. Moral dilemmas become transparent in terms of the roles attached and the complexity of the contexts illustrated, and sometimes for the small details that can change the meaning of everything.

4.7   Afterthought on method

Literature, films, stories, images – in short, popular culture and perception – will be essential sources for the process of developing ethical discourses about the mechanisms of desires, both as they really are now and how they could be in the future. They cannot replace rigorous philosophical argument, but without them these arguments may remain sterile and blind. In this chapter, I have acknowledged the truth value of popular perception, but want to explain why I found this move to be both necessary and reasonable. The opposing view holds that popular perceptions give only imperfect understandings. Truthful understandings must be produced by professional scientists, medical professionals, or bioethicists. Lay people can learn from them, but they themselves do not have their own *direct* access to the reality and the depths of the issues.

On the contrary, as argued in this chapter and exemplified above, popular and personal understandings do provide a source of understanding. Earlier in the chapter, we heard B carefully explaining what she believes that genes are and what they mean. For her world, her belief is what counts. For her perception of the ethical issues, it is her belief about the complexities of genetics and society that make the moral difference. If we consider seriously and without judgment what she tells us about her world, we have a chance of understanding the issues with which she as a subject is confronted. Then (and only then) does bioethics have a chance of communicating with those making these decisions.

This approach requires a dose of methodologic asceticism from scientific dogmatics. We should not be diverted by the flawed science we easily can find in B's assertions. We should start with accepting what she says and be interested in what she means by it. Public lessons in genetics are a separate task. The same holds for reading pop culture stories or images. They may be an easy target for criticizing their scientific accuracy, but they may still tell us something we did not know before. And very often, they are not straightforwardly wrong; they pose other types of questions. Anthropologist Paul Rabinow speaks of "biosociality," pointing to processes of co-production of knowledge between scientists and patients.[40] In this same sense of biosociality, we all belong to communities sharing fictions and narratives as hermeneutic tools which help us to "understand" our fate and our human challenges.

Acknowledgments

I thank the editors for the idea for this article, together with a very helpful and rich film/novel list compiled by Jason Tong (when he served as research assistant at the Unit for History and Philosophy of Science, University of Sydney). Rachel Ankeny gave many helpful comments on the first draft and improved the manuscript linguistically. Jackie Leach Scully's philosophical clarity helped to make my chapter comprehensible. Parts of this chapter are related to the research project "Perceptions of healing needs: Somatic gene therapy, disability and identity" funded by the Swiss National Science Foundation grant 4037-053073.[41]

NOTES

1   See Françoise Baylis and Jason Scott Robert, Crossing species boundaries, *American Journal of Bioethics* 3 (2003), 1–13.

2 Further references can be found in David A. Kirby, The new eugenics in cinema: genetic determinism and gene therapy in *GATTACA*, *Science Fiction Studies* 27 (2000), 193–215.

3 Manuela Rossini, Künstliche Reproduktion (in) der Science/Fiction: Neue Technologien – alte Geschichten? *Figurationen* 4/2 (2003), 65–83.

4 Anne Balsamo, Notes toward a reproductive theory of technology. In: E. Ann Kaplan and Susan Squier (eds.), *Playing Dolly: Technocultural Formations, Fantasies, and Fictions of Assisted Reproduction.* New Brunswick, NJ: Rutgers University Press (1999), 87–97.

5 Evelyn Fox Keller in her books *Refiguring Life: Metaphors of Twentieth-Century Biology.* New York: Columbia University Press (1996); *The Century of the Gene.* Cambridge: Harvard University Press (2000). Eva M. Neumann-Held and Christoph Rehmann-Sutter (eds.), *Genes in Development Re-reading the Molecular Paradigm.* Durham: Duke University Press 2005.

6 Nicole Hollander, untitled cartoon (1992), reprinted in: Ruth Hubbard and Elijah Wald (eds.), *Exploding the Gene Myth.* Boston: Beacon (1997), p. 115.

7 Translation my own; original quote: "Grundsätzlich habe ich keine Vorstellung davon, wie ein Gen aussieht. Wahrscheinlich würde man es von blossem Auge gar nicht sehen … Der Mensch besteht aus Genen. Sie bestimmen z.B. die Haarfarbe oder ob jemand an CF erkrankt oder nicht. Man kann ein Gen vererben … Ich weiss nicht, vielleicht ist ein Gen klein und rund?" in Catherine Löw, *Gentherapie aus der Sicht Betroffener: Eine empirische Untersuchung der individuellen Wahrnehmung von PatientInnen und Eltern von Kindern mit Cystischer Fibrose,* unpublished medical dissertation, University of Basel (2001), pp. 139ff.

8 "Vielleicht will aber dieser Mensch diese anderen Gene gar nicht", in Löw, *Gentherapie aus der Sicht Betroffener,* p. 140.

9 See Jackie Leach Scully, Inheritable genetic modification and disability: normality and identity (Chapter 10, this volume); Rosemarie Tong, Traditional and feminist bioethical perspectives on gene transfer: is inheritable genetic modification really the problem? (Chapter 9, this volume).

10 Max Delbrück, Aristotle-totle-totle. In: Jacques Monod and Ernest Borek (eds.), *Of Microbes and Life.* New York: Columbia University Press (1979), 50–5, p. 51.

11 Delbrück, Aristotle-totle-totle, p. 53.

12 Dorothy Nelkin and M. Susan Lindee, *The DNA Mystique: The Gene as a Cultural Icon.* New York: Freeman (1995).

13 Natalie Angier, Reading the book of life: the context; a pearl and a hodgepodge: human DNA, *New York Times* (27 June 2000), A1.

14 Lily Kay, *Who Wrote the Book of Life? A History of the Genetic Code.* Stanford: Stanford University Press (2000).

15 Colin F. Macilwain, World leaders heap praise on human genome landmark, *Nature* 405 (2000), 983–6.

16 M. Ridley on the Today Programme, BBC Radio 4, June 2000, reported in Priscilla Alderson, The new genetics: Promise or threat to children? *Bulletin of Medical Ethics* 176 (2002), 13–8.

17 August Weismann, Das Keimplasma: Eine Theorie der Vererbung (Jena: G. Fischer, 1892); for a discussion of Weismannism, see Françoise Baylis and Jason Scott Robert, Radical rupture: exploring biological sequelae of volitional inheritable genetic modification (Chapter 7, this volume).

18 Kim Sterelny and Paul E. Griffiths, *Sex and Death: An Introduction to Philosophy of Biology.* Chicago: University of Chicago Press (1999), p. 65.

19 Wilhelm of Ockham, Summa logicae (1324), translated as Summe der Logik: Über die Termini. Hamburg: Felix Meier Verlag (1984).

20 Compare Rachel A. Ankeny, No real categories, only chimaeras and illusions: the interplay between morality and science in debates over embryonic chimaeras, *American Journal of Bioethics* 3/3 (2003), 31–3.

21 Jean-Jacques Kupiec, Histoire d'être. In: Jean-Jacques Kupiec and Pierre Sonigo (eds.), *Ni Dieu ni gène: Pour une autre théorie de l'hérédité* Paris: Editions du Seuil (2000), 15–59.

22 John Frankenheimer (director), *The Island of Dr Moreau* (film), New Line Productions, 1996, after the novel of the same name by H.G. Wells, *The Island of Doctor Moreau* (1896), reprinted in H.G. Wells, *The Science Fiction.* London: Phoenix (1995), 1, 71–178. The novel used vivisection and interspecies transplantation surgery as technological elements. At the end of the nineteenth century, antiseptic surgery (with carbolic acid) was a crucial biotechnological innovation, and connections can be made between the content of the novel and current debates over xenotransplantation.

23 George Levine and U.C. Knoepflmacher (eds.), *The Endurance of Frankenstein.* Berkeley: University of California Press (1979); Steven Earl Forry, *Hideous Progenies: Dramatization of Frankenstein from Mary Shelley to the Present.* Philadelphia: University of Pennsylvania Press (1990); Fred Botting, *Making Monstrous: Frankenstein, Criticism, Theory.* Manchester: Manchester University Press (1991); Christoph Rehmann-Sutter, Frankensteinian knowledge? *The Monist* 79 (1996), 264–78; Langdon Winner, *Autonomous Technology: Technics-out-of-Control as a Theme in Political Thought.* Cambridge: The MIT Press (1997); Christoph Rehmann-Sutter, Hubris and Hybrids in the Myth of Frankenstein. In: Veikko Launis, Juhani Pietarinen and Juha Räikkä (eds.), *Genes and Morality.* Amsterdam: Rodopi (1999), 157–73.

24 More's Letter to Mother Nature is quoted in Gregory Stock, *Redesigning Humans: Our Inevitable Genetic Future.* Boston: Houghton Mifflin (2002), p. 158ff. See also www.extropy.org and www.transhumansim.org (last accessed 1 July 2005).

25 Johann Wolfgang Goethe, *Faust: Der Tragödie erster Teil* (1808), L.J. Scheithauer (ed.), Stuttgart: Reclam (1971), pp. 1334–6; Faust: "… Nun gut, wer bist du denn?" ("Well, who are you?"); Mephistopheles: "Ein Teil von jener Kraft, die stets das Böse will und stets das Gute schafft" ("A part of that force which always wants Evil and always generates Good").

26 Rita Hau, *PONS Globalwörterbuch Lateinisch-Deutsch,* 2nd edn. Stuttgart: Klett (1986), p. 634.

27 Judith Shklar, *Faces of Injustice.* New Haven: Yale University Press (1990).

28 Mary Shelley, *Frankenstein: Or The Modern Prometheus*. The 1818 Text (1818), Marilyn Butler (ed.), Oxford: Oxford University Press (1994), p. 1.

29 Shelley, *Frankenstein*, p. 105.

30 *Ibid.*, p. 96.

31 See Françoise Baylis and Jason Scott Robert, Radical Rupture: exploring biological sequelae of volitional inheritable genetic modification (Chapter 7, this volume); Scully, Inheritable genetic modification and disability.

32 James Whale (director), *Frankenstein* (film), Universal Pictures, 1931.

33 Sarah Kinney and Noel Van Horn, *Walt Disney's Mickey Mouse* (2000), translated by Susanne Walter, *Zwist der Zwillinge in Walt Disney's Micky Maus Magazin* 17 (18 April 2002), 22–31, cartoon number: D2000–129.

34 Harold Ramis (director), *Multiplicity* (film), Columbia Pictures, 1995.

35 Kirby, in his The new eugenics in cinema, observes that the genre of film, in contrast to novel, has remained, until quite recently, silent on the subject of genetic manipulation. My approach is to broaden the scope and to look also at other film themes that might as well be relevant in shaping the moral perception of IGM.

36 Roger Spottiswoode (director). *The 6th Day* (film), Columbia Pictures, 2000.

37 Andrew Niccol (director), *GATTACA* (film), Sony Pictures, 1997. See the discussion with further references in Kirby, The new eugenics in cinema.

38 See my own discussion of these issues in Christoph Rehmann-Sutter and Hansjakob Müller (eds.), *Ethik und Gentherapie: Zum praktischen Diskurs um die molekulare Medizin*, 2nd enlarged edn. Tübingen: Francke (2003), pp. 228ff.

39 Jimmy Margulies, untitled cartoon, 2000, on Daryl Cagle's Professional Cartoonists Index, section on "The Human Genome," http://cagle.slate.msn.com/news/gene/gene7.asp (last accessed 1 July 2002).

40 As Rabinow notes: "There already are, for example, neurofibromatosis groups whose members meet to share their experiences, lobby for their disease, educate their children, redo their home environment, and so on ... Such groups will have medical specialists, laboratories, narratives, traditions, and a heavy panoply of pastoral keepers to help them experience, share, intervene, and 'understand' their fate." *Essays in the Anthropology of Reason*. Princeton: Princeton University Press (1996), p. 102.

41 See Jackie Leach Scully, Christine Rippberger, and Christoph Rehmann-Sutter, Non-professionals' evaluations of gene therapy ethics, *Social Science and Medicine* 58 (2004), 1415–25.

Inheritable genetic modification as moral responsibility in a creative universe

Denis Kenny

The transformation of history begins with the history of transformations.[1]

Modern technology has introduced action of such moral scale, objects and consequences that the framework of former ethics can no longer contain them.[2]

5.1 Introduction

In February 1997, Ian Wilmut of Edinburgh's Roslin Institute introduced Dolly, the recently cloned ewe, to the world.[3] President Bill Clinton and Pope John Paul II responded with caution to the success of this project and took initiatives to prevent any future attempts to clone human beings.[4,5] The President and the Pope were, of course, responding from within two quite different moral universes. Clinton, the classical sophist, tailored his response to the dictates of his pollsters and spin-doctors, and fashioned his rhetoric to appeal to the dominant mood and fears of the American people. The Pope responded from within the long tradition of natural law theory in which human beings are morally subject to the natural order of things ordained by God. Both were responding on the basis of what can be argued to be a scientifically outmoded cosmology.

All moral orientations and theories arise from one or another conception of the structure and operation of the universe. We call the theoretical account of the nature of the universe "cosmology." The morality of society changes when the cosmology of a society changes. According to the philosopher Alasdair MacIntyre, shards of older moral traditions persist, sometimes for many centuries, emerging to challenge the validity of any new morality, even though these traditions have outlived the context within which they originally made sense.[6]

The techno-scientific prowess of the human race seems now to be expanding exponentially. Nearly every day brings news of some ever more dramatic breakthrough in biotechnology. Each new development seems to pose a new and difficult moral choice for society. The choice, however, is not necessarily between good and evil, right and wrong, or virtue and vice, though some insist on describing it in these terms, but between two very different ideas of and approaches to morality, each arising out of radically different cosmologies.

To appreciate this kind of moral conflict, that is, between different ways of understanding the very nature of morality, it is necessary, to recognize, at least in outline, how changes in cosmology over the centuries have led to changes in morality, and, more importantly, to appreciate the challenges to traditional morality posed by the new scientific cosmology that have emerged in the closing decades of the twentieth century.

Pope John Paul II, many Christian moral authorities, and adherents to other religious traditions, as well as many secular humanists, live in a conception of an essentially static universe which demands a morality of obligation and, hence, of obedience to what they interpret as the timeless laws of that universe, sacred or secular. In the closing decades of the twentieth century, however, many branches of science have converged to reveal a conception of the universe, a cosmology which is evolving and self-organizing, and which seems to demand of us a morality of creative responsibility, a morality for which there are no timeless laws.

Over the more than 100,000 year history of the human species, human beings have inhabited four quite different universes, in the cosmologic sense, and now seem to be on the threshold of a fifth kind which is radically different from all previous ones. Humans have lived successively, and sometimes concurrently, in an enchanted universe, a sacred universe, a mechanical universe, and an organic universe, as I will illustrate through a necessarily brief and selective historical narrative. We are now standing on the threshold of what I term a creative universe. To cross that threshold will require recognition of the unique cosmology with which contemporary science now confronts us, as well as a willingness to embrace the moral implications of that cosmology.

I will argue that, in the light of the scientific cosmology that has emerged in the closing decades of the twentieth century, our moral universe is undergoing a profound shift along two of its defining axes. In the first place, we can no longer think of our world as governed by fixed, timeless entities, laws or essences. In the second place, our relationship to this world can no longer be governed by unchanging moral imperatives which demand obedience and submission. In the new cosmology of an evolving and creative universe, our relationship to that universe must be governed by a morality of creative responsibility for the human and planetary future. Opposition to advances in biotechnology in general and to inheritable genetic modification (IGM) in particular, is often based on the conviction that the order of creation or nature is given, once and for all, and that human beings have no right to intervene in this order in any significant way. A morality based on the cosmology of the creative universe has implications for IGM because within the terms of this cosmology human beings have a responsibility intelligently and carefully to expand and transform this order. In this context we have a responsibility seriously to consider IGM as part of our creative responsibility despite the current regulatory consensus that our responsibility is not to implement it.[7]

I will suggest a number of strategic and procedural protocols that might serve as useful methodologic bases for taking moral initiatives in an undetermined future and assist us in crossing the threshold from the organic to the creative universe.

Finally I will examine IGM in the context of the creative universe.

5.2   The cosmologic context of morality in the western tradition

5.2.1   The enchanted universe

For tens of thousands of years the human species lived in what could be called an enchanted universe. Most preliterate cultures were animistic. The world was alive with forces, powers, and influences, often personified as gods, which were thought capriciously to toy with the lives of human beings. In coping with these forces, pre-literate cultures resorted to carefully transmitted experience, craft ingenuity, group solidarity, rituals of celebration, sacrifices of appeasement, and the manipulation of the natural world by magic. The cosmology of the enchanted universe lives on in the many forms of New Age romanticism.

With the cultivation of crops, the domestication of animals, and the spread of villages, towns, and commercial activity, a new order of greater stability began to emerge. One of the key features of this new order was the rise of literacy and numeracy, perhaps the most dramatic transformation in human technical and cultural evolution. This development launched the long historical process of the internalization and individuation of consciousness, and provided the human species with the means of philosophically establishing a critical and hence potentially creative distance from the physical and biologic world in which it had previously been immersed.

The demand for order, and perhaps also for security, could be seen as having been crucial in settling one of the earliest philosophical debates in ancient Greece, based on the limited source materials available to us. Heraclitus, on the one side, claimed that being is becoming, that reality is a relentless state of change. Parmenides, on the other side, claimed that change is only a superficial manifestation of reality, that at a deeper level there are abiding structures or forms immune to change. Plato favored the latter view, asserting the existence of eternal forms not obvious to our untutored senses, but accessible, nevertheless, to the carefully cultivated mind.[8]

With the rise of imperial Rome, the unique intellectual energy and curiosity manifested in Athens went into decline, as did the ideal of a democratic society. While the gods of the enchanted universe officially lived on in Roman culture, it was Rome itself that provided the central organizing focus of life. Although the people of imperial Rome lived in a highly ordered world, an increasing number of its citizens, progressively deprived of effective political participation in that world, many of the old patrician class among them, sought intelligibility, meaning, and purpose in the private domains of Stoicism, Epicureanism, or a variety of mystery religions. Stoicism, the cultivation of imperturbability, and Epicureanism, the cultivation of taste, though quite different from each other, did nevertheless agree on one important point – both defined freedom as the recognition of and submission to necessity. They both accepted that the world could not be changed.

5.2.2 The sacred universe

When Paul, the Christian missionary, arrived in Athens, he encountered Stoic and Epicurean philosophers. They conducted him to the Areopagus and invited him to preach his new religion. Paul opened his address by pointing to an altar dedicated to "an unknown god."[9] He proceeded to identify and describe this God. Unlike the gods of the ancient world and of Greece and Rome, who were often capricious and cruel in their treatment of men and women, this Christian God was a loving Father who sent his own son to die for all humankind and thus to ransom them from the slavery of sin, the human condition, and from the power of death itself.

Over the next two centuries, allegiance to this God spread dramatically, not just among slaves and the poor, but also among the upper classes. With the conversion of the Emperor Constantine in the early fourth century, the Roman empire and the now extensive Christian church, engaged in a reciprocal conversion process.[10] Rome became Christian and the church became Roman. This merger initiated the 1000-year reign of Christendom and the triumph of the cosmology of the sacred universe.

This sacred universe was the first comprehensive, fully integrated theory of everything in human experience. It reconciled the intelligibility of the world with the meaning and purpose of human beings within it. In its dramatic narrative of fall, redemption, and salvation, it provided a compelling account of the origin, identity, and destiny of mankind, including a clearly identifiable path to eternal salvation. The cosmology of the sacred universe introduced a new order of freedom: the freedom of the individual person to choose or to reject the promise of eternal life offered by this benevolent Father. This cosmology did not, however, provide the freedom to change either the order of the cosmos or the social order, but only to accept or reject the terms of liberation from sin and death.

In the fifteenth century, however, the sacred universe and order of Christendom began to disintegrate in the face of its own internal theologic conflicts, a renewed fascination with this world engendered by the Renaissance, the rise of nation states and powerful monarchs jealous of both their political and religious authority, the proliferation of vernacular literatures and cultures, the relentless growth of trade and commerce, the expanding technologic prowess of the human species, and the widening of the narrow horizon of European consciousness to the rest of the world. It was science, however, that provided the crucial catalyst for change.

5.2.3   The mechanical universe

Isaac Newton, following Galileo and Copernicus, vindicated empirically an entirely new cosmology and provided a fresh approach to the intelligibility of the world. He achieved the unprecedented feat of what the astronomer John Barrow has called "algorithmic compressibility."[11] Into a small number of mathematical formulae or algorithms, Newton was able to compress an extraordinary amount of complicated information about the universe and how it operates. It was the role of the French astronomer Pierre Laplace, however, to define the new cosmology of the mechanical universe, a cosmology that would dominate the early modern era. In this understanding of the world, everything within it could, in principle, be finally explained in mechanistic terms.

Although the work of Newton was one of the most spectacular achievements in the history of human thought, what the human race had gained in terms of the intelligibility of the universe it had correspondingly lost in the meaning and purpose of it all.[12] A world governed by deterministic laws seemed to leave little room for the domains of religious, moral, or artistic endeavor.[13] The world had become disenchanted and deconsecrated. Uncertainty and skepticism became more persuasive, and a harsh new realism came to prevail in scientific, political, and economic affairs.[14]

The French philosopher, René Descartes, proposed a workable, if a not entirely satisfying compromise: while deterministic laws govern the external material world, the internal world of the human spirit is a qualitatively different domain not entirely accounted for by these mechanical laws. The practical result of this compromise was to separate the realms of politics, economics and science governed by principles of functional rationality from the realms of religion, morality and aesthetics governed by their specific principles, criteria and forms of discourse.[15]

5.2.4   The organic universe

By the closing decades of the nineteenth century, however, the ghost of Heraclitus was returning to haunt the very fixed and stable structures and timeless laws of the clockwork universe. It manifested itself in the Promethean dynamic of the industrial revolution. It appeared in the evolutionary writings of Hegel, Marx, and Darwin. Some slowly began to suspect that the philosophers and the scientists were only interpreting the world while the engineers were beginning to change it, and radically.

Charles Lyell and Charles Darwin demonstrated that evolutionary change had been one of the key features in the history of our planet and its life forms.

But though this evolutionary perspective allowed considerable progress in the field of biology, it took over a hundred years before it had very much impact in the field of the physical sciences. Heraclitus' ghost was, nevertheless, beginning to make its spooky presence felt in physics.

At the beginning of the twentieth century, Sigmund Freud challenged the Enlightenment ideal of human rationality by exposing the turbulent psychic substrate of the order of rational consciousness. At about the same time, in positing quanta as the explanation of the peculiar behavior of black body radiation, Max Planck revealed the turbulent quantum substrate of the tangible order of the Newtonian universe. Earlier in the nineteenth century, Michael Faraday had introduced the idea of fields of force, demonstrating that electricity, magnetism, and light are closely related phenomena, and recognized that fields of force play an important role in the interactions of the material universe. At the beginning of the twentieth century Einstein surpassed even Newton in the search for algorithmic compressibility. The formula $E = mc^2$ compressed an enormous amount of information about the world, and established the equivalence of matter and energy. Einstein linked time and space in a single manifold, and recognized that, far from being a neutral arena in which the events of the world transpired, space and time constitute integral components of the events themselves. The universe began to appear as a cosmic dance of energy in which the distinction between the material and the spiritual no longer seemed to make much sense, as Paul Davies and John Gribben have argued.[16]

Throughout the twentieth century, while the physicists explored the frontiers of the subatomic, microcosmic universe, the astrophysicists mapped the frontiers of the macroscopic universe. Biologists established the genetic continuity and connectedness of organisms throughout biologic history, and the new science of ecology demonstrated the extent to which the multiplicity, diversity, complexity, and interconnectedness of organisms was indispensable for the survival and health of all living systems. Gradually a vast new scientific mosaic began to come into focus. Instead of the atomistic, mechanistic cosmology of Newton and Laplace governed by timeless laws, a dynamic, interconnected universe began to emerge – an organic universe or cosmology. In the second half of the twentieth century, what the quantum physicists were discovering about the subatomic world in their particle accelerators began dramatically to complement what the astrophysicists were discovering in their observatories about the composition and origin of the cosmos.

In 1927 a Belgian Catholic priest, George Lemaître, claimed to have found a solution to Einstein's cosmologic equations by proposing what would later be called the "Big Bang" theory of the origin of the universe. Two years later, the observations of American astronomer Edwin Hubble confirmed that the universe was, indeed, expanding, and reinforced the suspicion that it had a singular, dramatic beginning. This suspicion became scientifically confirmed when Arno Penzias and Robert Wilson discovered microwave radiation coming from every direction in the universe in 1964.[17]

In the closing decades of the twentieth century, all of these avenues of scientific investigation finally converged in what we can now recognize as a vast, integrated, though diversifying, evolutionary process – the first universally valid and scientifically-based cosmology in the history of human consciousness and culture. The physicist Brian Swimme and the poet Thomas Berry have called this vast saga, quite simply, "The Universe Story!"[18] Although there are still some unsolved problems and deep mysteries in this story, it weaves all of the components of cosmic, planetary, and biologic history into a single narrative of the organic universe. The cosmology of the organic universe, and the very strong sense that the destiny of all of the components living and non-living of the planet earth are intertwined, forms the basis for the morality and politics of the environmental movement.[19]

5.2.5   The emergence of the creative universe

The organic universe, however, is not the end of the story. It brings us, rather, to a new threshold, and to the challenge of another cosmology. For Erich Jantsch, Ilya Prigogine, and Paul Davies, among others, the universe is itself engaged in a self-organizing, creative process.[20] What is meant by the term "creative" in this context? Creativity is a formidably difficult phenomenon to pin down and define. It can be briefly described, however, as the progressive interaction of energy and structure, of dynamism and form, which results in more comprehensive, elaborate, enriched, and coherent forms, relationships, or ideas. Dynamism without form exhausts itself in entropy, resulting in a state of equilibrium. Form without dynamism suffers from a form of sclerosis and can suffocate from lack of vital energy. Many contemporary cultural forms suffer from entropy, and many traditional institutions suffer from this type of sclerosis.

Prigogine, who won the Nobel Prize for chemistry in 1977 for his theory of dissipative structures, conclusively explained in this theory how simple substances become more complex, and how inorganic compounds can become organic. With this theory he is widely thought to have significantly closed the mysterious gap between the organic and the inorganic domains of the evolutionary process.[21] He has subsequently become one of the leading advocates of the cosmology of the creative universe, a cosmology that describes the universe as not just evolving, but as *creatively* evolving.

Two other developments bring us to the threshold of the creative universe. The first is the dramatic growth of biotechnologies, of which the cloning of Dolly is just one of the more controversial achievements. This advance confronts us with a fundamental moral question about what justification we as human beings have for intervening in, and attempting to direct, the future of the evolutionary process. The second development is the contemporary study of the human mind and consciousness. Two conclusions seem to be emerging from this very broad, and still controversial, field of study. The first is that the mind is not the prisoner of our biology, as many religious traditions have believed. It is, rather, an emergent product of biology. The second conclusion is that the mind is not merely passive in the act of knowing. It is active and creative. The brain is not merely an organ for mirroring the world, as the early empiricists and positivists asserted: it is an instrument for changing it. As Gerald Edelman, one of the leaders in the field of neural science has insisted in light of his studies, the mind is not ultimately the prisoner of description. It is the master of meaning. We are not just political animals, as Aristotle thought; instead we are semantic animals. We are meaning-creating and purpose-creating animals.[22]

The biologist Steve Jones has argued that evolution has tactics but no strategy.[23] By this he means that while the evolutionary process has tactical mechanisms for creating ever more diverse and complicated forms and entities from atoms to molecules, to organisms and galaxies, these tactical initiatives have no conscious direction or purpose. This is where we humans enter the picture. After 100,000 years of cultural evolution, we are discovering that we are the only organisms on the planet Earth, and, as far as we can tell, in the cosmos, with the consciousness, knowledge, and capacity for creative responsibility to provide the evolutionary process with a strategic orientation or direction into the future. It is our task, in an evolutionary cosmos, to provide it with purpose and meaning.

Perhaps the greatest and most common odyssey of the twentieth century has been the search for meaning. In the cosmology of the creative universe we do not find meaning. We *create* meaning in taking responsibility for the future direction of the evolutionary process at every level, from the personal to the planetary. The Jesuit paleontologist, Pierre Teilhard de Chardin, aptly described our present relationship to the cosmos: "Man is not the center of the universe as once we thought in our simplicity, but something much more wonderful – the arrow pointing the way to the final unification of the world in terms of life."[24]

At the threshold of a cosmology of the creative universe we are therefore faced with a choice between two very different forms or conceptions of morality. The first is the traditional conception of the morality of obligation in which we are bound (from the Latin *ligare*) by the laws of God, nature, history, evolution, or the market. The second is the emerging morality of creative responsibility in which we are required democratically to participate, to the best of our knowledge, experience, and ability, in the design of our personal, social, and planetary future. In the design of this future there is, as the philosopher Richard Bernstein has argued, no "fixed Archimedean point … not God, philosophy, science or poetry … that satisfies our longing for ultimate foundations." Beyond the chronic dichotomy of "objectivism and relativism," we must "recover a sense of practical rationality," of prudent design which responsibly copes with both the accelerating pace of change and the exponential increase in the diversity and the complexity of life.[25] For believers in the cosmology of the creative universe, the complete reliance of any moral or political agent on some Archimedean fixed point is viewed as morally immature and irresponsible.

5.3   The protocols of creative responsibility

Many moralists, both sacred and secular, think that if there are no enduring and absolute moral principles or imperatives, the very fabric of morality itself will unravel and human society and civilization will revert to barbarism. Many commentators think that the postmodern condition, defined by Jean-Francois Lyotard as "incredulity towards metanarratives,"[26] or by Bernstein as the repudiation of Archimedean fixed points, leads inexorably to an entropic state of relativism, nihilism, and cynicism. This fear leads them to cling to some outmoded cosmology which, though it may provide clear moral guidelines for the present, I maintain invariably provides no methodology for moral initiatives in an undetermined future in an evolutionary context.

The cosmology of the creative universe, in fact, brings us to the threshold of a much deeper, more demanding, and more authentic morality. Though it does not dictate absolute and unchanging principles of moral action, I believe that it does suggest a set of protocols which constitute a flexible and evolving framework for moral discourse and behavior. This new cosmology demands that we look more closely at the very nature of morality and moral discourse. With careful analysis, we can begin to discover that the appeal to and reliance on one or another set of moral absolutes, while providing psychologic certitude and security, often results in various forms of irresponsibility.

A protocol is a set of terms of agreement, or conventional courtesies, about how negotiations are to be conducted among different groups of people or nations. They are designed to facilitate future agreement rather than specify the content or substance of the agreement. My purpose in suggesting them is to provide a methodology for taking moral initiatives in an undetermined and evolving future.

A morality of creative responsibility requires two levels of protocols: broad strategic protocols, followed by more specific procedural protocols.

5.3.1   Broad strategic protocols

Six broad strategic protocols follow from accepting the concept of creative responsibility: the need to accept

(a) the ontogenetic assumption;
(b) morality as unavoidably polycentric;
(c) the use of design rationality;
(d) reality as complex and emergent;
(e) the biologic capacity for the exercise of responsible moral agency as a specific and defining human characteristic; and
(f) some limitations on the exercise of creative responsibility.

5.3.1.1   Shifting to the ontogenetic assumption

The first of these broad protocols is concerned with the underlying assumption we as human beings make about our relationship to the world in which we live. We can operate on the basis of what can be called the *ontocratic* assumption, or alternatively, on the basis of what can be called the *ontogenetic* assumption. Acceptance of the notion of the cosmology of a creative universe seems to demand that we alter our basic orientation to the world in which we live from the pervasiveness of the former to the emergence of the latter.

In a passage in *The Adventure of Ideas*, Alfred North Whitehead argued that in the conflict of ideas over a long period of time there is often an unacknowledged and even unrecognized agreement about an even-deeper set of unarticulated assumptions about which all of the conflicting parties actually agree. There is often, he wrote, "a general form of the forms of thought ... so pervading, and so seemingly necessary, that only by extreme effort can we become aware of it."[27] The all-pervasive form of thought that has underpinned conflicting ideas throughout human history has been the ontocratic assumption. The key feature of this assumption is that we human beings live under the inexorable rule of "ontos" or being. The conflict over the variations of this general form includes the different versions of the *truth* about the nature, or the structures or the dynamics of being. Stories about the powers of nature or the gods, revelations about Yahweh, God, or Allah, mystical illuminations, philosophical systems, or scientific theories have all claimed to describe the nature of the reality to which we must submit and to which our behaviors must conform.

The alternative assumption, which differs fundamentally from the ontocratic assumption, is the ontogenetic assumption. On the basis of this assumption, although we are beings which emerge from cosmic evolutionary and personal developmental processes, in the last analysis we are not completely encompassed by these processes, nor entirely subject to them. We have the discretionary power consciously to go beyond what this 15 billion year process has precipitated in order to *direct* the future of the process. Biotechnology in general and IGM technologies in particular, are potent examples of the tools at our disposal. The shift from the ontocratic to the ontogenetic assumption is the unavoidable conclusion of the convergence of three late twentieth century phenomena: the emergence of the scientific universe story, the exponential growth of human technologic prowess, and the recognition that the human mind is not simply the mirror of nature but also is an organism for the transformation of nature and the creation of meaning and purpose.

A key feature of the shift from the ontocratic to the ontogenetic assumption as the basis for human moral agency is the broad contemporary shift in focus on an epistemic axis, oriented to the search for truth along which most human conflicts – religious, philosophical, or scientific – have occurred, to what can be termed the "praxis axis," oriented to the practice and design of the human and planetary future. This reorientation does not mean that the search for empirical truth about the reality that we inhabit is no longer relevant. It is rather that, as Jacques Derrida has argued, there is never just one truth, and no truth can be dogmatically represented as timeless certainty.[28]

5.3.1.2 Morality as unavoidably polycentric

The second broad strategic protocol establishes that morality is unavoidably polycentric. The writer Charles Hampden-Turner has noted that the Greeks in the era dominated by the Homeric epics believed that human beings were influenced by, and had to come to terms with, a wide variety of natural, human, and divine influences.[29] With the rise of literacy, natural philosophy (roughly what we now call science), and philosophy, however, a fundamental cultural sea change began to occur that profoundly influenced the subsequent history of western civilization. In the Homeric order, the Greeks were required to worship at the shrines of a wide variety of gods, and establish a practical balance among the different and often conflicting characteristics and demands that each of the gods represented. Their moral practice was, therefore, polycentric. With the rise of scientific and philosophical literacy, and with the concomitant shift from mythos to logos, however, western culture and civilization embarked upon a significantly different odyssey.

This new odyssey was the search for the truth about our human condition and it became what Richard Tarnas has called "the passion of the western mind."[30] Over 2500 years of history the search has taken many forms and directions. One of the key features of this search, however, has been the attempt to establish what is currently being called a "theory of everything." Each form of the search has sought to find a superordinate principle in terms of which subordinate principles and considerations can be coordinated and integrated. Until the time of the scientific revolution launched by Newton, the superordinate principle was the Christian God and his laws. In the modern era, the holy grail of science has been to discover a fundamental law in terms of which all phenomena can finally be explained. The governing ethos and goal of this search has, nevertheless, been monocentric. The history of ethical theories and of moral systems reflects this general odyssey.

In the light of the cosmology of the creative universe, a morality of creative responsibility is based on reviving the polycentric style of the Homeric era and taking into consideration, in a constantly changing constellation of imperatives, concerns, priorities, and values, most of the key ethical principles of the traditional moral systems without, however, attributing to any of them the privileged status they respectively enjoyed within each system. The great paradox of the scientific advances of the closing decades of the twentieth century is that, instead of bringing us to the triumph of "logos" in the uncovering of the ultimate truth of our world, science has returned us to the domain of mythos, but with a difference. Joseph Campbell has defined myth as the story people tell themselves about their origin, their identity, and their destiny.[31] Put in these terms, therefore, the myth that the contemporary universe story suggests is that there is no one truth that can illuminate our life or provide the terms by which we can live it. It suggests, rather, that there are many partial truths that we must configure into a mosaic best suited both for our survival and for an enhanced future. It does tell us that our origin is in the 15 billion year process of physical and biologic evolution. But it also tells us that our identity as human beings is that of conscious citizens of the cosmos, intelligent moral agents, who have the unavoidable responsibility for the future direction of this evolutionary process, and that our destiny is in our own hands.

5.3.1.3   Design rationality

The third broad strategic protocol concerns the nature of human rationality that emerges from the cosmology and mythos of the creative universe. Since the time of Plato there have been four broad categories of rationality which have at different times dominated the societies of the western world: theologic, philosophical, scientific, and technologic. The key characteristics of the first three has been internal coherence, consistency, and a predominantly linear reasoning process, although all have been radically different from each other in most of their other features. The key characteristic of technologic reasoning, on the other hand, has been the blending of divergent, dissident components into a functional whole to achieve a specific purpose. This involves reaching an outcome, not by a linear, logic, Euclidian process, but by the imaginative juxtaposition of the necessary components or functional imperatives. This is design rationality, which is the most difficult teaching task in an engineering degree. Almost without our noticing it, technologic (or design) rationality has been, for a long time, the dominant form of rationality of the western world. Although science has provided the solid base for the modern technologic enterprise, technologic rationality is a qualitatively distinct form of rationality from those that preceded it.

Practical moral reasoning has much more in common with technologic reasoning and design rationality than it does with the other traditional forms of human rationality. The crucial difference between morality and technology is that in the latter the purpose of the exercise is specified in advance, and need not be an integral part of the reasoning process. In practical moral reasoning, the purpose, both immediate and strategic, is an inescapable or integral part of the moral design or reasoning process. For Aristotle, moral reason was qualitatively different from speculative reason. The latter was "theoria," a form of contemplation. The former was "phronesis," a form of practical action. This kind of practical action does not simply involve the application of fixed principles to varying circumstances, but demands the creative process of devising an ingenious configuration of priorities, values, and imperatives under the given circumstances to achieve the best outcome.

5.3.1.4   Reality as complex and emergent

The fourth broad strategic protocol is the recognition that the reality we inhabit is a complex of emergent phenomena. The notion of "emergence" is a very recent and still developing set of ideas. Put very simply, it is the growing conviction in both the physical and biologic sciences that the whole is greater than the sum of its parts. It arises from the fact that complex mixtures of chemicals can spontaneously stimulate, or catalyze, the production of more complex substances which cannot be accounted for simply in terms of the properties or the laws of interaction of the individual chemicals involved. Expressed more generally, at different levels of scale and complexity, new properties and characteristics of substances and organisms emerge that are qualitatively different from the sum of their component parts. At different levels of scale and complexity, moreover, new laws and algorithms governing the behavior of substances and organisms emerge.[32] The laws governing reality, in other words, are sensitive to scale and complexity.

The moral significance of emergence theory is that it potentially eliminates the gap and the conflict between reductionist and dualistic accounts of reality. In the search for scientific certitude, the reductionist impulse sought to explain complex phenomena as "nothing but" more intricate combinations of basic chemical and physical laws. In attempting to preserve the uniqueness and integrity of complex phenomena such as life, consciousness, and the realms of art and morality, the dualists sought to explain them in terms of non-material or spiritual forms or forces, qualitatively different from physical forms or forces. Dualism emerged in ancient Greece as an attempt to anchor our understanding of reality in abiding, unchanging forms, natures, or essences in the face of change and contingency. In dualism, these philosophically or religiously constructed forms, natures, or essences provided the allegedly solid foundations for the fixed moral laws which were derived from them. Cosmology, the physical sciences, and biology, however, now provide us with accounts of reality that seem to make both reductionism and dualism obsolete.[33]

There is now a growing consensus that the human mind and consciousness, and all its diverse activities, cannot be reduced to, nor simply explained in terms of, the basic laws of physics and chemistry, nor in terms of a meticulous mapping of the dynamics of stimulus and response. In this consensus, the mind is no longer the prisoner of biology, as ancient Orphic religion believed and the various forms of dualism perpetuated, but is the product of biology. It is an emergent phenomenon resulting from a long process of cosmic and biologic evolution, and from the complicated developmental process involved in the gestation of an individual human being. In this consensus, while nothing is absolute, not everything is contingent. There are patterns, regularities, algorithms, and laws, but they are functions of scale and complexity.

5.3.1.5   Respect for responsible moral agency as a defining human characteristic

The fifth broad strategic protocol is respect for the unique quality of moral agency and potential for creative responsibility of the human person. The uniqueness of human beings lies not in some abstract nature or essence, nor in a special election or creation by a divine power, but in the empirical fact that alone (as far as we can currently tell) among the products of the evolutionary process, human persons have the ability not only to transform their external physical and social environment, but also in the light of the exponentially expanding biotechnologies, to transform the internal environment of the human genotype and phenotype.

This is a qualitatively different understanding of the moral status of the human person from what the sociologist Robert Bellah has described as "ontological individualism," an attitude and a conviction that the fulfillment of the individual is a moral absolute.[34] Daniel Bell, doyen of American sociologists, has identified and deplored the sea change in moral consciousness that has rhetorically established the ego, the self, as the "lodestar of consciousness" and made it the center of the moral universe.[35] In this moral universe the self is the subject of rights and entitlements, not a source of creative responsibility. The ego becomes obsessed with its own "self-infinitization," as Bell terms it, and this obsession is the antithesis of becoming, in Teilhard de Chardin's words, "the arrow pointing the way to the final unification of the world in terms of life".[36] Ontologic individualism fosters omnivorous consumers in the global supermarket, not creative and responsible citizens of the planet Earth.

This moral protocol, which emerges from the universe story of human persons as free, moral agents exercising creative and cooperative responsibility for their personal and planetary future, is the most plausible source of human rights and of the demand for authentic democracy. This understanding of the dignity and value of a human person is not an exercise in species arrogance. It is rather recognition of the creative and comprehensive responsibility of human beings not to do injustice to other animal species by treating them as if they have no value beyond their subordination to the interests and needs of humans.[37]

5.3.1.6   Limitations on the exercise of creative responsibility

The sixth moral protocol is a corollary of the fifth. The logic of the universe story, of biologic evolution, and of what we now know of the creative potential of human consciousness persuades us thus to acknowledge the dignity and value of each human person. It follows, therefore, that any institution or force – physical, military, political, economic, social, cultural, or psychologic – that seriously curtails the scope or exercise of creative responsibility by any citizen is in serious violation of the value, rights, and dignity of that citizen. By the same token, however, the creative scope of each citizen is qualified and curtailed by this very protocol. The exercise of creative responsibility by one person, in other words, is modified by the limitation that it does not significantly impair its exercise by other people.

5.3.2   Specific procedural protocols

The six broad protocols suggested above thus serve as a flexible, interactive framework for moral discourse and action within the cosmology of the creative universe. But it is also necessary to specify more detailed procedural protocols for the exercise of creative responsibility. The changed cosmologic context of morality does not mean that we can simply make relatively minor adjustments to the traditional forms of moral thought and discourse. It demands a serious reconceptualization of the very form of moral thought, discourse, and action. Before spelling out the procedural protocols for a morality of creative responsibility it is important, briefly, to summarize the key elements of the transformation of morality implied by the cosmology of the creative universe as I have presented it thus far.

First, the context of moral discourse has changed from one based on the various forms of the ontocratic assumption and consciousness to one based on an ontogenetic assumption and consciousness.

Second, the scope of moral discourse has expanded from the personal and the interpersonal to the social, the political, and the planetary. The cosmology of the mechanical universe reduced morality to the personal domain and proclaimed all other realms to be subject to the amoral laws of functional rationality. The environmental movement and the electronically-wired global village in particular have made it increasingly clear that the planetary and the political are inescapably personal, and that the personal is inescapably political and planetary.

Third, the new cosmology demands a shift in the nature of moral discourse from one of obligation and obedience to pre-established moral imperatives and laws, to one of responsibility. In addition, it demands a changed orientation from timeless, perennial normative structures – from "moral truth" – to an open future in which imperatives and values, indeed morality itself, must constantly be re-evaluated and reconceptualized. It demands a changed orientation to moral design. It also demands changed idioms of moral discourse; the idioms of virtue–vice, good–evil, and legal–illegal must be replaced with the language of responsible–irresponsible design and management of the behavior or the projects in which we engage.

The new cosmology demands a radical shift in emphasis from the epistemic axis along which often lethally competitive conflicts about the truth of reality occur to the praxis axis along which cooperative negotiation for the design of a more just and peaceful future can occur.

Finally, it demands a changed moral psychology from one that either explicitly or implicitly fosters dutiful, conformist consumers of inherited norms and values, or disabled, dependent victims of heredity or circumstances, to one that fosters free moral agents and confident citizens responsible for their personal and planetary future.

But what are the criteria for responsible behavior at any level of human activity? How do we determine, on the other hand, that behavior has been culpably irresponsible? Six key words (the six "p words"), can be used to specify the procedural protocols for assessing responsible behavior: priorities, probability, proportion, purpose, prolepsis, and prudence. The careful observation of all of these protocols is the hallmark of moral responsibility. The neglect of any one of them leaves any consequent action vulnerable to the accusation of moral irresponsibility.

5.3.2.1   Priorities

Every person, society, and institution holds, either implicitly or explicitly, a set of priorities or values that are ranked, once again either implicitly or explicitly, in a hierarchical order. In the age of public relations and spin doctoring, it is often difficult to determine what the rank ordering of priorities and values really is behind the self-serving rhetoric of ambitious people, greedy institutions, and expansionist nations in hot pursuit of their own advantage. But this is a separate issue. For a genuinely responsible moral decision, moral agents must be reasonably explicit about the rank ordering of their priorities and values.

The ordering of priorities is not just a matter of individual choice. The order depends to a very large extent on a social consensus, legitimation, and support. It is clear, moreover, especially in the contemporary context of accelerating change, that new priorities and values emerge, and their rank ordering is subject to constant change. Individual human life is now of much more value than in previous ages. Human happiness and fulfillment, and the autonomy of the individual, are now important priorities. As a result of the environmental movement, other species and the wilderness now are conceded to have value which was not recognized in the first surge of modern industrialization that reduced them simply to their commercial value. As new priorities and values are espoused, cultural conflict intensifies. The priority of sexual freedom and expression conflicts with the traditional puritan values of sexual obligations and reticence. The demands of the social order conflict with the demands of the autonomy of the self. In the last analysis, however, individual moral agents are at least morally, if not legally, accountable for the choices they make and priorities they give to the competing demands that can arise in making a moral decision.

5.3.2.2   Probability

The second procedural protocol is the level of probability of the factual data involved in the process of making a decision. In the era of Newtonian physics it was hoped that science would finally provide us, using the appropriate means of empirical reason, with a very high level of certitude. This hope was undercut by Heisenberg who established that at the heart of reality the best we could ever achieve in establishing the facts of any case was higher or lower levels of probability. This has proved to be particularly true of the domain of biologic reality. In nearly every field of study now, observations and descriptions of phenomena are recognized as distributed across a Gaussian curve of probability, and particularly with regard to human nature and behavior. This development in western intellectual history, in principle, curtailed dogmatic religious and philosophical assertions about the fixed nature of things. Hence, calculating the level of probability of a phenomenon, a conceptual tool that had little use in absolute, ontocratic moral systems, becomes an important tool in the ontogenetic morality of creative responsibility.

5.3.2.3 Proportion

A sense of proportion is one of the most important of the moral ideas or tools we have inherited from the ancient Greeks in general, and from Aristotle in particular. Many of the great evils of the twentieth century arose because leaders, and the people who followed them, became so obsessed with an ideal that they lost all sense of proportion, harmony, and balance in the decisions they made. For Aristotle, moral virtue stands in the middle between two or more extremes. It seems, moreover, that in both biology and ecology there is a kind of imperative that demands a sense of balance, of proportion, and of limits, which, if flouted, can lead to serious environmental consequences. This protocol can be understood in the more concrete terms of cost–benefit analysis though not one that is purely economic. In a complex, fast-changing universe, in which multiple factors and imperatives often conflict with each other, moral decisions inevitably involve a calculus of costs and benefits. There are, today, almost no cost-free possibilities or alternatives. Moral decisions, therefore, must involve a proportional balance among the conflicting moral design imperatives.

5.3.2.4 Purpose

The historian and philosopher of technology, Lewis Mumford, observed that "you cannot get rid of purpose" even though mechanistic science attempted to exclude it in the pursuit of objective truth. Purpose, Mumford claimed, always creeps back through "the institutionalized purposes that are actually controlling our society."[38] While the purpose of the moral exercise must be made as explicit as possible, it can also be the point of serious vulnerability for moral rationality. Purpose has two dimensions. The external dimension is the publicly articulated objective. The internal dimension is the private motive of the moral agent that, as Freud and his epigones have established, may be subject to a significant range of unconscious influences. Ambition and greed can often be the driving forces behind an otherwise impeccably honorable proposal. Be this as it may, both dimensions of the moral protocol of purpose must be made as explicit as possible in the procedure of making a responsible moral decision.

5.3.2.5 Prolepsis

As the pace of change accelerates, and as our focus is increasingly oriented towards the future, the proleptic aspect of moral agency becomes increasingly important. The economist Kenneth Boulding remarked that while all experience is about the past, all decisions are about the future.[39] Experience, after all, is a poor teacher. It provides us with the lesson only after we have had the test. The accelerating pace of change, and our growing recognition that we alone have creative responsibility for the direction of change and the shape of the future raises the critical problem of how we make responsible decisions burdened with the realization that the future, however it emerges, is not going to be very much like the past, and that we cannot rely entirely on past experience for the future we attempt to create.

The proleptic protocol for making moral decisions, therefore, demands a careful analysis and assessment of, and balance between, both the possibilities and the risks involved in the exercise of creative responsibility.

5.3.2.6 Prudence

The final protocol is prudence. Indeed, this is not so much a moral protocol or tool as the very central act of decision-making, the act of practical moral reasoning. It is an old-fashioned term that, unfortunately, currently conveys a sense of prissiness or overcautiousness. It was previously described in moral discourse, however, as "the charioteer of the virtues," because it steered all the divergent energies, priorities, and demands in a coherent and practical direction. A moral decision is prudent, be this at the personal level or at the social and political level, when it has taken all the relevant design factors into consideration, and has decided upon the best balance among a whole range of competing values and demands, in order, under the circumstances, to use the best available means to achieve a worthy purpose. The careful observance of all of these protocols is the hallmark of moral responsibility. The neglect of any one of them leaves any consequent action vulnerable to the accusation of moral irresponsibility.

5.4 The morality of IGM

A morality of creative responsibility, on the basis of the ontogenetic assumption within a creative cosmology, in principle, legitimates the human technologic enterprise of transforming both its external and internal environment. This constantly expanding enterprise continues to be problematic for most ethical theories and moral systems based on the various forms, sacred and secular, of the ontocratic assumption. This in-principle legitimation or sanctioning, however, does not absolve specific technologic projects from the difficult task of moral analysis and assessment. This is especially true of biotechnology in general and IGM in particular because they may require us to revise our traditional concepts of morality and justice as genetic attributes which were once given and inalterable become modifiable and distributable.[40]

In the face of a high level of often justified technophobia, a fear that often complicates rational discussion of technologic enterprises, it is important to clarify, initially what is meant by the term "technology." By "technology" I mean scientifically-based, systematic thought and discourse about the responsible deployment of matter, energy, and information for human purposes. When described in these inclusive and neutral terms technology becomes an essentially moral enterprise. That it has fallen into such disrepute in the closing decades of the twentieth century is due largely to the fact that engineering, both mechanical and biologic, has far too often been hijacked by, and subordinated to, crassly commercial and military purposes.

It is useful, in approaching this issue, to summarize the various ways in which genes have functioned in the evolutionary process and can now be manipulated for human purposes.

First, evolution can be understood in terms of its genetic underpinnings; the fundamental mechanisms for biologic change are the processes of the segregation, mutation, diversification, and recombination of genes.

Second, there has been traditional craft-based manipulation of genes. As the biologist, Richard Lewontin has noted, human beings have, for many millennia, sought through the selective breeding of animals and plants, to improve the quality or characteristics of subsequent generations.[41] The selection of mates, among human beings, moreover, was at least implicitly often concerned to maintain the quality of the breeding, especially among social elites.[42] As Lewontin points out, however, this traditional craft method of gene manipulation, though often based on shrewd experience, was unscientific, and thus a hit and miss exercise likely to produce as many undesirable as desirable outcomes.

Third, and most important in the context of IGM, we now have science-based genetic engineering. The great advantage of science-based genetic engineering over the craft-based tradition of breeding practices is the accuracy, specificity, and precision the former brings to the task of improving the phenotype through manipulation or alteration of the genotype. For the purpose of moral discrimination and assessment, it is necessary, then, to discuss different kinds of activity in this area of biotechnology in some detail.

There is now a high level of consensus among medical researchers and bioethicists that somatic cell gene transfer (SCGT) for disease conditions, provided it conforms to the standard norms for medical research and practice, does not offer serious moral problems. This procedure aims to cure a pathologic condition through the alteration of a single gene or a combination of genes in the non-germ or somatic cells of the body. This therapy does not purposefully result in the transmission of the new genes to subsequent generations (though there are some concerns with inadvertent transmission). The moral validity of its use depends on the satisfaction of the usual medical criteria of its safety, effectiveness, reasonable cost within the context of the overall allocation of medical resources in a society, informed consent of the patient, and on decisions and debates about what are appropriate conditions to target (i.e., which conditions are diseases). IGM, however, involves more ethically contentious issues, particularly with regard to the ramifications it has not just for the individual involved but also for future generations.

IGM is a unique biotechnology since it explicitly and purposively alters the genetic composition of inheritable material carried by the recipient and thus potentially affects not just the health of the individual, but the genetic composition of subsequent generations through the offspring that might be later produced. This raises the proleptic dimension of biotechnology quite directly and emphatically. What are the likely consequences of IGM for subsequent generations? What is the responsibility of those utilizing this kind of intervention for those future generations? How does one do a cost–benefit analysis when the ramifications of an intervention conducted in a contemporaneous time frame potentially extend to people living in the future?

It is important, first of all, to recognize the potential benefits of IGM. Unlike SCGT, its aim is to correct a defect in all the cells of the unborn fetus and in the earliest stages of development. It also has the potential to be much more specific and direct in its targeting and substitution of genes. For parents who oppose abortion, moreover, it could provide a morally acceptable alternative to embryo screening and diagnosis of a suspected serious genetic defect followed by termination, assuming the technique is proven to be safe and effective.

This leaves us, therefore, with the two questions specific to IGM. What is the degree of risk of this kind of intervention for future generations? Do parents, or does anyone else have the authority to make a decision of this kind?

While it is true that IGM is a historically unprecedented form of intervention in the direction and shape of the human evolutionary future, human beings have been making decisions, either advertently or inadvertently, about the genetic composition of the human evolutionary future ever since human beings began reproducing. Couples almost routinely, sometimes knowingly, run the risk of passing on genetic defects to their children and subsequent generations. The only traditional protection against this has been prohibitions against the various degrees of consanguineous marriages.

Until now there have been no significant formalized requirements that men and women check the risk that their begetting of children will have serious consequences for posterity although there are social and informal mechanisms, especially in high-risk communities. Indeed, because modern medicine is keeping many people alive who previously would have died in infancy because of genetic defects, and because no subsequent restrictions are legally imposed on these survivors to insure that they do not randomly beget children, some geneticists worry about the decline in the quality of the human gene pool. Other than specified risks such as insertional mutagenesis, which may be overcome in the future,[43] the development of the technology of IGM it could be argued, therefore, may pose no greater risk to the genetic quality of future generations than the persisting traditional practice, currently reinforced by the ethos of individual rights, of random couplings of human beings who are mostly oblivious to the genetic content of their gametes, and to the future consequences of their combination.

Yet another positive consideration about this kind of intervention is that it could foster, with much greater scientific expertise and moral care, what the natural evolutionary process has fostered as the basis for the survival of species, namely genetic variation. This consideration could, of course, be a double-edged sword. In the long haul of the evolutionary process, what could today be regarded as an undesirable gene might turn out to be, in changed circumstances, one which helps promote adaptation and survival (the example of the selective advantage of a single dose of the gene associated with sickle cell anemia for malaria protection is well-recognized). The advantage we enjoy today, however, with our vastly expanded repertoire of scientific knowledge and technical expertise, is that the level of risk to later generations has been significantly reduced, though not entirely eliminated, from that which prevailed in the prescientific situation of random couplings.

The risks of IGM to subsequent generations are also diminished by two biologic facts. The first is that the human population is now over 6 billion and rising. This kind of intervention will be available, in the foreseeable future, to only an extremely small proportion of that population. The second is that if the replaced gene is dominant, it will manifest itself in only half of the descendants, and if it is recessive, will manifest itself only rarely. If it is dominant, and turns out to cause disease, subsequent advances in medicine should be able to detect and correct the defect in future generations, though perhaps not in the individuals originally affected.

The issue of risk itself needs to be assessed. Every historical change has involved enormous antecedent risks whether it has been the movement of tribes, voyages of discovery, the colonizing of new lands, the domestic use of powerful chemicals, the deployment of nuclear power, space exploration, the imposing of new economic orders such as globalization, or the overthrow of older social orders in political revolutions. It is only over the past 40 years that we have come to recognize the vast environmental risks that the human race fecklessly took in the process of global industrialization, the indiscriminate use of fertilizers and insecticides, and in the application of advances in private and public health that resulted in the earth's population increasing by a factor of five or six in just over a century.

The exercise of human adventurousness and ingenuity has always been a high-risk enterprise. What is unique about biotechnology in general and IGM in particular is that it is crossing new frontiers in human experience qualitatively different from previous projects of exploration, scientific discovery and technologic ingenuity. The recent awareness of the consequences of human biologic depredation has resulted in a growing demand for environmental impact studies which highlight the proleptic dimension of creative responsibility. But while studies of this kind lower the level of the risk involved in expanding the range of human ingenuity, they do not eliminate it. This is especially true in the field of bioengineering.

Of course careful research is an essential component in the evolving moral calculus. In fact, the whole enterprise of gene modification, whether it is conducted on somatic cells or germ cells, has been developed much more carefully and responsibly than most other modern technologic enterprises which have had enormous impacts on human health and wellbeing. For instance, we might never know the extent of the genetic mutations inadvertently caused by the vast array of chemical agents routinely used in modern life. The argument that Lewontin makes against the opponents of genetically modified food is precisely that we are now much more scientifically aware, better technologically equipped, and much more morally responsible about the use of biotechnology than when strains of plants and animals were crossed on the basis of prescientific conjecture and folk wisdom about hereditability.

To ask whether prospective parents, in consultation with medical professionals have the *right* to make a decision that will affect future generations is to overlook the fact that although increasing numbers of prospective parents use genetic technology as a basis for decision-making about having children, many make the decision to have children with little consideration of the genetic content they are likely to contribute to future generations. Faced with the possibility and potential benefit of IGM, they could, in the future, be confronted with a *moral obligation* to consider the issue of their responsibility for the health of future generations which is currently usually ignored in typical childbearing which is based on impulse or romantic love.

The key threats to the responsible use of biotechnology in general, and IGM in particular, are greed and ambition. The moral protocol of purpose applied to research and therapy in the context of the institution of medicine demands that they be governed by the key imperative of the promotion of private and public health. The ethics and morality of creative responsibility requires that all of the strategic and procedural protocols be meticulously observed. When medical research and therapeutic practice become dominated by the motives of corporate profit or personal or institutional ambition and competition, however, key moral protocols can be neglected and serious problems can arise.

This is by no means a distant threat. As numerous commentators have noted in recent years, universities, medical and scientific research institutions are being forced to become more "entrepreneurial" and enter into commercial partnerships with biotechnology and pharmaceutical companies, the traditional scientific imperatives of open disclosure and peer review of research findings can become deeply compromised by the commercial imperatives of industrial secrecy, product promotion, and marketing strategies.[44,45] Ultimately, responsibility in any enterprise of biotechnology, and its moral validity, rests on maintaining the integrity and openness of the scientific community of researchers, and the obligation of this community to insure that both the positive and negative results of research be readily available to peer review and public scrutiny. The role of legislators and of the research community, therefore, is not precisely to dictate what kind of research can or cannot be conducted, but to ensure that biotechnologic research conforms to the norms of open scientific disclosure and scrutiny.

James Watson, co-discoverer of the structure of DNA, seemed to reflect a consensus among scientists and ethicists at a 1998 conference on the future of germline gene transfer when he said that any attempt to impose restrictive legislation governing research in this field, at either the national or international level, would be a complete disaster.[46] What is called for at this stage of knowledge and experience is careful research, accurate reporting of results, and open and cooperative sharing of findings. In this way it will be possible to build both a scientific and moral consensus about the best way to proceed in this challenging field of biotechnology and to take creative responsibility for the future health of the human species.

5.5 Conclusions

Biotechnology in general and IGM in particular, pose revolutionary challenges to the boundaries and the structures of traditional ethical theories, and moral systems and traditions. These radically new initiatives in the exercise of human technologic and moral agency force us to recognize the new scope of our scientific understanding and technologic prowess. The convergence of formerly separate streams of the physical, biologic, and cognitive sciences have resulted in the emergence of a historically unique cosmology, the cosmology of the creative universe. As I have argued, this new cosmology demands a correspondingly new morality of creative responsibility. It is only within the context of this new cosmology, and following the strategic and procedural protocols that are implied by them, that the morality of IGM can be adequately assessed. On these terms it can, in principle, be justified. But these terms also define the conditions for the responsible conduct of both research and therapy in this challenging enterprise.

NOTES

1 William Irwin Thompson, *Pacific Shift*. San Francisco: Sierra Club Books (1985), p. 3.

2 Hans Jonas, *The Imperative of Responsibility*. Chicago: University of Chicago Press (1984), p. 6.

3 Ian Wilmut, A.E. Schnieke, J. McWhir, *et al.*, Viable offspring derived from fetal and adult mammalian cells, *Nature* 385 (1997), 810–3.

4 William J. Clinton, Directive, *The White House, Office of the Press Secretary* 4 March 1997, as posted on 2 November 2000 on the National Institutes of Health Office of Extramural Research web site at http://grants.nih.gov/grants/policy/cloning_directive.htm (last accessed 30 March 2005).

5 John Paul II, "Address," *18th International Congress of the Transplantation Society*, 29 August 2000, http://www.vatican.va/holy_father/john_paul_ii/speeches/2000/jul-sep/documents/hf_jp_ii_spe_20000829_transplants_en.html and http://www.xenotransplan. ineu.org/xenotrans/news/20000829.htm (last accessed 30 March 2005).

6 Alasdair MacIntyre, *After Virtue: A Study in Moral Theory*. Notre Dame: University of Notre Dame Press (1981), pp. 1–5.

7 For example the National Institutes of Health (NIH) Recombinant DNA Advisory Committee (RAC) "will not at present entertain proposals for germ line alterations but will consider proposals involving SCGT," in "Points to consider in the design and submission of protocols for the transfer of recombinant DNA molecules into one or more

human research participants (points to consider)," *NIH Guidelines For Research Involving Recombinant DNA Molecules*, Appendix M, amended April 2002, http://www4.od.nih. gov/oba/rac/guidelines_02/APPENDIX_M.htm (last accessed 28 February 2004).

8 Karsten Friis Johansen, *A History of Ancient Philosophy: From the Beginnings to Augustine*. London: Routledge (1991), trans. Henrik Rosenmeier, pp. 33, 47.

9 "Acts of the Apostles," in *The Holy Bible: Revised Standard Version*. London: Thomas Nelson and Son Ltd. (1966), Chapter 17, verses 22–5.

10 See Albert Mirgeler, *Mutations of Western Christianity*. London: Burns and Oates (1961), trans. Edward Quinn, Chapter 2, pp. 6–15.

11 John Barrow, *Theories of Everything*. London: Vintage (1992), p. 10.

12 Georges Dicker, *Descartes: An Analytical and Historical Introduction*. New York: Oxford University Press (1993), p. 6.

13 Newton's own view was that his scientific theories provided a foundation for demonstrating a generally provident deity. See James E. Force, Hume and the relation of science to religion among certain members of the Royal Society. In: John W. Yolton (ed.), *Philosophy, Religion and Science in the Seventeenth and Eighteenth Centuries*. New York: University of Rochester Press (1990), Chapter XV, p. 233.

14 The revival of skepticism began in the late sixteenth century, prior to Newton. See Georges Dicker, *Descartes: An Analytical and Historical Introduction*. New York: Oxford University Press (1993), pp. 6–7.

15 For further analysis of the cultural aspects see Susan R. Bordo, *The Flight to Objectivity: Essays on Cartesianism and Culture*. Albany: State University of New York Press (1987), pp. 13–43.

16 Paul Davies and John Gribben, *The Matter Myth*. New York: Simon and Schuster (1992), pp. 10–29.

17 Brian L. Silver, *The Ascent of Science*. New York: Oxford University Press (1998), pp. 453ff., 469ff.

18 Brian Swimme and Thomas Berry, *The Universe Story*. New York: Harper Collins (1994).

19 See J. Baird Callicott, The metaphysical implications of ecology, *Environmental Ethics* 8 (1986), 301–16; Edward Goldsmith, The way: an ecological world-view, *The Ecologist* 18 (1988), 160–85.

20 Ilya Prigogine, *From Being to Becoming*. San Francisco: W.H. Freeman and Co. (1979); Erich Jantsch, *The Self-Organizing Universe*. New York: Pergamon Press (1980); Ilya Prigogine and Isabelle Stengers, *Order Out of Chaos: Man's New Dialogue with Nature*. New York: Bantam (1984); Paul Davies, *The Cosmic Blueprint*. London: Unwin (1987).

21 Paul Davies provided a brief account of this phenomenon in The creative cosmos, *New Scientist* (17 December 1987), 41–4. Physicist Lee Smolin describes the role of Prigogine and others in closing this gap in *Life of the Cosmos*. New York: Phoenix (1997), pp. 191ff.

22 See Gerald Edelman and Guilio Tonini, *A Universe of Consciousness*. New York: Basic Books (2000), pp. 220ff; Gerald M. Edelman, *Bright Air, Brilliant Fire: On the Matter of Mind*. New York: Basic Books (1992).

23 Steve Jones, The set within the skull, *The New York Review of Books*. (6 November 1997), p. 15.

24 Teilhard de Chardin, *The Phenomenon of Man*. London: Wm. Collins & Sons and New York: Brothers (1959), p. 224.

25 Richard Bernstein, *Beyond Objectivism and Relativism: Science, Hermeneutics and Praxis*. Philadelphia: University of Pennsylvania Press (1983), p. 230.

26 Jean-Francois Lyotard, *The Postmodern Condition: A Report on Knowledge*. Minneapolis: University of Minnesota Press (1993), trans. Geoff Bennington and Brian Massumi, p. xxiv.

27 Alfred North Whitehead, *The Adventure of Ideas*. New York: Mentor (1956), pp. 13–4.

28 Richard Appignanesi and Chris Garratt, *Introducing Postmodernism*. New York: Totum (1995), pp. 80–1.

29 Charles Hampden-Turner, *Maps of the Mind*. New York: Collier Books (1982).

30 Richard Tarnas, *The Passion of the Western Mind: Understanding the Ideas that Have Shaped Our World View*. New York: Ballantine Books (1991).

31 Joseph Campbell, *The Power of Myth*. New York: Doubleday (1988), pp. 22–4, 39.

32 See for example Stuart Kauffman, *At Home in the Universe*. New York: Oxford University Press (1995), pp. 23–4.

33 Charles Birch, Five axioms for a postmodern worldview. In his: *On Purpose*. Kensington: NSW University Press (1990), pp. 128–36. In this paper Birch describes how previous debates about dualism and reductionism seem no longer useful in the emerging organic understanding of our reality.

34 Robert N. Bellah, Ann Swidler, Steven M. Tipton, *et al.*, *Habits of the Heart: Individualism and Commitment in American Life*. Berkeley: University of California Press (1985), p. 334.

35 Daniel Bell, *The Cultural Contradictions of Capitalism*. New York: Basic Books (1975), p. 47.

36 From de Chardin, *The Phenomenon of Man*, p. 224.

37 Peter Singer, *Animal Liberation: A New Ethics for Our Treatment of Animals*. London: Jonathan Cape (1976), pp. 1–27.

38 Lewis Mumford, Closing statement. In: Robert Disch (ed.), *The Ecological Conscience*. Eagle Cliffs, NJ: Prentice Hall (1970), p. 93; see also Lewis Mumford, *Technics and Civilization*. Orlando: Harcourt Brace and Co. (1963).

39 Kenneth Boulding, Foreword. In: Fred Polak, *The Image of the Future*. London: Elsevier Scientific Publishing Co. (1973), pp. v–vi.

40 Allen Buchanan, Dan W. Brock, Norman Daniels, *et al.*, *From Chance to Choice: Genetics and Justice*. New York: Cambridge University Press (2000), pp. 61–103.

41 Richard Lewontin, Genes in the food! *The New York Review of Books* 48 (21 June 2001), pp. 81–4.

42 For a discussion of the relevance of eugenics to the current technology see Allen Buchanan, Dan W. Brock, Norman Daniels, *et al.*, Eugenics and its shadow, in their *From Chance to Choice*, pp. 27–60.

43 Donald B. Kohn, Michel Sadelain and Joseph C. Glorioso, Occurrence of leukaemia following gene therapy of X-linked SCID, *Nature Reviews Cancer* 3 (2003), 447–88.

44 For example see Ray Moynihan, Dangerous liaisons, *The Australian Financial Review Magazine* (April 2002), 49–54.

45 James Robert Brown, Privatizing the university – the new tragedy of the commons, *Science* 290 (2000), 1701–2.

46 Quoted in Meridith Wadman, Gene therapy must be spared excessive regulation, *Nature* 392 (1998), 317.

Ethics and welfare issues in animal genetic modification

Gabrielle M. O'Sullivan

6.1 Introduction

Unlike the situation in human animals, inheritable genetic modification (IGM) is currently implemented in non-human animals. Targeted mutants (transgenic animals) and random mutants are widely created in medical research.[1] A number of animal species have already been cloned, with plans underway to clone many others, including pets, species on the verge of extinction, and species that are already extinct.

Genetically-modified non-human animals (hereafter, "animals") are used in basic and pre-clinical research as well as in product development and agriculture research. They are used as disease models, as sources of organs for experimental xenotransplantation, as bioreactors for the production of therapeutic proteins ("pharming"), and as test animals for vaccines and toxins. Thus, while we might hope to be designers in human IGM, we are already designers in animal IGM.

Although animal IGM deserves ethical consideration in its own right without necessarily referring to human IGM, it can be instructive for human IGM, as some of our fears and hopes for human IGM might already be realized in animal IGM. Indeed, the major concerns in animal genetic modification are similar to those voiced in connection with potential human IGM technology, namely concerns about animal welfare and risks to human health and the environment. For example, there are fears that genetically-modified animals might escape into the environment and alter evolutionary balances or be somehow involved in the modification of the human genome. There is also some debate about whether or not gene modification research using animals causes more animal suffering than non-gene modification research, and about whether or not it raises new ethics and welfare issues in animal research generally.[2]

The purpose of this chapter is not to answer this question, but to examine the ethics and welfare issues associated with animal IGM in the medical research context. Before exploring these issues, I outline how animal genetic modification is achieved and regulated, and examine the available statistics that show that the landscape of animal research is changing as a result of genetic modification. I will also explore the role of animal genetic modification in the future development of human IGM and the impact that one might have on the other. Commercialization and the potential limits of legal remit in chimera production will also be discussed, as these are two areas in which genetic modification causes new tensions.

6.2 Techniques for genetically modifying animals

Targeted IGM is achieved by a process known as transgenesis, whereby functional exogenous DNA (or a transgene) is introduced into the germ cells of an organism using artificial gene transfer techniques. The goal is to delete specific phenotypic characteristics from, and/or to introduce new phenotypic characteristics into, the organism's progeny. The resulting progeny are known as transgenic organisms (e.g., transgenic animals). A "gene knockout" organism (e.g., a gene knockout animal) is the term used to denote a transgenic organism in which the transgene that is substituted for a functional gene in the unmodified organism is a non-functional gene. Cloning can also be viewed as a type of IGM, in the sense that the clone's genetic identity is conferred by a manipulation (i.e., nuclear transfer) and is inheritable. But in another sense, cloning might not be viewed as IGM if the transferred nucleus is not itself genetically modified in some way. Cloning can be performed as an additional step during the transgenesis process, although transgenesis does not necessarily involve cloning. IGM can also be achieved by random mutagenesis by treating mouse gametes or embryonic stem (ES) cells with chemical mutagens.

The technical interventions that are used to genetically modify animals include the microinjection of DNA into a pronucleus in a fertilized egg; the manipulation of ES cells (for gene targeting, gene knockout, or homologous recombination); the application of conditional targeted mutagenesis systems (for controlling when and where transgenes will be expressed); the inhibition of gene expression using antisense DNA or RNA; gene transfer using viral vectors; cytoplasmic transfer (e.g., ooplasm); the manipulation of primordial germ cells; nuclear transfer; and the manipulation of spermatogonial cells. The first three methods are most commonly used. Gene addition and random insertion of mutations can be achieved by all these methods.

6.3 The regulation of genetic modification of animals

The creation and use of genetically-modified animals is regulated by the same legislation that regulates scientific procedures involving non-genetic modification in animals and also, in a number of countries, such as Australia and the U.K., by legislation regulating gene technology from a biosafety perspective.

The use of animals in scientific procedures is regulated by legislation governing the use of animals in research, animal welfare,[3] and/or the prevention of cruelty to animals.[4] Compliance with the regulations is supported by guidance principles,[5] research funding policies,[6] and accreditation agencies.[7] The regulations generally apply to any research using any vertebrate animals regardless of the source of funding, except in the U.S.A., where they do not apply to privately-funded research on mice, rats, and birds.

Regulatory compliance oversight systems differ between countries. In Canada, the U.S.A., Sweden, and Australia there are local institutional animal ethics committees; in Germany there are regional committees; and in the U.K. and France there are national agencies. All of these committees are charged with "ensuring that the pain and distress experienced by animals in research is avoided or minimized."[8]

The priority granted to human interests over animal interests differs between the various national regulatory systems. A weak human priority position is embodied in the U.K. and Swedish regulations, whereby human benefit must be sufficient to justify animal suffering in research. A stronger human priority position is embodied in the legislation of other European countries that follow the 1986 European Directive that human benefit must be sufficient to justify severe animal suffering in research. The strongest human priority position is embodied in the U.S.A. and Canadian legislation, whereby animal interests do not ever outweigh human interests.[9]

Animal welfare regulatory systems and authorities are just beginning to examine the ethics and welfare implications of the use of genetically-modified animals in research[10] and some countries now keep specific statistics and welfare guidelines on genetically-modified animals.[11]

6.4 The effects of genetic modification on the use of animals in scientific procedures

Despite widely acknowledged problems in estimating the number of animals used in scientific procedures,[12] it appears that the total number of animals being used annually is decreasing slightly, or remaining constant, while the number of genetically-modified animals being used is increasing rapidly.[13] In this chapter, I refer primarily to the U.K. Home Office annual *Statistics of Scientific Procedures on Living Animals* (*Great Britain*),[14] as they provide the most comprehensive national picture of the scale of animal genetic modification in the world to date. They show that between 1995 and 2003 the use of genetically-modified animals in regulated scientific procedures increased from

8% to 27%, while the use of non-genetically-modified animals fell from 84% to 63%. Other indicators reflect a worldwide growth in the use of genetically-modified animals. These include a reversal of a 6-year decline in the use of mice in Canada that was attributed to the increased use of transgenic mice;[15] the expansion of transgenic services facilities at Charles River Laboratories in Europe and Japan in response to increasing demand for animal research models;[16] and predictions of increasing growth in the use of transgenic mice in the U.S.A.[17] and from the Organisation for Economic Co-Operation and Development (OECD).[18]

While it is difficult to project how many genetically-modified animals will be used in the future, it is expected that the trend of increasing use of genetically-modified animals will continue.[19] It will be driven by the fact that gene modification is considered to provide the ultimate confirmation of a gene's function[20] and by the opening of promising new avenues of research, collaborative efforts to systematically characterize the phenotypes (phenomes) of various species (especially the mouse),[21] a patent "rush" on genes[22] and genetically-modified animals,[23] spin-off commercial and contract opportunities, and regulatory requirements.[24] Although biologic research is increasingly becoming an engineering science, current transgenic and genetic research is largely a descriptive science with a limited engineering base: genomes are altered to a very limited extent (at the level of genes) and descriptively compared with unaltered genomes so that functions can be ascribed to genes. In order to "complete the picture," the scales of current descriptive exercises are enormous (as exemplified by the various phenome projects) and are likely to increase as background genetic constitution, environmental factors, and various interactions become experimental variables in gene modification research.

Rodents constitute the majority of all animals used, with mice and rats predominating. Of the 27% of all scientific procedures in 2003 in Great Britain that involved the use of genetically-modified animals, 97% involved mice. About two-thirds of all genetically-modified animals were used to maintain breeding colonies and one-third were used for further scientific purposes. Of those used for further scientific purposes most (about 80%) were used as models for human disease or for research into gene function and the rest were mainly used in applied work such as toxicity or carcinogen testing.[25]

Non-human primates are also used, although in much fewer numbers than rodents. The number of non-human primates used for the first time fell by 24% between 1995 and 2003, reflecting the facts that they are accorded special protection under the U.K. Animals (Scientific Procedures) Act 1986 and cannot be used unless there is no other suitable species, and that they are often reused for minor procedures in the areas of pharmaceutical research development or safety.[26] However, it is expected that their use in these areas, as well as in basic research and in gene therapy, will increase in the future in response to regulatory requirements and research developments derived from the human genome project.[27]

Genetically-modified animals are used for different purposes at different stages in the development of new pharmaceuticals, therapeutic, and/or enhancement regimes that could include IGM in the future. In the initial discovery stage, the emphasis is on creating models of human disease or normality. In the pre-clinical phase, the emphasis is on determining effective dose parameters, predicting potential adverse events, and satisfying regulatory requirements with respect to toxicity. The more closely an animal model "models" the human condition of interest and the more effective the developing therapeutic is, the more that animal use can be refined. This has special implications for non-human primates, especially macaques, as non-human primates are considered to provide the best models of human biology and cognition,[28] and macaques are currently one of the non-human primates of choice for use in research.

Regulatory authorities normally require at least two test species to be used in the pre-clinical phase of therapeutic development: a species of rodent as the first, and dogs or non-human primates as the second. Although the regulations do not specify that non-human primates must be used as the second species, they are often preferentially chosen as a precaution against the imposition of further testing requirements by the regulatory authorities. It is expected that they may become the only species for fundamental research and regulatory testing in the growing areas of human degenerative diseases and neuroactive drug development.[29]

Between 1990 and 2000 there was a move towards using marmosets, tamarins, and macaques and away from prosimians, other old and new world monkeys, and baboons. In the U.K., no great apes have been used since the current legislation (the 1986 Act) banning their use was introduced in 1987, and no baboons have been used since 1999. The current animal welfare regulatory environment is likely to consider the use of transgenic higher non-human primates to be "in principle unacceptable."[30] But it is difficult to predict if this line will prevail in the future, especially if there are moves towards human IGM research. Some consider that an important step on the way to human IGM has already been made, with the creation of the first genetically-modified primate, a macaque named ANDi, who was born on October 2, 2000 at the Oregon Regional Primate Research Center in Portland, Oregon.[31] ANDi carries a green marker transgene from a jellyfish.

6.5   The role of genetically-modified animals in human IGM

Although intentional human IGM is currently prohibited by the combined effects of various laws,[32] regulations,[33] and policies,[34] and inadvertent human IGM is viewed as a serious potential side effect in somatic cell gene transfer (SCGT),[35] it is believed that theoretical paradigms for proceeding with intentional human IGM are beginning to emerge.[36] Improved gene repair technologies, new knowledge about the functions of genes, new methods of assessing safety, and the existence of candidate disorders for initial clinical application have contributed to their development.

Even though the strategies currently used in animal IGM would not be acceptable for application in human reproduction, it is clear that results from research on animals have contributed to the development of these theoretical paradigms. It is also apparent that animals will be used as one of the main testing grounds for any future human IGM enterprise. Therefore the course of development of human IGM, in terms of its extent and type, has important implications for animal ethics and welfare. Indeed lessons learnt from animal IGM have already affected that course. They have changed the scientific view of what can and cannot be done in human IGM. For example, new knowledge about the role of imprinting in embryonic development has tempered earlier discussions that presupposed that someday IGM, of the kind then imagined, would be inevitable.

Even if human IGM technology improved, as is expected, to the point where it was considered acceptably safe for intentional application, it is difficult to estimate how widespread its application would ever be. Estimates vary from limited potential therapeutic application for monogenic disorders,[37] to more widespread application in the modification of susceptibility genes in complex polygenic disorders.[38]

The American Association for the Advancement of Science (AAAS) report on IGM written by Audrey Chapman and Mark Frankel summarized the present-to medium-term view when it stated that it:

Identified few scenarios where there was no alternative to IGM for couples to minimize the prospect that their offspring will have a specific genetic disorder... The further development of SCGT, moreover, will offer more options for treating one's offspring.[39]

The report recommended that:

At this time, the investment of public funds in support of the clinical development of technologies for IGM is not warranted. However, basic research should proceed in molecular and cellular biology and in animals that is relevant to the feasibility and effects of germ line modification.[40]

Christopher Evans presents a more distant future view than the AAAS report when he suggests that, once safe methods of inserting genes using relatively straightforward IGM protocols have been achieved, the cost–benefit arguments might turn in favor of IGM, for the prevention or therapy of expensive polygenic inheritable disorders such as breast cancer, familial adenomatous polyposis, cardiovascular disease, and Alzheimer disease.[41] He suggests that "safe docking sites" might be engineered into the genome for the activation of inducible extra chromosomal elements as required. In this scenario it is not difficult to envisage that the therapeutic application of IGM in families with inheritable mutations predisposing them to serious disease could then be extended to a wider population to provide gene products that are known to assist in protecting from the morbidity associated with more common diseases. For example, he suggests that inducible extra copies of appropriate interleukin molecules might be provided to combat certain types of arthritis.[41] The application of IGM techniques for enhancement could also be envisaged, such as introducing growth factor genes for increased muscle strength. Indeed, Mark Frankel argues that the prospect of enhancement and market forces are more likely to determine the path of IGM than therapy.[42]

Even if the extent of explicitly human IGM research is never large enough for its refinement to have a significant impact in reducing the overall numbers of animals used in research, refinements that result in the reduction of the number of animals used in most types of gene research are relevant to the human IGM enterprise. This is because many different kinds of gene modification experiments in animals will be needed to provide basic and pre-clinical trial information before any attempts at human IGM could be contemplated. Transgenic animals will be required to define pathogenic and therapeutic molecular mechanisms and targets; cloning research will be required to elucidate the mechanisms of nuclear programming, and embryonic and adult growth and development; and pre-clinical research in animal models will continue to be one of the essential means of reducing the degree of moral offense in stem cell and embryo research, which potentially could converge into IGM in the future.[43]

In addition to gene modification changing the scale and purposes of animal usage as discussed earlier, there are other ways (that are all connected to human research) in which animal usage might change in response to scientific advances and limitations, regulations, commercial interests, and societal attitudes. For example:

(a) The prevalence of using "natural" death as an experimental endpoint might increase as a consequence of increasing research into long-term development and aging.

(b) The use of genetically-modified non-human primates in pre-clinical research might increase in response to progress in applied research, using other animals, that indicates that safe human IGM is potentially feasible.

(c) Gene modification research and development might move away from countries that continue to ban any scientific procedures in great apes (such as the U.K., Eire, or New Zealand), if apes become the species of choice in developing gene modification therapies, as is likely in the area of neurodegenerative disorder research.[44]

(d) Certain kinds of animal experiments might be bypassed in some human IGM protocols because traditional clinical trial routes might not suffice due to non-parity between humans and animals, and different consumer expectations for IGM compared with other therapeutics. Ultimately, longitudinal epidemiologic studies in humans might become the biosafety/ efficacy test for such protocols.

(e) There might be different types of ethics assessment for animal gene modification protocols that are designed with human application in mind, compared to protocols that are designed to create animal models of human diseases. For example, the effect of genetic modification on experimental animal integrity might be considered in greater depth in the former than in the latter, because the information gained might be relevant to the application of the protocols in humans.

(f) For some conditions, there may be limited potential benefits to be derived from genetic interventions because redundant, conserved, compensatory biologic mechanisms already make up for deleterious gene mutations.

In summary, while it is difficult to predict the potential future course of human IGM research, it is clear that animal research and probably almost all genetic research will provide essential background information for its consideration. Therefore, at this point in time, the reduction, refinement, and replacement of animals in many types of research (especially gene modification research) are relevant to any future human IGM enterprise, regardless of whether or not the research is specifically geared towards human IGM.

6.6   Welfare issues in animal genetic modification

As discussed earlier, there has been some debate about whether or not animal genetic modification is associated with unique welfare issues that need to be addressed by special welfare assessment and ethics review procedures, or by the application of extra rigorous evaluation.[45] The reports of the European Center for the Validation of Alternative Methods (ECVAM),[46] the BVAAWF/FRAME/ RSPCA/UFAW Joint Working Group on Refinement,[47] and others,[48] identify factors in gene modification procedures that may adversely affect animal welfare. They provide detailed refinement and reduction proposals (including special welfare monitoring schemes), the implementation of which require special welfare assessment and ethics review procedures. As more details about these factors become available, it is to be expected that these proposals will be increasingly integrated into the norms and standards of gene modification-specific welfare assessment and ethics review procedures. One consequence of this could be an increased potential for researchers, and ethics review committees, to be the subjects of non-compliance and/or negligence proceedings.

The factors in genetic modification procedures that may adversely affect animal welfare include:

(a) Initial reproductive interventions such as surgery, hormonal stimulation, embryo collection, and *in vitro* culture: microinjection and gene transfer can result in embryonic and fetal losses, growth anomalies, and/or distress in mothers and foster mothers; vasectomies can cause pain in males; and matings and biopsies for genotyping can cause distress in males and females.

(b) Pronuclear microinjection, which can lead to unpredictable mutation of host genes due to random integration of the donor gene into the host genome.

(c) The biologic effects (intentional or unintentional, predictable or unpredictable) of the transgene construct and its products, tissue expression pattern, secretory pathways, expression level, and interactions with other gene products.

(d) Environmental conditions, such as germ-free conditions, housing, social conditions, husbandry, transport, and production systems that may not meet the behavioral needs of animals (e.g., space, companionship, routing material, and so on).

(e) The scale of animal usage, as discussed earlier.

(f) The scale of animal numbers consigned to waste because of great inefficiencies in current techniques, whereby large numbers of animals are needed to generate the small numbers of animals that are of actual scientific value (i.e., founders).

While there are very limited data on the prevalence of welfare problems in genetically-modified animals generally, one can get a sense of the kinds of problems that they may experience by examining the Jackson Laboratories databases.[49] A more objective sense can be obtained from an inventory study of reports regarding genetically-modified animals to the Animal Experiments Inspectorate in Denmark.[50] This indicated that 36% of genetically-modified strains of mice experience discomfort, with 21% experiencing minor discomfort, and 15% experiencing severe discomfort; and that increased mortality, disease incidence, and/or susceptibility occurred in 30%. Information about particular welfare effects are provided by Miriam van der Meer et al.[51] and Patrizia Costa.[52] The fact that the majority of cloned animals have serious welfare problems[53] is cited as being a significant factor in the basis of moral objections to human cloning.[54]

Even if the factors that adversely affect genetically-modified animal welfare also occur in non-genetically-modified experimental animals (and many of them do), and it is only the greatly increasing scale of genetically-modified animal usage that raises the ethics and welfare issues associated with them, they could be important. Indeed, the Canadian Council on Animal Care has acknowledged this by taking a precautionary approach and differentiating genetically-modified animals from non-genetically-modified animals by making it mandatory for the creation of new transgenic strains to be initially classed as experiments that cause moderate to severe distress or discomfort (Category D). It directs local

Animal Care Committees to only grant provisional approvals for a 12-month period, subject to reports on phenotype, pain, and distress.[55] These measures have been mandated to ensure that appropriate monitoring is implemented, despite the absence of definitive adverse welfare prevalence data.

The kinds of welfare monitoring that have been recommended for transgenic animals include case-based assessment, as the welfare issues will depend on the experimental methods and objectives (e.g., a transgenic disease model would by definition be expected to have welfare problems); detailed half-sibling comparisons (transgenic versus non-transgenic); breeding to homozygosity for a number of generations while maintaining non-transgenic controls; agreed protocols for identifying adverse health effects including cryptic effects; ongoing assessments and reporting; pre-transgenesis research to determine the likely effects of transgene expression (e.g., treatment with gene product or SCGT); and the publication of negative and positive effects on a publicly-accessible database.

The study of Rikke Thon *et al.* indicates that the current forms used to collect information about welfare-related parameters in genetically-modified animals are inadequate.[56] Similarly, the ECVAM report concluded that "existing regulations and legislation for animal experimentation do not adequately provide for the development and varied applications of genetically-modified animals."[57] Perhaps this is partly because until relatively recently, most scientific procedures have involved the treatment of animals with exogenous agents that have known effects and a long and evolved history of experience of use from which to draw guidance, whereas with gene modification many experiments have unpredictable welfare effects that, when manifested, pose questions about whether the creation of a particular animal constitution might be a form of unacceptable cruelty that should be prevented.

6.7   The effects of genetic modification on animal natures, ethics, and welfare

Gene modification can alter an animal's "nature." By this I mean that it can alter an animal's opportunities to employ and develop capabilities that are considered inherent and normal in its unmodified state. In its Biotechnology Report, the U.K. Animal Protection Committee (APC) expressed this capability as the capacity of gene modification to violate an organism's "integrity" or "telos" – that is it can violate the form of life that allows best fulfillment of the goals of its powers and organs.[58] Included in this definition are an organism's molecular structures and capabilities, as well as its natural history (i.e., unimpeded development of natural capabilities and adaptations), as constituent parts of its natural embodiment (nature). This concept of nature is useful because it allows some degree of objective assessment of what animal flourishing is, even in circumstances where references to a "species norm" are absent. It also facilitates consideration of the extent of harms caused by modifications that do not cause suffering. The special environmental requirements for genetically-modified animals can additionally violate animals' natures. Of course, gene modification technology is not the only way to alter an animal's nature. The same effect can be achieved by non-gene-modifying scientific procedures or by conventional selective breeding programs. Selective breeding has been undertaken for thousands of years. The natures of the non-genetically-modified ancestors of genetically-modified animals have also been changed through selective breeding, often with the aim of being used as models of disease. Thus our notions about individual and species integrity, and about what is natural and what is normal, have been contested for quite some time. These already familiar "nature-altering" approaches may require no less ethics and welfare assessment than gene modification approaches. But laboratory-based gene modification technologies such as transgenesis greatly increase the pace, scale, and types of purposeful alterations of animals' natures through the systematic transfer, modification, ablation, and recombination of genes or parts of genes (such as novel human–animal gene combinations) that would not be achieved in a similar time scale, or possibly ever, by any other method. It therefore could potentially consolidate further the notion of animals as models of processes and conditions in humans, and in so doing, lead some people to regard the entitlements of model animals as being somewhat different (perhaps less) than those of other animals. Thus gene modification technology further challenges our notions of what is "natural," what is a species,[59] and what should constitute the bases for concepts of animal welfare and its scope.

Societal support is an important factor in setting the scientific and ethics agendas in gene research, biotechnology, and human and animal experimentation. Shared concepts of what constitutes animal well-being and how these relate to welfare and naturalness have important implications for animals. They help regulators, scientists, and society generally to determine what welfare is, what is beyond welfare, and what are acceptable and unacceptable animal experimentation practices. The extent of alignment between the public's and researchers' definitions of animal welfare will be important in determining public support for scientific research using animals.

Some consider the public's view of animal welfare to be more holistic than that of scientists and farmers. It takes account of indicators of good health (e.g., normal growth, physiologic, and behavioral functions); of natural history (i.e., the unimpeded development of natural capabilities and adaptations embodied in "objective welfare"); and of subjective experience (i.e., "free from prolonged and intense fear, pains, and other negative states" embodied in "subjective welfare").[60] Scientists and farmers, on the other hand, tend to rely more on indicators of biologic function (i.e., good health and subjective experience).[61] This suggests that the public expects animal flourishing to be accommodated (perhaps even promoted) within animal welfare and that some scientists and farmers might consider animal flourishing to be beyond the scope of animal welfare. While there is some dissonance within the public view, particularly as it relates to agriculture,[62] evidence from opinion polls suggests that the public would be concerned by the use of technologies that could modify animals' natures.[63]

There also appears to be dissonance in the scientific community's view of welfare. This is shown by the facts that standard biologic indicators are applied as measures of animal welfare in standard laboratory settings across species regardless of strain, and species-specific differences are often ignored in the application of tests.[64] In addition, different institutions and countries vary greatly in their reporting of the proportion of animals experiencing pain;[65] there is evidence of "under-reporting of animal research that involves unrelieved pain and distress in the U.S.A."[66] Research scientific validity,[67] relevance to humans,[68] and animal behavioral influences on validity[69] are beginning to be critically examined. Validity and relevance are essential precursors to cost–benefit assessments, and necessary, though not sufficient, conditions for the justification of animal experiments.[70] Other evidence comes from the facts that economic costs, the requirements for germ-free environmental conditions, and experimental tradition are frequently cited as reasons for the slow pace of change in animal research in response to animal welfare considerations.

Animal flourishing might not be difficult for an empathetic person who is experienced with animals to recognize, but it is difficult to describe and evaluate scientifically. Therefore its role in welfare, and thus whether or not particular genetic modifications undermine welfare, is prone to contestation, misappropriation, and marginalization in narrow views of welfare. Richard Haynes provides an example of this when he describes how the use of the concept of psychologic well-being as a state of mind as the basis of welfare for non-human primates has shifted the burden of proof about welfare status unreasonably from animal users onto welfare advocates and regulators: in essence, welfare advocates and regulators have to prove to animal users that animals have minds that can be abused and that the abuse can be measurably demonstrated. This facilitates the misappropriation of welfare by scientific experts and ultimately by animal users. In practice, it has turned out that the meaning of "promoting the psychological well-being of non-human primates has been reduced to 'attempting to satisfy the psychological needs of non-human primates.'"[71]

To circumvent this type of misappropriation Haynes proposes that access to opportunities to engage in enjoyable activities with relative ease–not necessarily with the sole purpose of satisfying essential needs–should be the basis of welfare, as these are the primary goods that an animal can choose between in a good animal life.

The capacity of IGM to violate an animal's integrity and natural history affects its ethical assessment, because there is potential in its application for the intrinsic values of animals to be not fully respected. Albert Musschenga describes the duties derived from taking account of the non-moral intrinsic values of animals as duties that are "other duties than just duties to others."[72] According to this view, experimental animals' access to opportunities to engage in enjoyable activities, or to lead natural lives, does not depend on the moral status of the animal, but on these other duties.

Musschenga criticizes the emphasis on limiting conceptions of welfare to "subjective welfare," whereby it is mostly internal factors that are taken into account such as freedom from pain and stress. He proposes that our concept of welfare should be expanded to also include "objective welfare" so that there should be opportunities to lead a "natural life" and welfare would be indicated by animal "flourishing," an objective criterion.[73] He argues that for opportunities to lead a "natural life" to occur, the integrity of an animal must be maintained and this integrity must include the animal's possession of all the elements of wholeness and completeness: balance with its species and capacity to independently maintain itself. His underlying thesis, in contrast to that of Peter Singer,[74] is that there are complex criteria for inclusion in the moral community; and that sentience is just one criterion. The reasons Musschenga gives for proposing objective welfare are that "naturalness is a component of the intrinsic goodness of animals" and "care for an animal's naturalness provides those who adopt a particular conception of the good, moral reasons for action." His views are that welfare concerns are not the only valid moral reasons for action in our relation with animals (some of the reasons go beyond welfare) and that flourishing "is much more that not to suffer."[75] Thus, we have objective reasons that do not depend on the moral status of animals, to care for animals in the kinds of IGM we apply and animal suffering is clearly not the only type of cost: there are also moral issues that involve costs.[76]

Care for animals' natures is increasingly being considered as a valid concern in mainstream biotechnology ethics guidance discussions. For example, the Swedish Committee on Xenotransplantation based all its considerations on the principal that experimental animals should live a "good animal life" and that the fundamental preconditions required for this to occur are:

that animal protection legislation be complied with; that animals must be in good health and have a reasonable opportunity to exercise their natural behavior; and that genetic modifications of the source animal shall not as such in themselves result in discomfort, pain or illness or alter the behavior of the animal and that the animal is monitored following gene modification by a specially trained staff.[77]

However, because of the difficulties in defining an animal's nature and therefore what constitutes an unacceptable alteration of it, there is still some way to go before this concern is translated into regulatory practice. This is apparent in the Home Office's response[78] to the APC recommendation that genetic modification of animals "with the intention of (a) stripping them of their biological integrity, or (b) rendering them incurably insentient" should not be allowed regardless of any potential benefit.[79] The Home Office considered that such experiments would be controlled by the current 1986 Act; that any relevant applications would be required to satisfy the cost–benefit assessment in the same way as other applications; and that the lack of a definition for what constitutes an unacceptable alteration of an animal's nature makes it preferable for any relevant applications to be evaluated in the usual way, on a case-by-case basis, with the advice of the APC. However, the APC disagrees with this assessment. Its view is that cost–benefit assessments are irrelevant to such applications because these kinds of genetic modifications should never be allowed, regardless of benefit.[80]

The real ethics assessment challenges occur with genetic modifications that are not intended to cause radical phenotypic affects on animals, but do. Genetic modifications and the creation of transgenic animals or clones are usually experiments (in the research context) that are intended to determine the functions of genes and gene products, and their mechanisms of action by examining the effects of a particular genetic change on an animal's phenotype. However, the difficulty in estimating prospective harms supports an argument for careful monitoring of new transgenic lines, on a case-by-case basis, for welfare problems. It does not necessarily follow that transgenic lines whose phenotypes are radically affected by their genetic alterations will be used less frequently than those that are not. It is likely that they will be used more frequently if they are of greater scientific interest. Special monitoring will enable ethically acceptable (humane) endpoints and conditions to be set for the use of such animals.

6.8   Other ways in which genetic modification affects ethics

There are aspects of IGM (other than its capacity to alter animals' natures, as discussed above) that also have an impact on the type of ethics assessments that apply. First, in IGM experiments, the experimental subjects (progeny) are modified endogenously, whereas in most non-IGM experiments, experimental subjects are modified exogenously. In IGM, intrinsic properties of animals are prevented from ever forming, and/or extrinsic elements are interiorized as intrinsic properties. Subjects are not allowed any experience of an unmodified ("natural") embodiment, even if phenotypic expression of the modified genotype only becomes apparent late in life. Although welfare agencies do not normally attribute any kind of "personhood" to animals, except perhaps in the case of the great apes, it may not be over anthropomorphizing to imagine that the "person" of an animal is altered by genetic modification; as an animal's construct of its own "selfhood," whatever that might be, is connected to its specific embodiment through its effect on relations with others. Thus, by this reasoning, the violation of animal "integrity" by genetic modification might be considered somewhat analogous to descriptions of the "disruption of identity" in modified humans discussed by Jackie Leach Scully[81] and Christoph Rehmann-Sutter.[82]

Second, IGM experiments are irreversible. Although there can be some control over phenotypic expression – through the use of conditional targeted mutagenesis systems – the long-term effects of genetic modification will depend on when and where in the organism's life cycle gene expression is induced or ablated.

Third, IGM affects cost–benefit assessments. Ethical justification of research involves proportionally balancing costs and benefits. In all animal research the cost is generally conceived to be animal suffering (conceived of as a welfare issue) and the benefit is conceived to be new knowledge leading (proximally or distally) to a human or animal life-saving benefit, medical or otherwise. Balancing costs and benefits in animal research is complicated by the fact that these parameters are measured in different terms. Costs are usually easier to measure than benefits, particularly in exogenous scientific procedures: they occur in a shorter time frame, they can be estimated for individual animals, and their likelihood is definable in terms of expectedness. However, as mentioned earlier, the cost is more than just suffering: it can also be the harm done to the animal whereby the animal is made worse off, even if it is not aware of this. Benefits are less obvious than costs; they occur much further downstream from the experiment at hand, they rely on aggregated benefits from other experiments on other animals or humans, and their likelihood is less definable in terms of expectedness.

IGM costs can occur over a more extended time frame (e.g., in a second generation) than they might in exogenous scientific procedures (with the exception of teratogen testing). They can be multiplied across many subsequent generations. They include exogenous scientific procedure costs in the initial creative steps, iterative costs in the breeding stages, and possibly further exogenous scientific procedure costs in experiments. It can be difficult to estimate costs for individual animals (e.g., the pattern of inheritance or unknown exogenous factors might cause variable expressivity). As discussed earlier, their likelihood can often be not clearly definable in terms of expectedness, and quality, until at least a few generations have passed. As also discussed before, integrity of body and being can be compromised, for example by constitutively reducing opportunities for "joy" or "ease," possibly leading to disrespect of animals as "goods in themselves."

IGM benefits can occur near or well downstream from the original experiments. They can be both independent of, and dependent on, aggregated benefits from other experiments on other animals or humans (e.g., phenome projects). Their likelihood can be both more or less definable in terms of expectedness. While they can be increased in individual fields of research, because IGM animals provide sharper experimental tools that can ultimately reduce the numbers of animals used to answer a particular question, the scale of animal research overall (a cost) can be substantially enlarged, as new research opportunities are presented.

Fourth, IGM science is evolving quickly and there is potential for it to become too complex for many local ethics committees to fully evaluate it with respect to justifying the use of animals. This can lead to increased committee reliance on the integrity and ability of the scientist who intends to perform the work to give a proper account of the proposed research in terms of the balance between the benefit to humans and the harm to animals. In this respect and others, it is interesting to note that the problems encountered in the ethical oversight of animal gene modification research are similar to those described for the ethics oversight of human research,[83] and have led to calls for the formation of overarching independent bodies to provide oversight in each area.[84]

In summary, the above four characteristics of IGM experiments – namely, their effects on animals' social and self development; on experimental reversibility; on the prospective estimation of potential harms and the estimation of harms that occur in the absence of suffering (e.g., molecular structure integrity violations); and on the cost–benefit assessment overall, including the level of expertise required for local ethics review committees to be able to fully evaluate proposals – raise important ethical issues about how the costs of IGM to animals can, and should, be proportionally balanced against the benefits to humans in justifying animal IGM.

6.9   Other tensions in animal genetic modification

Genetic modification causes tensions in the areas of commercialization and the limits of legal remit, each of which will be examined separately.

First, the newly increased efficiencies that transgenic technology offers science[85] have potential to be used to further facilitate animal production, use, and specification as a bespoke manufacturing process, that is driven by age-old commercial and technologic motivations. Previous experience with somatic cell genetic research suggests that commercial pressures are likely to have a prominent influence on the scope and direction of IGM research[86] and may stymie reduction, refinement, and replacement of animals.[87]

The extent to which this potential will be realized will depend to some degree on the structures of national regulatory systems and research approaches. For example, the higher ratio of commercial, public, and government research in the U.K. (60:20:20) compared with Canada (22:65:13) and the U.S.A. (40:30:30), coupled with a move towards using targeted approaches (*in vitro* screening) in drug discovery in the 1970s, were implicated as factors in reducing total animal numbers used in the U.K. compared with Canada and the U.S.A. in the 1980s.[88] Countries that have more stringent animal welfare regulations for publicly-funded research than for privately-funded research (such as the U.S.A.) could have increased potential for animal production to be developed as a pure manufacturing process. The same might also be true wherever the breeding process is not regulated as a scientific procedure, such as in Europe.[89] In this situation, the breeding process becomes a type of farming and the welfare problems associated with the presence of modified genes might not be subject to the same controls as the welfare problems associated with the experimental procedures that were used to initially modify them.[90]

All this is not to say that commercial enterprises necessarily have lower animal welfare standards than public enterprises. Some animal production companies, such as Charles River Laboratories, voluntarily adhere to codes of higher standards than those required by law. Indeed, the expertise and efficiencies inherent to commercial production systems can refine animal use, through the reduction of waste and the contracting out of technologic functions that are not the prime interests of research organizations. But commercialization is not just a manifestation of the simple outsourcing of functions that have been deemed necessary on scientific grounds after full ethics justification. Commercial entities are self-perpetuating and seek to manufacture demand for their own services. Thus there can be obvious tensions between the profit-making motives of companies and the ethical motives of regulatory systems that view animals as having a good of their own and rely on the case-by-case assessment process for justification.

For example, potential burdens to industry and the Inspectorate were the prime considerations behind the Home Secretary's rejection of an APC recommendation that the Home Secretary require study-by-study justification for the use of old world non-human primates in toxicology studies of greater than mild severity. The current policy of issuing large generic project licenses to companies carrying out regulatory toxicology tests was instituted to facilitate the ability of contract research organizations to bid for contracts in a relatively short time-scale. This policy obviates the need for companies to specify which compounds will be tested or to justify the use of primates on a study-by-study basis, other than in generic terms. It could render the cost–benefit assessment for the testing of materials that have been developed in jurisdictions with less rigorous approaches to cost–benefit analyses inadequate, as benefits might be assessed purely in terms of safety, rather than utility.[91] Presumably this could also be a potential concern in the use of primates for testing the safety of human gene therapy and IGM protocols.

The increasing trend to shorten the period prior to Phase I clinical trials places increased pressures on companies to schedule rodent and non-rodent toxicity tests at the same time, thus potentially leading to a waste of non-rodent animals if toxic effects become apparent in rodents. The concern is that the current regulatory system might not result in the use of primates only when fully justified, particularly in the way that species are selected and scheduled for use in regulatory toxicologic purposes.[92] It has been suggested that industry's preference for using non-human primates as the second non-rodent species in pharmaceutical safety testing, in the absence of stipulation in the regulations, is partly driven by industry's fears of litigation and of being required by regulators to repeat studies.[93]

Ethical analyses of commercial genetically-modified (and non-genetically-modified) animal production require a shift from the case-based approaches used in evaluating individual scientific research proposals to population-based approaches, in which potential aggregation effects on cost–benefit estimates, and changing motivation effects on benefit estimates, must be considered. Questions must be asked such as how the cost–benefit evaluation for the provision of a profit-making service differs from that for the provision of a non-profit-making service (e.g., a repository) or from that for a scientific research proposal; and what kinds of inter-institutional reduction and refinement arrangements should be made.

A second major concern is for the fate of hybrid animals produced from the potential application of gene modification to overtly humanize animals or animalize humans, through the creation of human/animal embryo aggregation chimeras using established human embryo stem cell lines.[94] Such derived cell lines might not fall under the remit of human embryo research regulatory authorities (such as the Human Fertilization and Embryology Authority in the U.K.), but might be allowed to be considered for licensing under the terms of legislation regulating the use of animals in scientific procedures.[95]

This concern prompted the APC to recommend to the Home Office that the "production of embryo aggregation chimeras, especially not cross-species chimeras between humans and other animals, nor of hybrids which involve a significant degree of hybridization between animals of very dissimilar kinds"[96] should not be allowed regardless of the potential benefit.[97]

6.10   Conclusions

Animal IGM raises important ethics and welfare issues that need to be addressed. These issues arise because of the ability of IGM to alter animals' natures and to provide new opportunities for humans to realize the motivations behind, and to alter the scale, type, and purposes of, animal experimentation. They relate to ethics; welfare problems; the meanings of welfare, harm and nature; challenges to assessing and balancing cost–benefit; the extent of animal waste; and regulatory challenges that arise from the blurring of legal boundaries between species, primary cells, and derived cell lines.

NOTES

1 John J. Sharp, Larry E. Mobraaten and Hendrick G. Bedigian, Mutant mouse resources. In: Jerrold M. Ward, *et al.* (eds.), *Pathology of Genetically Engineered Mice*. Ames, IA: Iowa State University Press (2000), p. 5.

2 For example, the House of Lords *Select Committee on Animals In Scientific Procedures Report* (2002) states that "our witnesses disagreed over the extent to which GM animals suffered," and that "in the reports by the Royal Society, the Animal Procedures Committee (APC) and others, there is at least a consensus that there is not enough information about the actual levels of suffering, if any, experienced by GM animals," (Chapter 8, paragraph 8.9). See http://www.publications.parliament.uk/pa/ld200102/ ldselect/ldanimal/150/15011.htm (last accessed 4 January 2005). The Royal Society's *Report on the Use of Genetically Modified Animals* states that "although genetic modification is capable of generating welfare problems, in the view of the Royal Society, no qualitative distinction in terms of welfare can be made between genetic modification using modern genetic modification technology and modification produced by artificial selection, chemicals, or radiation. Indeed, the targeted character of modern genetic technology may provide fewer welfare problems than older techniques," Policy Document 5/01 (London, 2001), paragraph 123, p. 24. It should be noted that the Royal Society Report was considered by some to underplay the problems with genetic modification; see the criticisms by Mae-Wan Ho, "The Royal Society's soft sell of GM animals," Institute of Science in Society (ISIS), London, June 2001, http://www.i-sis.org.uk/royal_society.php (last accessed 4 February 2004).

3 In the U.S.A.: (1) the Animal Welfare Act (AWA) (1966 as amended), which does not cover mice, rats, and birds and is enforced by the Animal and Plant Health Inspection Service (APHIS) of the United States Department of Agriculture (USDA) and local Institutional Animal Care and Use Committees (IACUC); (2) the Health Research Extension Act 1985, which mandates compliance with the Public Health Service Policy on Humane Care and Use of Laboratory Animals by any experimenter or institution using any vertebrate animal and is enforced by the Office of Laboratory Animal Welfare (OLAW), which has the power to withhold federal funds; and (3) voluntary accreditation by the Association for Assessment and Accreditation of Laboratory Animal Care (AAALAC) which is a non-governmental organization. In the U.K., the Animals (Scientific Procedures) Act (1986), which covers all non-human vertebrates and the common octopus (*Octopus vulgaris*) and is enforced by the Secretary of State on advice provided by an Inspectorate and an independent APC and European legislation as applies in the U.K. (i.e., Directive 86/609). In Europe: (1) the European Council Directive 86/609/EEC of November 24, 1986 on the approximation of laws, regulations, and administrative provisions of the Member States regarding the protection of animals used for experimental and other scientific purposes, *Official Journal of the European Communities L 358, 18/12/1986 P. 0001–0028*; (2) the Council of Europe, European Convention for the Protection of Vertebrate Animals used for Experimental and Other Scientific Purposes, Strasbourg, 18.III.1986, http://conventions.coe.int/treaty/en/treaties/html/123.htm (last accessed 29 October 2004); (3) national laws that for European Union Member States must meet the requirements of European Council Directive 86/609. In Australia, individual state legislation regulating the use of animals for scientific purposes and common guiding principles are set out in the National Health and Medical Research Council (NHMRC), *Australian*

*Code of Practice for the Care and Use of Animals for Scientific Purposes 7th Edition
2004*, http://www.nhmrc.gov.au/publications/synopses/ea16syn.htm (last accessed 1
April 2005).

4 In Australia, this occurs via state and territory legislation in Victoria, South
Australia, Western Australia, and the Northern Territory.

5 For example, NHMRC, *Australian Code of Practice for the Care and Use of Animals for
Scientific Purposes*.

6 For example in the U.S.A., the Public Health Service (PHS), Policy on Humane Care
and Use of Laboratory Animals, applies to all species and to all research and research
facilities funded by the National Institutes of Health (NIH); non-compliance could
result in the withdrawal of federal funds.

7 For example, in the U.S.A., the Association for the Assessment and Accreditation of
Laboratory Animal Care (AAALAC) is an independent, peer-review accreditation
agency.

8 Ann Fitzpatrick, Ethics and animal research, *Journal of Laboratory Clinical Medicine*
141 (2003), 89–90.

9 Anders Nordgren, Moral imagination in tissue engineering research on animal
models, *Biomaterials* 25 (2004), 1723–34.

10 In the U.K., the U.K. Parliament, House of Lords Session 2001–02, *Animals in
Scientific Procedures Report* by the Select Committee on Animals in Scientific
Procedures, 16 July 2002, Chapter 8, paragraph 8.12 recommends that "a welfare
assessment of all new strains of animals used in experiments (whether produced by
new technologies or by more traditional methods) should be made as a matter of
course," http://www.publications.parliament.uk/pa/ld200102/ldselect/ldanimal/150/
15001.htm (last accessed 18 October 2004). In Canada, the Canadian Council on
Animal Care (CCAC), *Guidelines on Transgenic Animals* (1997) require investigators to provide information about the use of transgenic animals in the "Animal
Use Data Form" and to assign a category of invasiveness level "D" (i.e., moderate to
severe stress) to proposals to create novel transgenics initially. Approvals granted by
animal care committees (ACC) for such proposals "should be provisional, limited to
a 12-month period, and subject to the requirement that the investigator report back
to the ACC as soon as feasible on the animals' phenotype, noting particularly any
evidence of pain or distress," http://www.ccac.ca/en/CCAC_Programs/Guidelines_
Policies/GDLINES/TRANSGEN/TRANSGE1.HTM (last accessed 24 September 2005).
In Australia, the NHRMC *Australian Code of Practice for the Care and Use of Animals
for Scientific Purposes* requires investigators to monitor and report the details of
unexpected side effects of genetic modification of animals to local animal ethics
committees. See Sections 3.3.56–3.3.64, pp. 29–30.

11 For example, the U.K. currently produces the most comprehensive national statistics
on the use of genetically-modified animals in scientific procedures.

12 The reasons have much to do with definitional differences. For example, the definition of an "animal" for the purposes of the U.S. Animal Welfare Act of 1966 (Public
Law 89–544) (CFR Parts 1–9 as amended on 1 June 2004) excludes mice (*Mus*)

and rats (*Rattus*) bred for use in research. See http://www.aphis.usda.gov/ac/rmbde-fine.pdf (last accessed 18 October 2004). Therefore figures for animal use reported to the USDA and the U.S. Congress by APHIS do not include the two species that constitute the majority of animals used in research. Accounting problems due to differences in the definition of the term "use" are explained in U.S. Congress, Office of Technology Assessment (OTA), *Alternatives to Animal Use in Research, Testing, and Education* (Washington, DC: U.S. Government Printing Office, OTA-BA-273, February 1986). Although the Congressional Office of Technology Assessment closed on 29 September 1995, its published analyses are still useful today and are available at http://www.wws.princeton.edu/~ota/ (last accessed 18 October 2004).

13 Clément Gauthier, Overview and analysis of animal use in North America, *Resource* 26 (2002–3), 3–7, http://www.ccac.ca/en/Publications/Facts_Figures/pdfs/DrGauthier Article.pdf (last accessed 24 September 2005); Diane J. Gaertner, Lela K. Riley and Dale G. Martin, Reflections on future needs in research with animals, *ILAR Journal* 39 (1998), http://dels.nas.edu/ilar_n/ilarjournal/39_4/39_4Reflections.shtml (last accessed 24 September 2005); Erik Stokstad, Humane science finds sharper and kinder tools, *Science* 286 (1999), 1068; Organisation for Economic Co-Operation And Development (OECD), *Why Mice Matter: Novel Systems For The Study Of Human Disease From Basic Research To Applications*, Key points from an OECD Workshop held in Rome in December 1996. OECD: Paris (1998), 7, http://www.oecd.org/dataoecd/34/13/2097798.pdf (last accessed 12 November 2004).

14 Home Office, *Statistics of Scientific Procedures on Living Animals Great Britain 2003*, Command paper (Cm) 6291. London: HMSO (7 September 2004), 1–100. See http://www.official-documents.co.uk/document/cm62/6291/6291.htm (last accessed 13 November 2004).

15 Clément Gauthier and Gilly Griffin, *The Use of Animals in Scientific Research and as Sources of Bioengineered Products*, Report prepared for the Canadian Biotechnology Advisory Committee, Project Steering Committee on Intellectual Property and the Patenting of Higher Life Forms, Industry Canada, 2001, http://cbac-cccb.ic.gc.ca/epic/internet/incbac-cccb.nsf/vwapj/AnimalResearch_Gauthier_Griffin_e.pdf/$FILE/AnimalResearch_Gauthier_Griffin_e.pdf (last accessed 30 March 2005).

16 *Charles River Annual Report 2003* (p. 9) and *Charles River Laboratories International, Inc. Annual Report on Form 10-K* (pp. 3, 22), http://ccbn.mobular.net/ccbn/7/588/637/print/print.pdf (last accessed 14 December 2004).

17 IACUC Assessment of Mutant, Transgenic, and Knock-out Mice, Dr M.B. Dennis, American Association for Laboratory Animal Science, 1999 National Meeting, Indianapolis, IN, cited in Canadian Biotechnology Advisory Committee, "Use of Animals in Scientific Research and as Sources of Bioengineered Products," http://cbac-cccb.ca/epic/internet/incbac-cccb.nsf/en/ah00440e.html#5 (last accessed 13 December 2004).

18 OECD, OECD proceedings: Novel systems for the study of human disease: from basic research to applications, *Science and Information Technology* 2 (1998), 13–14.

19 Select Committee on Animals in Scientific Procedures, *Animals In Scientific Procedure – Report*, U.K. Parliament, House of Lords Session 2001–2, 16 July 2002, http://www.publications.parliament.uk/pa/ld200102/ldselect/ldanimal/150/15001.htm (last accessed 18 October 2004), 1.6–1.9.

20 APC, *Report on Biotechnology*, June 2002, 1–54.

21 The Mouse Phenome Project aims "to establish a collection of baseline phenotypic data on commonly used and genetically diverse inbred mouse strains through a coordinated international effort," http://aretha.jax.org/pub-cgi/phenome/mpdcgi?rtn=docs/home (last accessed 18 October 2004).

22 James Meek, The race to buy life – carve up of the human heart: private firms, universities and charities are rushing to isolate and patent human genes before it is even understood what they do, *The Guardian*, 15 November 2000, http://www.guardian.co.uk/genes/article/0,2763,397827,00.html (last accessed 31 March 2005).

23 See *Patenting of Higher Life Forms and Related Issues – Canadian Biotechnology Advisory Committee – Report to the Government of Canada Biotechnology Ministerial Coordinating Committee*, June 2002, http://cbac-cccb.ca/epic/internet/incbac-cccb.nsf/en/ah00188e.html#sec2 (last accessed 31 March 2005).

24 For example, the U.S. Environmental Protection Agency's (EPA) High Production Volume Chemicals Testing Program and the European Union's proposal for a new regulatory system known as REACH (Registration, Evaluation, and Authorisation of Chemicals), see http://www.epa.gov/opptintr/chemtest/view.htm (last accessed 24 October 2004).

25 These percentages were estimated from figures provided in *Animals and Biotechnology – A Report by The Agriculture and Environment Biotechnology Commission (AEBC)*, U.K. Department of Trade and Industry Publication 6228, September 2002, pp. 11–12.

26 Great apes (gorillas, orangutans, and chimpanzees) are not allowed for use under any circumstances under the U.K. Animals (Scientific Procedures) Act 1986, and none have been used since the Act was introduced in 1987. In 2003, no scientific procedures were performed on prosimians, baboons, great apes, gibbons, non-specified new world primates, or non-specified old world primates, or *Octopus vulgaris*, the single cephalopod species protected by the Act (Home Office, *Statistics of Scientific Procedures 2003*, p. 14).

27 APC, *The Use of Primates under the Animals (Scientific Procedures) Act (1986) – Analysis of Current Trends with Particular Reference to Regulatory Toxicology*, December 2002, http://www.apc.gov.uk/reference/primates.pdf (last accessed 9 December 2004), 1–39.

28 Anthony W.S. Chan, Transgenic nonhuman primates for neurodegenerative diseases: review, *Reproductive Biology and Endocrinology* 2(39) (2004), 1–7. http://www.rbej.com/content/2/1/39 (last accessed 17 November 2004).

29 APC, *The Use of Primates under the Animals (Scientific Procedures) Act (1986).*

30 T. Ben Mepham, Robert D. Combes, Michael Balls, *et al.*, The use of transgenic animals in the European Union: the report and recommendations of ECVAM Workshop 28, *Alternatives to Laboratory Animals (ATLA)* 26 (1998), 21–43.

31 APC, *Report on Biotechnology.*
32 Laws to restrict embryo research, for example, the U.S. Congress amendment to the Health and Human Services Appropriations Law 111 Statutory 1467, Sections 513 and 107 P.O. 116; 115 Statutory 2177, Section 510 (10 January 2002). For one analysis of the effects of laws to protect embryos on research see Kathryn L. Miehl, Pre embryos: the tiniest speck of potential life carrying the seeds for sweeping change, *Journal of Technology Law and Policy*, VI (1) (Fall 2003), available at http://www.pitt.edu/~sorc/techjournal/articles/Vol6Miehl.pdf (last accessed 15 October 2004). Laws to ban human cloning: for example, the Human Cloning Prohibition Act of 2003 (H.R. 534 (Weldon)), which bans the process of human cloning for any purpose and the importation of any product derived from an embryo created via cloning, was passed by the U.S. House of Representatives on 27 February 2003; see Judith A. Johnson, *Human Cloning, Report for Congress*, Congressional Research Service, The Library of Congress, updated 10 March 2003, http://usinfo.state.gov/usa/infousa/tech/biotech/rl31358.pdf (last accessed 15 October 2004).
33 Regulations to protect human subjects: for example, the U.S. Code of Federal Regulations, Title 45, Public Welfare, Department of Health and Human Services, National Institutes of Health (NIH), Office for Protection from Research Risks, Part 46, Protection of Human Subjects (revised 23 June 2005; effective 23 June 2005), http://www.hhs.gov/ohrp/humansubjects/guidance/45cfr46.htm (last accessed 24 September 2005).
34 Funding policies to regulate research: for example, U.S. federal government (NIH) funding of recombinant DNA research is contingent on institutional compliance with the *NIH Guidelines* and the *Recombinant DNA Advisory Committee's (RAC) Guidelines* and *"Points to Consider in the Design and Submission of Human Somatic Cell Gene Therapy Protocols,"* which exclude consideration of human IGM. See Compliance with the *NIH Guidelines for Research Involving Recombinant DNA Molecules*, April 2002, http://www4.od.nih.gov/oba/rac/guidelines_02/NIH_Gdlnes_lnk_2002z.pdf (last accessed 15 October 2004), Section I–D.
35 "The RAC continues to explore the issues raised by the potential of *in utero* gene transfer clinical research. However, the RAC concludes that, at present, it is premature to undertake any *in utero* gene transfer clinical trial. Significant additional preclinical and clinical studies addressing vector transduction efficacy, biodistribution, and toxicity are required before a human *in utero* gene transfer protocol can proceed. In addition, a more thorough understanding of the development of human organ systems, such as the immune and nervous systems, is needed to better define the potential efficacy and risks of human *in utero* gene transfer. Prerequisites for considering any specific human *in utero* gene transfer procedure include an understanding of the pathophysiology of the candidate disease and a demonstrable advantage to the *in utero* approach. Once the above criteria are met, the RAC would be willing to consider well rationalized human *in utero* gene transfer clinical trials," NIH, "Appendix M. Points to consider in the design and submission of protocols for the transfer of recombinant DNA molecules into one or more human research

participants (Points to consider)," *NIH Guidelines for Research Involving Recombinant DNA Molecules*, p. 94.

36 Kenneth W. Culver, Gene repair, genomics, and human germ-line modification. In: Audrey R. Chapman and Mark S. Frankel (eds.), *Designing Our Descendents: The Promises and Perils of Genetic Modification*. Baltimore: John Hopkins University Press (2003), 77–92.

37 R. Michael Blaese, Germ line modification in clinical medicine: is there a case for intentional or unintended germ-line changes? In: Audrey R. Chapman and Mark S. Frankel (eds.), *Designing Our Descendents: the Promises and Perils of Genetic Modification*. Baltimore: John Hopkins University Press (2003), 68–76.

38 Christopher H. Evans, Germ-line gene therapy. In: Audrey R. Chapman and Mark S. Frankel (eds.), *Designing Our Descendents: the Promises and Perils of Genetic Modification*. Baltimore: John Hopkins University Press (2003), 93–101.

39 Audrey R. Chapman and Mark S. Frankel, *Human Inheritable Genetic Modifications: Assessing Scientific, Ethical, Religious and Policy Issues*, prepared by the American Association for the Advancement of Science, Washington, DC, September 2000, http://www.aaas.org/spp/sfrl/projects/germline/report.pdf (last accessed 20 October 2004), p. 7–8.

40 Chapman and Frankel, *Human Inheritable Genetic Modifications*, p. 10.

41 Evans, Germ-line gene therapy.

42 Mark S. Frankel, Inheritable genetic modification and a brave new world: did Huxley have it wrong? *Hastings Centre Report* 33 (2003), 31–6.

43 John Fletcher, The moral impasse in human embryo research: bypasses in the making? In: Audrey R. Chapman and Mark S. Frankel (eds.), *Designing Our Descendents: The Promises and Perils of Genetic Modification*. Baltimore: John Hopkins University Press (2003), 105–29.

44 APC, *The Use of Primates under the Animals (Scientific Procedures) Act (1986)*.

45 For example the U.K. Home Office disagreed with the APC's request for its ethical review procedures to be particularly sensitive to the welfare costs to animals of genetic modification research, on the basis that the review system should be applied with the same rigor to all animal procedures. See APC, Letter from Bob Ainsworth to Michael Banner of 4 February 2003 about the APC's recommendations on biotechnology, in the *Report of the Animal Procedures Committee for 2003*, The Stationery Office, HC 1017, London, 7 September 2004, http://www.apc.gov.uk/reference/APC_03.pdf (last accessed 7 December 2004), Annex E, p. 29.

46 Mepham, Combes, Balls, *et al.*, The use of transgenic animals in the European Union.

47 Vicky Robinson, David B. Morton, David Anderson, *et al.*, Refinement and reduction in production of genetically-modified mice, *Laboratory Animals* 37 (Supplement 1) (2003), 1–51. This is the report of the British Veterinary Association Animal Welfare Foundation (BVAAWF), Fund for the Replacement of Animals in Medical Experiments (FRAME), Royal Society for the Prevention of Cruelty to Animals (RSPCA), and the Universities Federation for Animal Welfare (UFAW) Joint Working Group on Refinement.

48 Rikke Thon, Jesper Lassen, Axel Kornerup Hansen, *et al.*, Welfare evaluation of genetically modifed mice: an inventory study of reports to the Danish Animal Experiments Inspectorate, *Scandinavian Journal for Laboratory Animal Science* 29 (2002), 45–53.

49 For example, the Induced Mutant Resource at http://www.jax.org/imr/notes.html (last accessed 24 October 2004).

50 Thon, Lassen, Kornerup Hansen, *et al.*, Welfare evaluation of genetically modifed mice.

51 Miriam Van der Meer, Patrizia Costa, Vera Baumans, *et al.*, Welfare assessment of transgenic animals: behavioural responses and morphological development of newborn mice, *Alternatives to Laboratory Animals (ATLA)* 27 (1999), 857–68.

52 Patrizia Costa, Production of transgenic animals: practical problems and welfare aspects. In: L.F.M. van Zutphen and Miriam Van der Meer (eds.), *Welfare Aspects of Transgenic Animals, Proceedings of EC Workshop, 30 Oct 1995, Utrecht, Netherlands.* Berlin: Springer Verlag (1997), 68–77; Patrizia Costa, Neuro-behavioural tests in welfare assessment in transgenic animals. In: *Proceedings of the 6th FELASA Symposium on International Harmonisation of Laboratory Animal Husbandry Requirements at Basel, 19–21 June 1996.* London: Royal Society of Medicine Press (1997), 51–3.

53 See Rudolf Jaenisch, Nuclear cloning, embryonic stem cells and gene transfer (Chapter 3, this volume).

54 Richard Mollard, Mark Denham and Alan Trounson, Technical advances and pitfalls on the way to human cloning, *Differentiation* 70 (2002), 1–9.

55 CCAC, *Guidelines on Transgenic Animals*, http://www.ccac.ca/en/CCAC_Programs/Guidelines_Policies/GDLINES/TRANSGEN/TRANSGE1.HTM (last accessed 4 January 2005), Section 1, b, iv.

56 Thon, Lassen, Kornerup Hansen, *et al.*, Welfare evaluation of genetically modifed mice.

57 Mepham, Combes, Balls, *et al.*, The use of transgenic animals in the European Union, p. 35.

58 APC, *Report on Biotechnology*, paragraph 48, p. 17.

59 See Jason S. Robert and Françoise Baylis, Crossing species boundaries, *The American Journal of Bioethics* 3 (2003), 1–13.

60 Albert W. Musschenga, Naturalness: beyond animal welfare, *Journal of Agricultural and Environmental Ethics* 15 (2002), 171–86.

61 Suzanne T. Millman, Ian J.H. Duncan, Markus Stauffacher, *et al.*, The impact of applied ethologists and the International Society for Applied Ethology in improving animal welfare, *Applied Animal Behaviour Science* 86 (2004), 299–311.

62 Hein Te Velde, Noelle Aarts and Cees Van Woerkum, Dealing with ambivalence: farmers' and consumers' perceptions of animal welfare in livestock breeding, *Journal of Agricultural and Environmental Ethics* 15 (2002), 203–19.

63 Eric Marlier, INRA Europe, *Biotechnology and Genetic Engineering. What Europeans Think about it in 1993, Eurobarometer,* 1993, http://europa.eu.int/comm/public_opinion/archives/ebs/ebs_080_en.pdf (last accessed 4 January 2005), 39.1; Anonymous, Europe ambivalent on biotechnology, *Nature* 387 (1997), 845–7.

64 I. Anna S. Olsson, Charlotte M. Nevison, Emily G. Patterson-Kane, *et al.*, Understanding behaviour: the relevance of ethological approaches in laboratory animal science, *Applied Animal Behaviour Science* 81 (2003), 245–64.

65 The Humane Society of the United States, E. Statistics on Pain and Distress, http://www.hsus.org/ace/11397 (last accessed 25 October 2004).

66 Andrew Rowan, *Letter to Top 50 Research Institutions*, The Humane Society of the United States, January 24 2002, http://www.hsus.org/ace/13884 (last accessed 28 October 2004).

67 Harry Olson, Graham Betton, Denise Robinson, *et al.*, Concordance of the toxicity of pharmaceuticals in humans and in animals, *Regulatory Toxicology and Pharmacology* 32 (2000), 56–67.

68 Pandora Pound, Shah Ebrahim, Peter Sandercock, *et al.*, Where is the evidence that animal research benefits humans? *BMJ* 328 (2004), 514–17.

69 Olsson, Nevison, Patterson-Kane, *et al.*, Understanding behaviour.

70 APC, *Review of Cost–Benefit Assessment in the Use of Animals in Research* (June 2003), 1–104.

71 Richard P. Haynes, Do regulators of animal welfare need to develop a theory of psychological well-being? *Journal of Agricultural and Environmental Ethics* 14 (2001), 231–40.

72 Albert W. Musschenga, Naturalness: beyond animal welfare, *Journal of Agricultural and Environmental Ethics* 15 (2002), 171–186, p. 180.

73 My use of the term "animal flourishing" is the same as in Musschenga, "Naturalness: beyond animal welfare," p. 173.

74 Peter Singer writes: "So the limit of sentience (using the term as a convenient if not strictly accurate short hand for the capacity to suffer and/or experience enjoyment) is the only defensible boundary of concern for the interests of others," in "All animals are equal," in *Writings on an Ethical Life*. London: Fourth Estate (2001), p. 35.

75 Musschenga, Naturalness: Beyond animal welfare, p. 179.

76 APC, *Review of Cost–Benefit Assessment*.

77 Swedish Ministry of Health and Social Affairs, *From One Species to Transplantation from Animals to Humans, Summary And Statutory Proposal, A Report by the Swedish Committee on Xenotransplantation*, Swedish Government Official Report No. 1999: 120, Stockholm, 1999, http://www.oecd.org/dataoecd/28/36/2397231.doc (last accessed 12 November 2004), p. 9.

78 APC, Letter from Bob Ainsworth to Michael Banner of 4 February 2003 about the APC's recommendations on biotechnology.

79 APC, *Report on Biotechnology*, recommendation 4, paragraph 51, p. 18.

80 APC, *Report of the Animal Procedures Committee for 2003*, paragraph 23, p. 6.

81 Jackie Leach Scully, Inheritable genetic modification and disability: normality and identity (Chapter 10, this volume).

82 Christoph Rehmann-Sutter, Controlling bodies and creating monsters: popular perceptions of genetic modifications (Chapter 4, this volume).

83 National Bioethics Advisory Commission (NBAC), *Ethical and Policy Issues in Research Involving Human Participants*, Bethesda, MD, August 2001,

http://www.georgetown.edu/research/nrcbl/nbac/human/oversumm.pdf (last accessed 4 November 2004), 1–19.

84 "To ensure the protection of the rights and welfare of all research participants, federal legislation should be enacted to create a single, independent federal office, the National Office for Human Research Oversight (NOHRO), to lead and coordinate the oversight system," NBAC, *Ethical and Policy Issues*, recommendation 2.2, p. 9.; see also the Farm Animal Welfare Council (FAWC), *Report on the Implications of Cloning for the Welfare of Livestock*, London, 1998, http://www.fawc.org.uk/reports/clone/clonetoc.htm (last accessed 5 January 2005), paragraphs 49–51.

85 Kenneth Paigen and Janan Eppig use the example of a human hypertension study that cost one hundred times more money and took five times the amount of time to find similar chromosomal locations of disease susceptibility genes as an equivalent study in mice to illustrate these new efficiencies; see A mouse phenome project (review), *Mammalian Genome* 11 (2000), 715–17.

86 Chapman and Frankel, *Human Inheritable Genetic Modifications.*

87 APC, *The Use of Primates under the Animals (Scientific Procedures) Act (1986).*

88 Gauthier, Overview and analysis of animal use, p. 3.

89 The Council of Europe (1992) does not necessarily regulate breeding as a scientific procedure and so the regulation of breeding depends on various national regulations, see Inger Jegstrup, Rikke Thon, Axel Kornerup Hansen, *et al.*, Characterization of transgenic mice – a comparison of protocols for welfare evaluation and phenotype characterization of mice with a suggestion on a future certificate of instruction, *Laboratory Animals* 37 (2003), 1–9.

90 Jegstrup, Thon, Kornerup Hansen, *et al.*, *Characterization of Transgenic Mice.*

91 APC, *The Use of Primates under the Animals (Scientific Procedures) Act (1986).*

92 Regulatory authorities (especially in U.S.A., Japan, and the European Union) normally require testing of pharmacologic compounds on two species – a rodent and a non-rodent species. The non-rodent species is usually a beagle dog or non-human primate (though sometimes mini-pigs, ferrets or, for veterinary products, the target species are used). See APC, *The Use of Primates under the Animals (Scientific Procedures) Act (1986)*, p. 18.

93 APC, *The Use of Primates under the Animals (Scientific Procedures) Act (1986).*

94 APC, *Report on Biotechnology*, paragraph 52, p. 18.

95 APC, *Report of the Animal Procedures Committee for 2003*, paragraph 23, p. 6.

96 APC, *Report on Biotechnology*, recommendation 5, paragraph 57, p. 20.

97 APC, *Report of the Animal Procedures Committee for 2003*, paragraphs 22–3, pp. 5–6.

Radical rupture: exploring biological sequelae of volitional inheritable genetic modification

Françoise Baylis and Jason Scott Robert

7.1   Introduction

In the late 1960s and early 1970s, there was considerable debate about the ethics of research involving the genetic modification of humans by inserting, repairing, or deleting genes. Opponents of gene transfer research argued that genetic interventions were dangerously different from other therapeutic interventions, while the proponents of such research insisted that somatic cell gene transfer (SCGT) was simply a logical extension of available techniques for treating disease. Those advocating gene transfer research argued, convincingly, that products of genetically modified somatic cells are similar to medications currently available (e.g., enzyme therapies for adenosine deaminase [ADA] deficiency) and that the techniques involved are similar to other widely used medical interventions (e.g., transplantation of tissues).[1] At the time, much ado was made about the fact that the proposed genetic modifications would affect only non-reproductive cells. Out of this debate emerged a moral demarcation line between SCGT and germ-line gene transfer (GLGT); under certain constraints and with appropriate oversight, it would be ethically acceptable to proceed with SCGT research, provided the proposed interventions would not affect the germ cells. The science moved forward on these terms; the ethical debate was, for some time, relatively quiescent.

In the late 1980s and early 1990s, however, with the move to clinical trials involving SCGT, debate about the ethics of gene transfer experiments resurfaced. Many began to question the entrenchment of the moral demarcation line between SCGT and inheritable genetic modification (IGM) and, in particular, to emphasize the potential benefits of research on IGM, especially GLGT.[2] Since then, with the "pre-proposal" for *in utero* gene transfer submitted to the U.S. NIH Recombinant DNA Advisory Committee (RAC),[3] and with the increasing awareness of the risks associated with the possibility of inadvertent IGM,[4] the ethical debate has intensified.

At this time, the ethics of IGM (whether intentional or inadvertent) remains contentious as people continue to debate both the potential benefits and harms of heritably modifying individual genomes. Arguments in favor of IGM and particularly GLGT are familiar and have been ably summarized by LeRoy Walters and Julie Palmer.[5] In very general terms, the arguments in support of intentional IGM aim to defend interventions directly intended to affect the germ line (either through the modification of early stage embryos or through the modification of parental germ cells) and also to diminish concern about unintended germ-line effects resulting from SCGT. To this end, it is argued that GLGT could potentially be an effective and efficient treatment for diseases that affect many different organs and their cell types (such as cystic fibrosis); it could also be an alternative to SCGT techniques for diseases expressed in non-removable or non-dividing cells (such as Lesch–Nyhan syndrome). Moreover, any genetic disease that damages, or is lethal to, the very early embryo could actually be prevented through IGM, an option impossible through somatic interventions (genetic or otherwise). Finally, arguments are elaborated in defense of the moral obligation to reduce the incidence of disease in subsequent generations using IGM, instead of continuing to treat successive generations with SCGT.

Arguments against GLGT/IGM experiments involving humans are also familiar, and well catalogued by David Resnik.[6] These arguments capture a range of concerns about physical and social harms, developed from both secular and spiritual perspectives. For example, some argue that there are significant safety concerns because of the known and as yet unknown short- and long-term harms to research participants and their progeny. As well, there are potential problems associated with the fact that, in principle, the offspring (potential beneficiaries of the research) are unable to provide informed consent; for some, this is a significant issue given the possible impact of such research on life opportunities. Added to this are potential problems of distributive and social justice given the likely high cost of any eventual therapy developed from the research. At issue is the moral acceptability of allocating health resources to expensive interventions with extremely limited applicability.

In addition to the above, there are worries about the ethics of tampering with our genetic inheritance, thereby possibly violating what some claim as the "right" of subsequent generations to inherit an "un-manipulated genome," and in so doing, according to some, "playing God." Finally, there are claims that IGM research may lead us down a slippery slope to genetic enhancement: while the initial goal may be the prevention or treatment of genetic disease, inevitably there will be efforts to alter humans for other, non-therapeutic purposes. One can easily imagine efforts to manipulate the genome to improve cognition, height, athletic ability, visual acuity, or skin color, in an effort to secure some kind of political, financial, social, or other advantage, thereby potentially introducing or exacerbating problems of social and economic inequality, prejudice, and discrimination.

In this chapter we are not concerned with the merits or limitations of these (and other similar) arguments for or against human IGM summarized above (and discussed elsewhere in this book). Our aim, instead, is to provide a new heuristic device for examining the prospect of volitional IGM (whether for therapeutic or enhancement purposes), grounded in the notion of rupture.

The first step in this project is to cleanse the term "rupture" of its negative connotations. "Rupture" (neutrally) denotes a "break," and breaks can either be positive, negative, or neutral. Our use of the term "rupture" may seem counterintuitive to some, however, inasmuch as ruptures are very often understood in negative terms: consider a ruptured appendix or spleen. Let us underscore that there is no necessary connection between "rupture" and its negative connotations. A rupture, understood narrowly as a break, might either be good or bad, desirable or undesirable, or simply neutral (neither good nor bad, neither desirable nor undesirable).

The idea behind the notion of rupture in discussions about genetics is not, in itself, original. Many of the anticipated consequences of various genetic interventions could easily be described as engendering rupture. Consider, for example, individuals who live in families with a long (sometimes traumatic) history of genetic disease. In recent years, with the advent of pre-symptomatic testing for susceptibility genes, some individuals have learned that they are at decreased risk for manifesting the familial illness, as compared with their relatives. One would reasonably expect that these individuals would be elated with this news. Recent data about predictive testing for Huntington disease, for instance, confirm this expectation; many individuals welcome this rupture with their past. But the data also confirm that some persons who receive "good news" about a reduced risk of Huntington disease experience a loss, as the personal risk was very much a part of their self-identity and as the shared risk was a significant element of the family narrative.[7] In being removed from the at-risk pool, what was once believed about one's self-identity is no longer secure, and what was once believed to be one's shared fate is no longer held in common. Rupture is thus manifest with predictive testing (at least in the case of Huntington disease) at the level of personal identity and familial relations, and can be construed either as positive (as when one is happy to be free of the family burden) or negative (as when one experiences a loss of membership and feels guilty about no longer sharing the familial narrative). As regards the issue of fate more generally, Anne Michaels asks provocatively in her novel *Fugitive Pieces*, "If you escape your fate, whose life do you then step into?"[8]

A further example of rupture, now in the realm of enhancement, might involve a family with distinct characteristics such as the red hair and black eyes of the MacDonald clan in Alisdair MacLeod's *No Great Mischief*.[9] In the novel, members of the clan are identified far and wide as MacDonalds specifically because of these distinguishing characteristics, and a particular history immediately attaches to each individual as a function of being so identified. Future generations of MacDonalds might, however, consider these distinguishing features, or the attention they draw, undesirable, and seek to modify them in subsequent offspring through IGM. The "beneficiaries" of these interventions, though genetically of MacDonald stock, are no longer so marked, and may experience this in positive, negative, or neutral terms. On the one hand, those offspring desiring relative anonymity in their life pursuits might welcome this rupture – not standing out in a crowd as red-haired and black-eyed, and, further, not standing out specifically as a MacDonald. On the other hand, other MacDonalds, proud of their long lineage back to Scotland, might reasonably experience this rupture with the "genetic narrative"[10] of the red-haired, black-eyed clan as negative. Then again, the rupture might not matter to the genetically-altered MacDonald offspring.

These kinds of ruptures resulting from genetic interventions, whether experienced in positive, negative, or neutral terms, are very interesting. They are not, however, the focus of our interest in the concept. Our interest in rupture is on a grander scale, as we imagine the widespread common use of intentional IGM. The presumption that IGM, *if* proven safe and effective, will be widely used, is neither arbitrary nor groundless.[11] Accordingly, this presumption underwrites our argument that volitional IGM should be characterized in terms of "radical rupture." In what follows, we introduce the notion of "radical rupture" and explore its usefulness in identifying and potentially elucidating a range of ethical concerns in several realms of biology.

7.2   Radical rupture: a definition and some caveats

From an evolutionary perspective, IGM that "corrects" mutations would typically be no more significant than currently available genetic interventions aimed at identifying and destroying "defective" embryos or aborting diseased fetuses. Similarly, and again from an evolutionary perspective, IGM that "enhances" certain features or abilities by inserting desirable genes would typically be no more significant than other eugenic measures directed at improvement.[12] Having said this, however, it is our contention that the *widespread use* of IGM could be more significant, in evolutionary terms, than previously imagined.

Intentional IGM as a common practice is not simply one more facet of gradual, if somewhat erratic, evolutionary change as has happened throughout the ages with the mixing of genetic material through reproduction and environmentally-mediated adaptation (or decay). It is, instead, very much about breaking with a familiar past and a delimited future to embrace both an indeterminate past and an uncertain and inherently unpredictable future where cultural norms, political interests, and market considerations will contribute in *new* ways to the human evolutionary story. These factors will not only continue to subtly shape mate preferences, personal decisions about establishing, continuing, or terminating pregnancies, and policies regarding same, but for the first time they will also play a substantial role in informing explicit decisions, practices, and policies about genetic options not previously in the realm of the possible. As such, the widespread use of IGM brings with it notable uncertainty, not only because of the vagaries of individual free choices about how best to improve individual genomes, but also because cultural, political, and economic forces will direct individual choices about new modes of human being and new ways of being human. For the first time, there will be the option of creating beings outside the range of what might otherwise be possible by stirring the gene pool, or within that range but at an unheralded pace, and with the prospect of considerably more precision than would otherwise be possible.

"From a secular point of view," H. Tristram Engelhardt Jr. argues, "the human biological nature that we possess, the genome that is ours, is the result of nearly 4 billion years of mutation, selective pressure, genetic drift, and haphazard natural events set within the constraints of physics, chemistry, and biology. The result is a constellation of biological characteristics that defines our human biological nature and could have been otherwise."[13] Significantly with widespread use of IGM, many of these facets of human evolution are sidestepped as individual or collective choices are made (in complex ways) about which diseases to eliminate, which abilities to enhance and, more radically still, which beings to create. This represents a phenomenal break (a radical rupture) with evolutionary processes as we currently understand them, in introducing contingency of a new order and in accelerating the pace and significantly altering the course of evolutionary change within humans.[14]

Let us be clear: we use the term "rupture" to mean "breach" or "break," of the sort through which, for instance, evolutionary changes (migration, mutation, speciation, extinction) have always, but contingently, occurred. As stated previously, no pejorative meaning attaches to this notion; that is, we use it merely descriptively as a useful heuristic to denote a dramatic break. In the specific case of widespread use of IGM, we qualify "rupture" with the adjective "radical" to refer (again, merely descriptively) to the possibility and sequelae of creating unprecedented beings, at an unheralded pace, with potentially tremendous precision, constrained almost exclusively by human volition.

The latter point is particularly important as it makes for a categorical change in the character of evolutionary contingency: from contingency primarily constrained by physics, chemistry, and biology to contingency now largely constrained by psychology and sociology. This is not to say that physics, chemistry, and biology would become explanatorily irrelevant if use of IGM were to become widespread, nor is it to say that psychology and sociology have not previously had explanatory force (culture has always helped shape biology). It is rather to suggest that whereas past evolutionary changes eventually leading to humans are largely explicable without reference to volition, future evolutionary changes in humans, presuming widespread IGM is adopted, are likely to be largely inexplicable without consideration of intentions and of how intentions are psychologically or sociologically shaped. And yet, as we suggest below, the very projects of explaining our past, our present, and our future, as selves and as members of *Homo sapiens*, may be intimately affected by this new order of contingency.

Finally, two caveats to avoid misunderstanding. First, the prospect of radical rupture to be addressed below is to be carefully distinguished from superficially similar accounts of genetic engineering that, unlike ours, rest on naïve views about genetic determinism. Genes are not causally foundational or primary in development; genomes do not contain blueprints for organisms.[15] Accordingly, the radical rupture we envision is not to be construed as resultant from tinkering with human genetic essence (a notion devoid of meaning, as we argue elsewhere).[16] Instead, radical rupture results from the intensification of volition where accident once reigned.

Second, this is not to deny that human volition of one sort or another has always shaped human evolution; it is, rather, to suggest that the adoption of IGM makes for a difference not only in degree but also in kind.[17] We anticipate that IGM, presuming its safety and efficacy, will be widely used.[18] Accordingly, we characterize volitional IGM in terms of radical rupture because of its inherent causal relationship with the complex of contingencies through the medium of human will, operating on a grand scale, with unprecedented precision (as compared, for instance, with matchmaking).

7.3   Rupturing inheritance?

Future widespread use of IGM portends the ability of humans to transform acquired characteristics into inheritable traits (as illustrated in an example below). This makes for radical rupture with the dominant view of heredity. In the final three decades of the nineteenth century, the German biologist August Weismann (1834–1914) introduced the distinction between germ plasm and soma; Brian Hall refers to this as one of the truly revolutionary ideas in the history of biology.[19] Weismann's position counted against the reigning view that acquired characteristics could be inherited because, while the germ plasm is continuous, the soma is mortal. In organisms in which there is an early separation of germ from soma, somatic modifications cannot heritably affect the germ plasm; consequently, following Weismann, since only the germ plasm is inherited, acquired traits cannot be transmitted across generations.[20] A widespread sense persists that the distinction between the continuity of the germline and the mortality of the soma is what undergirds a strong distinction between nature and nurture: though nurture (soma, environment) is required to realize nature (genes), nature is primary and necessarily so, given that nature is inherited and nurture is not.[21]

We imagine that volitional IGM has the potential to rupture the distinction between germ-line continuity and somatic mortality as the inheritance of acquired characteristics becomes a real possibility. A typical example of such inheritance might involve an athlete training hard to become a good sprinter; having succeeded, she does not thereby also succeed in conceiving children who are themselves fleet of foot. Fair enough. She might nonetheless encourage her children to be active, take them running with her, and foster in them the same drive to succeed athletically; after all, they inherit from her not only her genes but the environment in which they are reared. Yet we should not like to refer to this situation as one in which the acquired characteristics are themselves "inherited." This becomes newly possible, however, with IGM.

Acquired characteristics of the parent(s) that are desired characteristics have an increased probability of appearing genetically in future generations as a discrete function of volitional IGM. The athletic woman who wants an athletic child need not only rely on environmental enhancements to achieve her goal, but may also choose to alter her child's genetic constitution. We are, to be sure, not thinking here of a "gene for" sprinting ability; we are thinking, instead, of the developmental genetic resources involved in muscle determination, lung capacity, and blood-oxygen content, for example, which, properly "adjusted," might increase one's ability to succeed athletically. Similarly, the talented violinist who desires a musical child prodigy might elect to genetically (as well as environmentally) improve her offspring's dexterity, hearing ("having an ear"), and memory.[22]

The likelihood of some future scenario unfolding as described above should not be underestimated. There is a long and rich history of parents, throughout the ages, working hard to bestow on their children a range of benefits. With IGM, it is a foregone conclusion that valued acquired characteristics would become part of children's genetic inheritance as a result of technically executed visions of future children. Radical rupture, in this case, involves the exercise of unprecedented, willful, precise control over transgenerational continuity.

7.4   Rupturing history and anthropology?

Our second instance of radical rupture involves challenges to genetics and genomics as tools for historical and anthropological research. These challenges are contingent upon the widespread use of IGM and involve either the artificial acceleration of human evolution or the volitional introduction of evolutionary novelties.

In recent years, DNA testing has revealed some interesting facts at the level of peoples and at the level of persons as regards historical population migrations, ancestry and heritage of various ethnic groups, and kinship relations. For example, an analysis of the Y-chromosomes of present day Cohanim and Levites has been used to confirm the origins of Old Testament priests.[23] Y-chromosome research has also been used to support claims about the likely Jewish ancestry of the Lemba, a Bantu-speaking people in southern Africa.[24] As well, though somewhat more controversially, mitochondrial and other DNA testing has uncovered evidence suggesting that all humans' mitochondria are descended from one African woman, while our other genes likely trace to chromosomes of different ancient individuals.[25] Moving from the study of populations to the study of families, an analysis of the Y-chromosomes of Thomas Jefferson's male descendants has shown that the former U.S. President was the biologic father of Eston Hemings Jefferson, the last child of his slave mistress, Sally Hemings.[26]

These and similar findings have been reported in the media, contributing to the general public's awareness of the fact that their blood (i.e., their DNA) is an important source of historical and anthropological information. This is perhaps most evident now in the U.S.A. among African-Americans because of recent efforts by Dr Rick Kittles to trace African ancestry using mitochondrial and Y-chromosome DNA testing.[27] Mitochondrial DNA (mtDNA) is found in the cytoplasm of all body cells and eggs; mothers transmit mtDNA to their children more or less unchanged and their daughters transmit mtDNA to further generations. The Y-chromosome determines whether a child is male; fathers pass this chromosome directly to their sons. The mtDNA and Y-chromosomes escape most of the shuffling of genetic material that occurs between generations except for rare mutations in the DNA that accumulate slowly over time. For this reason, mtDNA and the Y-chromosome can be used to trace female and male lineages.[28]

From the perspective of those conducting genealogical research using DNA, any genetic intervention that results in a heritable modification to mtDNA or to the Y-chromosome is a significant potential threat to their research. A future in which individuals are able to tamper with their genetic lineage and thereby obscure the lines of individual descent is not a welcome prospect for DNA genealogists. This concern rests not on science fiction or idle musing, at least not with regard to mtDNA. In 1995 a group of researchers proposed a germ-line intervention they called *in vitro* ovum nuclear transplantation as an effective way to avoid the vertical transmission of mitochondrial disease.[29] The researchers outlined a project to assist women with serious mitochondrial disease to have genetically-related children. The protocol involved removing the nucleus from their ovum, discarding the cytoplasm with the diseased-linked mtDNA, and then fusing this nucleus with an enucleated donor egg with healthy mtDNA. The "combined" oocyte would then be fertilized and transferred to the uterus. Indeed, in 2001, researchers at the Institute for Reproductive Medicine and Science of St Barnabas, New Jersey, reported that they had produced nearly 30 babies worldwide using a variation on this technique for fertility treatment, which they labeled "ooplasmic transfer."[30] The researchers did not completely remove and replace egg cytoplasm, but rather modified the eggs of women with difficulties in establishing pregnancies by injecting small amounts of cytoplasm from other women's eggs to correct presumed deficiencies in the ooplasm. The resulting children had mitochondria from two women.

The major putative benefit of *in vitro* ovum nuclear transfer (and ooplasmic transfer) is that these techniques would safely perpetuate the woman's germ-line.[31] At present, women who want healthy children, but have either defects in the ooplasm of their eggs or have serious mitochondrial disease, must choose between adoption, embryo donation, or egg donation. These options allow infertile women with defects in the ooplasm of their eggs to sidestep their infertility and allow women with mitochondrial disease to avoid the vertical transmission of disease. In these instances, however, the children adopted or born following embryo or egg donation are not genetically related to the women who will be their social parent. In contrast, with either ooplasm transfer or *in vitro* nuclear transfer, the woman would be able to pass on her genes (i.e., her nuclear DNA) to her children. In doing so, however, the woman would have orchestrated a significant rupture in the genetic lineage of her descendants, despite continuity in nuclear DNA. Ooplasm transfer and *in vitro* ovum nuclear transfer affect inheritance because the mtDNA in the cytoplasm is passed from one generation to the next. It follows that any effort by subsequent generations to trace their ancestry through mtDNA would provide a false or confusing picture of where they come from. As such, this kind of IGM potentially represents a radical rupture in genealogic research. In the abstract, the potential for rupture could be minimized by choosing healthy female relatives as cytoplasm donors, but preserving the ability of DNA genealogists to do their research is unlikely to be a motivating priority in the choice of cytoplasm donor to correct infertility or mitochondrial disease.

As well, volitional IGM will radically transform historical and anthropological research on human population migration patterns and demographic history. As alluded to above, such research can presently be conducted through analysis of Y-chromosome polymorphisms[32] and mtDNA analysis,[33] and also through studies of human–viral co-evolution, such as with the human polyomavirus JC.[34] Such research is premised on the genetic continuity of humans from a single ancestral group, and facilitated by the remarkable conservation of gene sequences through evolutionary history. Accordingly, these studies can offer evidence not only of the geographical origins of humans, but also of likely population sizes, migration patterns and, in conjunction with other evidence, the timing of major migrations.[35]

It is only in the past decade or so that humans have achieved this knowledge; concurrently, we have achieved the ability to render it potentially useless in the future reconstruction of current human evolution. Volitional IGM has the potential to radically rupture the genetic legacy of humans, replacing its historical contingency on natural chance and physical law with willful contingency on unprecedented human procreative autonomy. Of course, humans have always exercised some degree of reproductive freedom, but within the bounds of the natural processes that scientists are only now finally uncovering. As these parameters are pushed or even ruptured through volitional IGM, genetic gaps of a likely stochastic nature may open, thereby potentially affecting genetically-based human evolutionary inquiry.

This latter instance of radical rupture involves not only the closing off of opportunities for evolutionary research (which might, we should note, be corrected for by the use of alternative genetic markers), but also the introduction of a rupture in the way that our descendants will construct their past, that is, the stories they will tell about who they are, where they come from, and where they are going.

7.5   Rupturing species?

Our final example of radical rupture involves the volitional creation of genuinely new "human beings." Imagine the volitional creation and rapid evolution of groups of pollution resistant "human beings" with genes for degrading polychlorinated biphenyls (PCBs);[36] poison-resistant "human beings" with genes coding for enzymes that help to break down poisons;[37] or "human beings" equipped with feathery gills to survive both on land and under the sea.[38] Here, we place "human beings" in scare quotes because these instances of radical rupture could well involve the willful generation of a new hominid species.

To begin, let us consider the insertion of non-human genes into the human germ-line to rectify actual deficiencies or to enhance perceived deficiencies. An example of the former would be the insertion into humans of genes responsible for synthesizing vitamin C from just about any other non-primate species (as discussed below); such an insertion, if it worked, would likely improve health prospects for those who do not consume enough vitamin C (such as those in the developing world suffering from scurvy), but might also prevent life-threatening complications in premature infants. An example of genetic enhancement through IGM would be expansion of the range of human color vision with the addition of rhodopsin synthesis capacities imported from animals capable of near ultraviolet or near infrared perception.[39] Such activities involve breaching species boundaries at the level of the germ-line, clearly instantiating our notion of radical rupture in intentionally generating (or accelerating the evolution of) naturally unlikely beings.

Though there are good reasons to be skeptical of the very idea of species boundaries,[40] we have in mind a very simple notion. Each individual human contains a genome, a specifically human genome. To be sure, it may not be a particularly representative human genome, and, moreover, thanks to evolution from a common ancestor, it will contain some DNA identical to that found in a wide range of other creatures. Nonetheless, it is a human genome. Next, consider some non-human animal or even a plant – your pet, a fern, a frog, or a lily pad. This living thing, too, contains a genome, which is a non-human genome. Again, it may not be representative, and it may not contain much, if any, unique DNA. Next, consider the application of standard genetic manipulation techniques to isolate a particular functional stretch of DNA from the non-human genome. Imagine that this particular sequence (i.e., gene) does not appear in the human genome and that some believe humans could benefit from having this gene; further imagine that there is the ability, and the will, to use standard gene transfer techniques to insert (across "species boundaries," as it were) the gene from the non-human genome into the human genome via the germ-line. Some of the human offspring born following this genetic manipulation would thereafter have genomes in which the gene from a non-human genome appears (and which was not present in the original human genome). They would be interspecific transgenic humans irrespective of whether the gene from the non-human genome is actually expressed.[41]

In order to strip this scenario of its philosophical abstractness, we can flesh it out in a variety of ways, some considerably more speculative than others. First, recall our example above of vitamin C synthesis. Many non-human creatures contain a gene or genes that enable those creatures to synthesize their own vitamin C. As vitamin C is crucial during embryonic development,[42] it may one day be desirable to insert non-human genetic resources involved in vitamin C synthesis into humans. As a second example, consider the following: imagine that a renowned international scientist returns from one of her research trips with a rare creature believed to contain a suite of genes that render it immune from measles, mumps, rubella, and other afflictions against which children are currently vaccinated. Gene therapy seems obviously desirable to a host of people, and so scientists sequence the relevant genes from this non-human creature. Having developed the appropriate vector, they then deliver the non-human genes into the germ-line of a human population.

Granting that the second example may well strain the reader's credulity, it nonetheless behooves us to seriously ask: how farfetched are these ideas about creating interspecific humans? At present, interspecific transgenic primates are in production. In 2001, the first one, a rhesus monkey dubbed "ANDi" (short for "inserted DNA" in a reverse transcribed direction), was engineered at the Oregon Regional Primate Research Center.[43] ANDi was engineered with a gene for green fluorescence (green fluorescent protein, GFP) originally isolated from jellyfish. The gene was inserted into mature rhesus oocytes via a retroviral vector, and so ANDi is clearly an interspecific transgenic product of IGM. ANDi does not, as it happens, glow green, but all tissues analyzed contain the transgene.

While this research success, and similar initiatives that eventually move beyond what might be described as "proof of principle" projects, will not immediately lead to the creation of interspecific transgenic humans, it would be naïve to think that the future will not include such heretofore impossible beings. The mixing of non-human animal and human genetic material has already occurred through the various media of *in vitro* fertilization and through stem cell research.[44] Should IGM be rendered safe and effective, and should potentially humanly beneficial genes be identified in non-human species, we have no doubt that the future will include willfully created interspecific transgenic humans, generated in pursuit of a range of objectives.

Somewhat more speculative is the prospect of volitional hominid speciation, the creation of new hominid species through IGM. Historically, according to the biologic species concept, the major driving force in speciation events in sexually-reproducing animals is geographical isolation, which generates reproductive isolation between two groups of animals belonging to the same species. Over time, the two groups diverge sufficiently that they can no longer successfully interbreed, and thus become two species. At present, geographical isolation does not characterize the human population, though it may at some point be achieved through environmental disaster or, less likely, through long-term space colonization where the colony loses contact with earth for many generations.[45] But reproductive isolation may be achieved through other means, IGM primary among them.

Though the intention of IGM may not be to purposefully create a new hominid species, a new hominid species may nonetheless accidentally result from the widespread use of IGM for other purposes. Or maybe humans will indeed choose to evolve a new species. R.C. Spier notes that, "The ten or so species that preceded modern humans came and went at a rate of about 200,000 years per species. Ours began some 130,000 years ago, so we could be just about due for a change."[46]

Presently, one of the technical challenges in IGM is to find ways to guarantee that a cell functionally incorporates inserted genes and expresses them appropriately. Some scholars foresee the use of artificial chromosomes as vectors to insert genes into gametes or embryonic cells and also to control gene expression.[47] But chromosomes interact with each other; and the reason that humans have 46 chromosomes compared to the 48 that simians have is that two of our simian ancestral chromosomes combined. It may well be that the next evolutionary step for humans involves the fusion of chromosomes. Spier sets out the possibility in a series of questions, assuming that artificial extra chromosomes are used as vectors for IGM: "What if bits of other human chromosomes that contain genes essential for survival joined with the newly inserted chromosome? Would not a condition emerge that is akin to the difference between the simian and human chromosomes, a difference that may have been involved in the speciation of humans? And if speciation did occur and a new species of human emerged that eventually became the only living hominid, would the situation differ from previous speciations in principle or in practice?"[48] Note that Spier's scenario involves the accidental joining of chromosomes. Presumably, the volitional joining of chromosomes could be seen as part of a recipe for generating a new human species. Why wait 70,000 years for the next species (or even genus) if we do not have to?

Any of the possibilities explored in this section are understandable as instances of radical rupture. IGM offers the prospect of intentionally creating interspecific transgenic humans, breaching the boundaries between humans and other species that many cherish for any number of reasons.[49] But even the insertion of *human* genes into other human genomes brings with it the possibility of directing and accelerating the evolution of a novel hominid species, especially if artificial extra chromosomes are used as vectors.

7.6   Conclusion: a heuristic to give us pause

We have shown that volitional IGM could potentially result in "radical rupture" in at least three domains: genetic inheritance, genetic history and legacy, and interspecific engineering and speciation. We have not addressed the potential appeal, acceptability, or undesirability of these radical ruptures, but have rather described them in order to facilitate a new moral discourse about IGM.

Recall our definition of "radical rupture": the creation of unprecedented beings, at an unheralded pace, with potentially tremendous precision, constrained almost exclusively by human volition. Our goal in introducing "radical rupture" as a heuristic device is twofold. First, we aim to move the current debate about the ethics of genetic engineering from the personal and the medical to the multi-generational and the cultural. In our view, it is important in identifying and weighing the potential harms and benefits of genetic engineering (in either secular or spiritual terms) that we attend not only to the interests of those with whom we will co-exist, but that we also seriously ponder concerns relevant to distant future generations of unprecedented beings that we will have willfully created in the image of some unknown but desired future being.

In particular, we want to ensure that ongoing debate about genetic modification focuses not only on concerns relevant to persons, but also on concerns relevant to peoples. IGM heralds the prospect of unprecedented, precise, willful control over transgenerational continuity, the introduction of rupture in our evolutionary history and, perhaps more dramatically, the distant but likely creation of new interspecific beings and possibly even new species. We need further debate about the moral significance of these sorts of ruptures, rather than further disputes about harms and benefits of the sort to which we allude at the outset.

Second, we aim to dispel the argument from precedent as critiqued by Eric Parens, an argument that moves from the laudability of using current techniques for preventing disease and improving the human condition, to the uncritical acceptance of any technology (including IGM) to achieve that goal (assuming that the technology engenders more good than harm).[50] That "we have always done it" does not imply that we should continue to do it by any means. The difference in means may well be a difference that matters morally.[51] Radical rupture is thus a heuristic to give us pause. Do the sorts of radical ruptures described in this chapter matter morally? To be precise, does it matter, from a moral point of view, if acquired traits are genetically engineered into future generations? Some will argue in support of efficiency achieving the same end with little effort through genetics trumps expending labor. Others may worry about how this approach to life may undermine valued social institutions, just as enhancement drugs undermine the competitiveness of sport. Still others simply will not see a moral issue here. Similarly, does it matter if we cannot genetically reconstruct genealogies of persons and histories of people because of widespread IGM? Some will argue that DNA genealogies are critically important for identity construction. Others will describe the current interest in one's roots as little more than a fad. Still others will suggest that other techniques will be developed to fill the genealogical gap. Finally, does it matter if we nimbly breach species boundaries in pursuit of health or enhancement, or in the quest for a new species? For some, volitional evolution is the "holy grail" of human evolution, for others it is fraught with moral peril, while for still others it is mere hubris.

In closing, we contend that the questions identified above are the ones that should inform public and scholarly discussion of IGM. If we choose to introduce IGMs, this should be a conscious choice to embrace radical rupture. Our first pass at sketching possible responses to these provocative questions only begins to map the moral terrain of radical rupture; considerable exploration and elaboration of these initial responses must be undertaken. Let us then pause to evaluate the moral importance of anticipated radical ruptures: are they good, bad, or indifferent, in which context, and from which perspective? Only by pausing to consider the morality of radical rupture can we begin to exercise the social responsibility to justly and wisely govern our evolution.[52]

Acknowledgements

We thank members of the Novel Genetic Technologies Research Team at Dalhousie University, especially Fern Brunger, Matthew Herder, and Josephine Johnston, for discussion of a draft of this chapter. W. Ford Doolittle also helpfully commented on a partial draft. We gratefully acknowledge financial support from the Canadian Institutes of Health Research (independently to both FB and JSR), and also from a grant to FB from the Stem Cell Network, a member of the Networks of Centres of Excellence (NCE) program. Finally, salary support is provided for FB through the Canada Research Chair Program.

NOTES

1   For example, LeRoy Walters and Julie G. Palmer, *The Ethics of Human Gene Therapy.* Oxford: Oxford University Press (1997), p. 36.
2   For example, Robert M. Cook-Deegan, Human gene therapy and Congress, *Human Gene Therapy* 1 (1990), 163–70; John C. Fletcher, Evolution of ethical debate about

human gene therapy, *Human Gene Therapy* 1 (1990), 55–68; LeRoy Walters, Human gene therapy: ethics and public policy, *Human Gene Therapy* 2 (1991), 115–22; John C. Fletcher and W. French Anderson, Germ-line gene therapy: a new stage of debate, *Law, Medicine and Health Care* 10 (1992), 26–39.

3   W. French Anderson, Letter submitted to the NIH Office of Recombinant DNA Activities, 31 July 1998; E.D. Zanjani and W. French Anderson, Prospects for *in utero* human gene therapy, *Science* 285 (1999), 2084–8.

4   Mark S. Frankel and Audrey R. Chapman, *Human Inheritable Genetic Modifications: Assessing Scientific, Ethical, Religious, and Policy Issues*. New York: American Association for the Advancement of Science (2000), available online at http://www.aaas.org/spp/sfrl/projects/germline/main.htm (last accessed 1 August 2005); N. King, Inadvertent germline effects in clinical research, *Hastings Center Report* 33 (2003), 23–30.

5   Walters and Palmer, The ethics of human gene therapy.

6   David Resnik, Debunking the slippery slope argument against human germ-line gene therapy, *The Journal of Medicine and Philosophy* 19 (1994), 23–40.

7   Susan M. Cox and William McKellin, "There's this thing in our family": predictive testing and the construction of risk for Huntington disease, *Sociology of Health and Illness* 21 (1999), 622–46; see also Joan Scott, Inherited genetic modification: clinical applications and genetic counseling considerations (Chapter 12, this volume).

8   Anne Michaels, *Fugitive Pieces*. Toronto: McLelland & Stewart (1996), p. 48.

9   Alisdair MacLeod, *No Great Mischief*. Toronto: McLelland & Stewart (1999).

10 In the sense explored by James Lindemann Nelson, Genetic narratives: biology, stories, and the definition of the family, *Health Matrix* 2 (1992), 71–83.

11 Françoise Baylis and Jason Scott Robert, The inevitability of genetic enhancement technologies, *Bioethics* 18 (2004), 1–26.

12 W. Ford Doolittle, personal communication.

13 H. Tristram Engelhardt Jr., Germline engineering: the moral challenges, *American Journal of Medical Genetics* 108 (2002), 169–75, 173.

14 Compare Denis Kenny, Inheritable genetic modification as moral responsibility in a creative universe (Chapter 5, this volume).

15 Jason Scott Robert, *Embryology, Epigenesis, and Evolution: Taking Development Seriously*. Cambridge: Cambridge University Press (2004).

16 Jason Scott Robert and Françoise Baylis, Crossing species boundaries, *American Journal of Bioethics* 3 (2003), 1–13.

17 See also Eric Parens, Should we hold the (germ) line? *Journal of Law, Medicine and Ethics* 23 (1995), 173–6.

18 Baylis and Robert, The inevitability of genetic enhancement technologies.

19 Brian K. Hall, *Evolutionary Developmental Biology*, 2nd edn. Boston: Kluwer (1998), p. 142.

20 James R. Griesemer and F.B. Churchill, Leopold Friederich August Weismann. In: M. Pagel (ed.), *Encyclopedia of Evolution*. New York: Oxford University Press (2002), vol. 2, pp. 1149–51; M. Hart, Germ line and soma. In: M. Pagel (ed.), *Encyclopedia of Evolution*. New York: Oxford University Press (2002), vol. 1, pp. 443–6. Around the

turn of the twentieth century, many early geneticists understood Weismann through the intermediary of E.B. Wilson, author of the influential textbook *The Cell in Development and Inheritance* (first published 1896; 2nd edn, 1900; 3rd edn, 1925). Wilson offered a pictorial representation of Weismann's view, a representation that was not strictly accurate but has come to be seen as authoritative and is known as "Weismannism," see James R. Griesemer, Tools for talking: human nature, Weismannism, and the interpretation of genetic information. In: Carl F. Cranor (ed.), *Are Genes Us? The Social Consequences of the New Genetics*. New Brunswick, NJ: Rutgers University Press (1994), 69–88; James R. Griesemer and William C. Wimsatt, Picturing Weismannism: a case study of conceptual evolution. In: Michael Ruse (ed.), *What the Philosophy of Biology Is: Essays for David Hull*. Dordrecht: Kluwer (1989), 75–137. Wilson's representation emphasized the importance of germinal continuity across generations, de-emphasizing soma as merely epiphenomenal within a single generation. Accordingly, this representation of inheritance led many early geneticists to infer that the developmental causes of inherited traits must be in the germs, as against Weismann's view that both soma and germ are required to explain heredity and development (Griesemer and Churchill, Leopold Friederich August Weismann). Strictly speaking, then, evolutionary biologists tend to follow "Weismannism" rather than Weismann himself.

21 John Maynard Smith, The concept of information in biology, *Philosophy of Science* 67 (2000), 177–94.

22 Françoise Baylis, Human cloning: three mistakes and an alternative, *Journal of Medicine and Philosophy* 27 (2002), 319–37.

23 Mark Thomas, Karl Skorecki, Haim Ben-Ami, *et al.*, Origins of Old Testament priests, *Nature* 394 (1998), 138–40; Mark G. Thomas, Tudor Parfitt, Deborah A. Weiss, *et al.*, Y chromosomes traveling south: the Cohen modal haplotype and the origins of the Lemba – the "black Jews of Southern Africa," *American Journal of Human Genetics* 66 (2000), 674–86.

24 Thomas, Parfitt, Weiss, *et al.*, Y chromosomes traveling south; Amanda B. Spurdle and Trefor Jenkins, The origins of the Lemba "Black Jews'" of southern Africa: evidence from p12F2 and other Y-chromosome markers, *American Journal of Human Genetics* 59 (1996), 1126–33.

25 Jorde L.B. Watkins W.S. Bamshad M.J., *et al.*, The distribution of human genetic diversity: a comparison of mitochondrial, autosomal, and Y-chromosome data, *American Journal of Human Genetics* 66 (2000), 979–88; Lluis Quintana-Murci, Ornella Semino, Hans-J. Bandelt, *et al.*, Genetic evidence of an early exit of *Homo sapiens sapiens* from Africa through eastern Africa, *Nature Genetics* 23 (1999), 437–41; S.A. Tishkoff, E. Dietzsch, W. Speed, *et al.*, Global patterns of linkage disequilibrium at the CD4 locus and modern human origins, *Science* 271 (1996), 1380–7; see also K. Owens and M.C. King, Genomic views of human history, *Science* 286 (1999), 451–3.

26 Eugene A. Foster, M.A. Jobling, P.G. Taylor, *et al.*, Jefferson fathered slave's last child, *Nature* 396 (1998), 27–8.

27 G. Wright, DNA helps find African roots: Howard University's genetic data match people with ancestors, *Cincinnati Enquirer*, 5 April 2000, http://enquirer.com/editions/2000/04/05/loc_dna_helps_find.html (last accessed 1 August 2005); see also http://www.africanancestry.com.

28 See Josephine Johnston and Mark Thomas, Summary: the science of genealogy by genetics, *Developing World Bioethics* 3 (2003), 103–8 for a summary of the basic science.

29 Donald S. Rubenstein, David Thomasma, E. Schon, *et al.*, Germ-line therapy to cure mitochondrial disease: protocol and ethics of *in vitro* ovum nuclear transplantation, *Cambridge Quarterly of Healthcare Ethics* 4 (1995), 316–39.

30 Jason A. Barritt, Carol A. Brenner, Henry E. Malter, *et al.*, Mitochondria in human off-spring derived from ooplasmic transplantation, *Human Reproduction* 16 (2001), 513–6.

31 Andrea L. Bonnicksen, Transplanting nuclei between human eggs: implications for germ-line genetics, *Politics and the Life Sciences* 17 (1998), 3–10.

32 Peter A. Underhill, Peidong Shen, Alice A. Lin, *et al.*, Y chromosome sequence variation and the history of human populations (letter), *Nature Genetics* 26 (2000), 358–61; Tishkoff, Dietzsch, Speed, *et al.*, Global patterns of linkage disequilibrium at the CD4 locus and modern human origins.

33 Quintana-Murci, Semino, Bandelt, *et al.*, Genetic evidence of an early exit of *Homo sapiens sapiens* from Africa through eastern Africa; Li Wang, Hiroki Oota, Naruya Saitou, *et al.*, Genetic structure of a 2500-year-old human population in China and its spatiotemporal changes, *Molecular Biology and Evolution* 17 (2000), 1396–1400.

34 Hansjürgen T. Agostini, Richard Yanagihara, Victor Davis, *et al.*, Asian genotypes of JC virus in Native Americans and in a Pacific Island population: markers of viral evolution and human migration, *Proceedings of the National Academy of Sciences – USA* 94 (1997), 14542–6; Angelo Pavesi, Detecting traces of prehistoric human migrations by geographic synthetic maps of polyomavirus JC, *Journal of Molecular Evolution* 58 (2004), 304–13.

35 See Elizabeth Culotta, Andrew Sugden and Brooks Hanson, Humans on the move, *Science* 291 (2001), 1721, the introduction to a special issue of the journal devoted to the various dimensions of this research; see also Rebecca L. Cann, Genetic clues to dispersal in human populations: retracing the past from the present, *Science* 291 (2001), 1742–8; Owens and King, Genomic views of human history.

36 W. Ford Doolittle, personal communication.

37 Anders Sandberg, Genetic modifications, *Transhumanist Resources* (n.d.), http://www.aleph.se/Trans/Individual/Body/genes.html (last accessed 1 August 2005).

38 Brian Stableford, *Future Man*. New York: Crown (1984).

39 Sandberg, Genetic modifications.

40 Robert and Baylis, Crossing species boundaries. In this article, we call into question the presumption that species boundaries exist. While there are many definitions of species in the literature, there is as yet no consensus on exactly what is being breached – beyond taboo – with the mixing of genetic material between different species.

41 Whether the gene from the non-human genome would be expressed is an open question. Even were it expressed, whether it would actually work as intended is also an open

question. No matter: should anyone ever attempt such a procedure, we have no doubt that she would make every effort to perfect every innovation to ensure its success.

42 Sotiria Sotiriou, Suzana Gispert, Jun Cheng, *et al.*, Ascorbic-acid transporter Slc23a1 is essential for vitamin C transport into the brain and for perinatal survival, *Nature Medicine* 8 (2002), 514–7.

43 A.W.S. Chan, K.Y. Chong, C. Martinovich, *et al.*, Transgenic monkeys produced by retroviral gene transfer into mature oocytes, *Science* 291 (2001), 309–12; Jonathan Knight, Biology's last taboo, *Nature* 413 (2001), 12–5; Gretchen Vogel, Transgenic animals: infant monkey carries jellyfish gene, *Science* 291 (2001), 226.

44 Advanced Cell Technology, Advanced Cell Technology announces use of nuclear transfer technology for successful generation of human embryonic stem cells, 12 November 1998, http://www.advancedcell.com/1998-11-12.htm (last accessed 1 August 2005); Nobuko Uchida, David W. Buck, Dongping He, *et al.*, Direct isolation of human central nervous system stem cells, *Proceedings of the National Academy of Sciences – USA* 97 (2000), 14720–5; Ying Chen, Zhi X. He, Ailian Liu, *et al.*, Embryonic stem cells generated by nuclear transfer of human somatic nuclei into rabbit oocytes, *Cell Research* 13 (2003), 251–63.

45 The latter possibility is expressed by Thomas Hayden, Jessica Ruvinsky, Dan Gilgoff, *et al.*, A theory evolves: how evolution really works, and why it matters more than ever, *U.S. News & World Report* 29 July 2002, 42–50, p. 50.

46 R.C. Spier, Toward a new human species? *Science* 296 (2002), 1807–8, p. 1807.

47 As discussed in Knight, Biology's last taboo; Spier, Toward a new human species?

48 Spier, Toward a new human species? 1807–8.

49 Robert and Baylis, Crossing species boundaries.

50 Parens, Should we hold the (germ) line?

51 For example, Baylis and Robert, The inevitability of genetic enhancement technologies; Daniel W. Brock, Enhancements of human function: some distinctions for policymakers. In: Eric Parens (ed.), *Enhancing Human Traits: Ethical and Social Implications.* Washington, DC: Georgetown University Press (1998), 48–69; Ronald Cole-Turner, Do means matter? In: Eric Parens (ed.), *Enhancing Human Traits: Ethical and Social Implications.* Washington, DC: Georgetown University Press (1998), pp. 151–61.

52 On this point, see also Parens, Should we hold the (germ) line?

"Alter-ing" the human species? Misplaced essentialism in science policy

Eric T. Juengst

8.1   Inheritable genetic modification as a science policy issue

For the last 20 years, the field of human gene transfer research has been bounded by two simple lines: the line between using gene-transfer techniques to cure disease or improve the human design, on one hand, and the line between applying gene-transfer techniques to somatic cells or germ-line cells, on the other.[1] The dominant view, received as wisdom in both formal science policies and in the rhetoric of scientists, has been that enhancement applications of gene transfer would be too morally problematic, and germ-line gene transfer (GLGT) would be too risky to prospective offspring, at least until the practice of safe and effective somatic cell gene transfer (SCGT) could be perfected.[2]

Today, both of these lines are being challenged, in unexpected ways. "Enhancement" turns out to be a matter of definition, and the relevant definitions all move the discussion away from objective description and into competing accounts of the values at stake.[3] Inheritable genetic modification (IGM), moreover, can be accomplished without using recombinant DNA gene-transfer techniques, and is thereby escaping scrutiny as "GLGT."[4] Moreover, even the anticipated modes of both enhancement and IGM have public advocates within the scientific and bioethical communities that would have been very surprising in 1985: mainstream theologians, prominent molecular biologists, distinguished philosophers, and senior bioethicists.[5] In short, the dykes against human genetic engineering are bulging against the tide of the "post-human," and much of the intellectual establishment on these matters seems to be leaning in the direction of letting them go.

This leaves a set of very strange bedfellows striving to maintain the science policy status quo. On the right are natural law theorists, both religious and secular, who continue to maintain that attempting to "direct evolution" is hubris, with consequences already foreshadowed in the eugenics movements of the past.[6] Most of the new apologists for genetic modification have felt compelled to address the challenge of the natural lawyers, and there are now a number of good critiques of the essentialism to which their views fall prey.[7]

On the left, however, are a collection of environmentalists, human rights activists, and communitarians, who have been active in attempting to prohibit IGM as a matter of public policy.[8] In this chapter, I offer a sympathetic critique of their views. Their policy arguments are superficially attractive to many who consider themselves progressive thinkers on social and environmental matters. But the price they pay for their rhetoric is a reliance on a set of assumptions that are ultimately more dangerous than the right wing's essentialism, and unnecessary to boot. Or so I shall argue below.

8.2   Preserving the species

An important example of the left-leaning concern is provided by work of the human rights lawyer George Annas and his collaborators. Over the last several years, Annas has been promoting the need for a new United Nations' (UN) "Convention on the Preservation of the Human Species," which would realize itself in an international treaty to ban "species-altering" research (at least, where the species involved is ours).[9] Annas defines the class of "species-altering" research as encompassing "any experimental interventions aimed at altering a fundamental beneficial characteristic of being human." He elaborates with a distinction:

There are at least two ways to change such characteristics. The first is to make a necessary beneficial human trait optional. Changing it in one member (who continues to be seen as a member of the species) would change the definition for everyone ... A second way to change a characteristic of being human is any alteration that would make the resulting person someone we (*Homo sapiens*) would no longer identify as a member of our species, or who could not sexually reproduce with a human.[10]

Under this rubric, the proposed treaty targets two kinds of research for prohibition: research involving human reproductive cloning, and research aimed at effecting IGM in humans. As Annas argues: "cloning and inheritable genetic alterations can be seen as crimes against humanity of a unique sort: they are techniques that can alter the essence of humanity itself (and thus threaten to change the foundation of human rights) by taking human evolution into our own hands and directing it toward the development of a new species sometimes termed the 'post-human.'"[11]

The core provisions of the proposed Convention expand on the dangers of such hubris:

The Parties to this Convention,
... *Noting* the increased power of genetic science, which opens up vast prospects for improving health, but also has the power to diminish humanity fundamentally by producing a child through human cloning or by intentionally producing an inheritable genetic change;

Concerned that experiments which for the first time would produce children with pre-determined genotypes, rather than novel genotypes, might cause these children to be deprived of their human rights;

Concerned that by altering fundamental human characteristics to the extent of possibly producing a new human species or subspecies, genetic science will cause the resulting people to be treated unequally or deprived of their human rights; ...

Have agreed on the following:
Parties shall take all reasonable action, including the adoption of criminal laws, to pro-hibit anyone from initiating or attempting to initiate a human pregnancy or other form of gestation using embryos or reproductive cells which have undergone intentional IGM.[12]

Annas' proposed convention is a good example of the left-leaning concern to preserve and formalize the existing moratorium on human IGM because it neatly folds together a number of important themes from that literature. On one hand, by framing the major danger of such interventions as the loss of human rights, the Convention puts species-altering interventions on a par with slavery, terrorism, and genocide as a legitimate topic for cross-cultural, inter-national legislation. The argument is that since "membership in the human species is central to the meaning and enforcement of human rights,"[13] the post-human progeny of genetic engineering may find themselves disqualified by definition. Annas writes that:

There are limits to how far we can go in changing our human nature without changing our humanity and our basic human values. As it is the meaning of humanness (our dis-tinctness from other animals) that has given birth to our concepts of both human dignity and human rights, altering our nature necessarily threatens to undermine both human dignity and human rights. With their loss, the fundamental belief in human equality would also be lost ... If history is a guide, either the normal humans will view the "bet-ter" humans as "the other" and seek to control or destroy them, or vice-versa. The better human will become, at least in the absence of a universal concept of human dignity, either the oppressor or the oppressed.[14]

The proposed draft Convention's text focuses on the political plight of the engineered as a potentially oppressed minority. What human rights advocates could be for the undermining of human dignity through taxonomical terror-ism? On the other hand, the Convention's title – "On the Preservation of the Human Species" – clearly alludes to the alternative: that the engineered would be our oppressors. As Annas writes:

Ultimately, it almost seems inevitable that genetic engineering would move *Homo sapi-ens* into two separable species: the standard-issue human beings would be seen by the new, genetically enhanced neo-humans as heathens who can properly be slaughtered and subjugated. It is this genocidal potential that makes species-altering genetic engi-neering a potential weapon of mass destruction and the unaccountable genetic engineer a potential bioterrorist.[15]

Raising this specter allows Annas and his collaborators to play two other attractive international policy cards in promoting his views: arms control concerns to forestall the extinction of our species at the hands of our own weapons, and the environmentalist concerns about the extinction of endangered species through the careless human introduction of eco-destabilizing, genetically-modified, biologic competitors. These are clever gambits: what humanitarians could be against additional curbs on humanity's reckless self-destruction? What environmentalists could resist extending their concerns about endangered species and genetically-modified organisms to ourselves? What better place to invoke, as Annas does, the environmental movement's "precautionary principle," and change the burden of proof by "outlawing potentially lethal activities, thus requiring proponents to change the law before proceeding"?[16]

A third theme captured in the convention is that interventions like IGM, because they might expand or transgress the current biologic boundaries of our species,[17] involve decisions in which the whole species has a stake. As Annas and his colleagues write:

As a baseline, if we take human rights and democracy seriously, a decision to alter a fundamental characteristic in the definition of "human" should not be made by any individual or corporation without wide discussion among all members of the affected populations … Altering the human species is an issue that directly concerns all of us, and should only be decided democratically, by a body that is representative of everyone on the planet.[18]

This position resonates well with the popular European view that the human genome is, like the sea-bed, a part of humanity's "common heritage," and should be explored and exploited only under the auspices of global agreements informed by what Vaclav Havel calls "species consciousness."[19] For Annas, private genetic decisions that affect the larger human gene pool "could all fit into a new category of 'crimes against humanity' in the strict sense, as actions that threaten the integrity of the human species itself."[20] This concern for the corporate human control of our species' boundaries provides common ground with both those who fear the consequences of disregarding "evolution's wisdom" in crafting our inheritance, and those who would seek to protect the rights of future generations by defending their "right to an untampered genome."[21] Thus, Annas et al. conclude that:

Opposition to cloning and inheritable genetic alteration is "conservative" in the strict sense of the word: it seeks to conserve the human species. But it is also liberal in the strict sense of the word: it seeks to preserve democracy, freedom, and universal human rights for all members of the human species.[22]

Casting human IGM research as "species-altering" experimentation is a clever strategy for international science policy-making. It enables policy-makers to invoke concern over the political oppression of minorities; human extinction; and ecologic recklessness, private exploitation of public resources, species integrity, the wisdom of nature, and the rights of future generations. But it is, as they say, too clever by half. I will argue that, as an international science policy approach to IGM research, banning "species-altering procedures" either does much too much or much too little, and on either interpretation sends much too muddled a message about the nature and grounding of the human values at issue in this research. The real moral concerns with the creation of neo-humans still lie far ahead of the science, but, sadly enough, they are not at all futuristic. Ultimately, what is at stake in genetic modification is our tolerance for human genetic diversity. Appeals to "species integrity" are about as helpful in that context as appeals to "racial purity" are in designing population genetic research.

8.3   "Altering" the species

Annas says that he draws his line at the nature of our species, because he thinks that of all the morally problematic uses of genetic technologies, interventions that go beyond "therapy" and beyond "enhancement," to "the extent of possibly producing a new human species or subspecies" will be seen by the widest range of cultures and countries as clearly "inhuman" or "de-humanizing." However, there are two different ways to interpret this, neither of which will be terribly helpful for international science policy.

First, this Convention cannot literally seek to preserve the human species from all species-altering procedures, because humans are doing things that change the species all the time. Species are not static collections of organisms that can be "preserved" against change like a can of fruit; they wax and wane with every birth and death, and their genetic complexions shift across time and space.[23] In our case, almost everything we do as humans affects that process. To argue, as some Europeans have, that everyone has the right to inherit "an untampered genome" only makes sense if we are willing to take a snapshot of the human gene pool at some given instant, and reify it as the sacred "genetic patrimony of humankind" – which some come close to doing.[24]

But putting some particular genetic version of our species on an altar and attempting to police human behavior in order to protect it is, from a human rights point of view, no better than the eugenicists' attempts to sanctify and promote a particular genetic ideal for our species: even if it were possible to do, it could not be done without widespread violations of basic human rights and liberties.[25] Under this interpretation, the draft Convention's ban on "species-altering procedures" would cover much too much, laying groundwork for the very kind of human rights abuses history has warned us of already. Even limiting prohibited alterations to changes in "fundamental beneficial characteristics of being human" does not help, since it merely shifts the problem to defining those characteristics. (Why, for example, is being the offspring of two-parent sexual reproduction a more fundamentally beneficial human characteristic than being the offspring of two-parent sexual reproduction involving coitus, or having two rearing parents of different genders?)

But if it is not artificial (i.e., human-caused) "genetic drift" within our species that is the true concern of this Convention, what does "species-altering" mean? Some language in the Convention suggests that "altering" is being used here not just to convey "modifying," but in the strong sense of "transforming" or "replacing." In other words, we are worried about interventions and experiments that might change the biologic classification of their subjects entirely: procedures that can produce what evolutionary biologists would call "speciation events."

Indeed, this is the only interpretation that allows the Convention's title to read as an environmentalist might, as referring to saving the species from extinction. The human species is not endangered by mere genetic change: but if a new species was generated that exterminated us, we might be endangered by a speciation event. If "fundamentally beneficial" traits are to be read as "taxonomically defining," then this interpretation might work. But then our treaty would cover only the most dramatic of genetic interventions: interventions that rendered the subjects biologically incapable of reproducing with human beings, but compatible with each other. Under this interpretation, even most IGM, genetic enhancements, and reproductive manipulations, like cloning, would be unproblematic, since their subjects are uncontroversially still taxonomically human. Since concerns over cloning and IGM are at the heart of this treaty, however, this interpretation would mean that banning "species-altering procedures" would not allow this convention to achieve its own goals.

8.4 What has species membership got to do with it, anyway?

Moreover, these definitional problems suggest a fundamental moral question about the "preservation of the human species" approach. What does peoples' species designation have to do with their moral status and their fundamental rights? There is a risk here of confusing the biologic sense of "human" as an taxonomic term (like "canine" or "simian") and the word's use in "human rights," where it serves as a synonym for "natural," "inalienable," or "fundamental" to distinguish that class of moral claims from other conferred, negotiated, or legislated rights.[26] Obviously it is not enough to be taxonomically human to be considered to have human rights: human tissue cultures and human cadavers show us that. Is it even necessary to be taxonomically human to enjoy human rights?

There are many candidates for the qualities that serve to give us our inalienable rights (the Convention singles out reason and conscience), but none hinge on a taxonomic designation.[27] So how is it that species-altering procedures "might cause the children to be deprived of their human rights"? As the draft Convention tellingly says, from most moral points of view on the derivation of human rights, even genetic speciation events would produce "new *human* species or subspecies." In fact, framing our concern about genetic threats to human rights in terms of "species-altering" makes the same mistake that some European analysts make when they seek to defend our "species integrity": it suggests that taxonomy might determine a creature's moral status, and that conceivably only those creatures displaying the motley collection of genes that human beings share (at some instant) warrant basic rights. Again, this is a form of "alter-ing" our gene pool that we should spurn as moral idolatry, an altar at which we should not bow.

But perhaps I am interpreting the draft Convention too literally. Perhaps, behind the ambiguous language, the intent is to warn us that, despite their evident moral status, the victims of species-altering procedures might be (wrongly) perceived by others to be "inhuman" and have their rights abused as a consequence. That interpretation would make sense of the Convention's opening appeals to our convictions about "rights based on the dignity and worth of the human person," the "equal rights of all persons," and "the inadmissibility of discrimination." But if it is actually genetic prejudice, or, in Annas' felicitous terminology, "genism," that is the real problem here, then the draft Convention has a deep problem. By focusing on "species-altering procedures" and the genetic interventions that might qualify as such, like radical IGM, the draft Convention actually distracts us from the vast bulk of real and imminent threats to human rights that genetic research can pose.

If we are worried about the threats of genism, the most dangerous products of human genetic research are not gene-splicing techniques: they are changes in what people think they know about each other that exacerbate existing prejudices between them. It is the social perception of genetic difference, not the actual biologic differences, which fuel human rights abuses. These perceptions, the prejudices they bolster, and the abuses they feed, will be coming for the foreseeable future not from the lunatic fringes of genetic research, but from its brightest hopes: from the new work in human genetic variation research, "public health genetics," and pharmacogenomics.

To the extent that this wave of post-genomic work accentuates perceived genetic differences between human groups already socially sorted by their mutual power relations (like the so-called "races"), it will be the primary engine for human rights threats because it is what will feed draconian "public health" infringements on reproductive freedoms, oppressive DNA identification and data banking programs, neo-eugenic immigration policies, economic discrimination practices, and, at the extreme, biologic warfare strategies. These are the problems that international policy-makers should be worried about long before they concern themselves with the moral merits of sexual reproduction. To the extent that the Convention's focus on "species-altering procedures" distracts us from the distinctly intra-species issues of genetic oppression, it is likely to be accused by the oppressed of being simply another smokescreen thrown up to hide the real, and more difficult, issues of how to keep manifestly beneficial research from being abused.

8.5   Conclusion: the alternative

So how *should* we frame a convention designed to protect human rights in an age of genetic technology? One approach would be to address the danger of genism directly, and present the initiative as simply a "Convention on Human Rights Abuses of Human Genetic Research." Here the word "abuses" does intentional double duty: we are worried about the ways in which (otherwise laudable) human genetic research can be abused to create social perceptions and practices that provoke human rights abuses. This reframing would take us back to the drawing board, admittedly. In addition to trying to prevent the genism that might attend reproductive cloning or IGM, the initiative would pay more attention to the messier and more mundane matters of limiting law enforcement and political uses of genetic profiling, defining appropriate public health uses of genetic screening tools, and combating genetic discrimination in insurance and employment.[28]

Framed explicitly as a human rights initiative, this Convention would direct international attention explicitly on the social and political assumptions about race, class, and group membership that continue to infect mainstream "normal science" in human population genetics, genetic epidemiology, and comparative genomics. In so doing, the real reasons why prohibitions against particular reproductive or IGM interventions might be warranted could be articulated in a cogent way: not because they alter the blend of humanity's gene pool or create new taxons within the genus *Homo*, but because they diminish the range of opportunities that human rights are designed to protect.

Of course, some IGM might also *expand* the range of opportunities available to their human recipients, and a regulatory framework based on human rights protections would not condemn them because of their modifications. As advocates for people with disabilities increasingly point out, to the extent that genetic interventions can be used to enhance strengths and compensate for weaknesses in creative ways that expand opportunity without "normalizing" their recipients, they could be a social force in improving tolerance for human diversity.[29] In other words, it is the opportunities for creativity that the human genome makes possible, not the genes themselves, that we should strive to preserve.[30] In the long run, that means that in contemplating IGM, the international community should focus on the promises we would like to make to our children, rather than fret about what we have (or have not) inherited from our parents. The human gene pool, unlike the sea, has no top, bottom, or shores: it cannot be "preserved." The reservoir of human mutual respect, good will, and tolerance for difference, however, seems perennially in danger of running dry. *That* is the truly fragile heritage that we should work to preserve in monitoring genetic research on behalf of the future.

NOTES

1 Eric Juengst and LeRoy Walters, Ethical issues in gene transfer research. In: Theodore Friedman (ed.), *The Development of Human Gene Therapy.* New York: Cold Spring Harbor Press (1999), 691–713.

2 LeRoy Walters and Julie G. Palmer, *The Ethics of Human Gene Therapy.* New York: Oxford University Press (1997).

3 Erik Parens (ed.), *Enhancing Human Traits: Ethical and Social Implications.* Washington, DC: Georgetown University Press (1998).

4 Erik Parens and Eric Juengst, Inadvertently crossing the germ line, *Science* 292 (2001), 397.

5 Compare Gregory Stock and John Campbell (eds.), *Engineering the Human Germ-Line.* New York: Oxford University Press (2000); Philip Kitcher, *The Lives to Come: The Genetic Revolution and Human Possibilities.* New York: Simon and Schuster (1997).

6 Francis Fukuyama, *Our Posthuman Future: Consequences of the Biotechnology Revolution.* New York: Profile Books (2002).

7 Allen Buchanan, Dan Brock, Norman Daniels, *et al., From Chance to Choice: Genetics and Justice.* New York: Cambridge University Press (2002); see also Roberta M. Berry, Can bioethics speak to politics about the prospect of inheritable genetic modification? If so, what might it say? (Chapter 13, this volume).

8 Council for Responsible Genetics, Position statement on human germ-line manipulation, *Human Gene Therapy* 4 (1993), 35–9; Bruce Jennings, The liberalism of life: bioethics in the face of biopower, *Raritan* 22 (2003), 132–46.

9 George Annas, Lori Andrews and Rosario Isas, Protecting the endangered human: toward an international treaty prohibiting cloning and inheritable alterations, *American Journal of Law and Medicine* 28 (2002), 151–78.

10 George Annas, The man on the moon, immortality and other millennial myths: the prospects and perils of human genetic engineering, *Emory Law Journal* 49 (2000), 753–82, p. 779.

11 Annas, Andrews and Isas, Protecting the endangered human, p. 153.

12 *Ibid.,* p. 154.

13 *Ibid.,* p. 153.

14 Annas, The man on the moon, immortality and other millennial myths, p. 773.

15 *Ibid.*

16 Annas, Andrews and Isas, Protecting the endangered human, p. 154.

17 See also Françoise Baylis and Jason Scott Robert, Radical rupture: exploring biologic sequelae of volitional inheritable genetic modification (Chapter 7, this volume).

18 Annas, Andrews and Isas, Protecting the endangered human, p. 153.

19 *Ibid.,* p. 152.

20 Annas, The man on the moon, immortality and other millennial myths, p. 778.

21 Council of Europe (Parliamentary Assembly), Recommendation 934: on genetic engineering, Council of Europe (Strasbourg, France, 1982).

22 Annas, Andrews and Isas, Protecting the endangered human, p. 173.

23 R.A. Wilson (ed.), *Species: New Interdisciplinary Essays*. Cambridge: MIT Press (1999).

24 Emmanuel Agius, Germ-line cells: our responsibilities for future generations. In: Salvino Busuttil, Emmanuel Agius, Peter S. Inglott and Tony Macelli (eds.), *Our Responsibilities Toward Future Generations*. Valleta, Malta: Foundation for International Studies (1990), 133–43.

25 Eric Juengst, Should we treat the human germ-line as a global human resource? In: Emmanuel Agius and S. Busutill (eds.), *Germ-Line Intervention and Our Responsibilities to Future Generations*. Boston: Kluwer Academic Publishers (1998), 85–102; see also Isabel Karpin and Roxanne Mykitiuk, Regulating inheritable genetic modification, or policing the fertile scientific imagination? A feminist legal response (Chapter 11, this volume).

26 Angela Campbell, Kathleen G. Glass and Louis C. Charland, Describing our humanness: can genetic science alter what it means to be human? *Science and Engineering Ethics* 4 (1998), 413–26.

27 Jason Scott Robert and Françoise Baylis, Crossing species boundaries, *The American Journal of Bioethics* 3 (2003), 1–14.

28 Compare Anita Silvers and Michael Stein, Human rights and genetic discrimination: protecting genomics' promise for public health, *Journal of Law, Medicine and Ethics* 31 (2003), 377–89.

29 Anita Silvers, Meliorism at the millennium: positive molecular eugenics and the promise of progress without excess. In: Lisa S. Parker and Rachel A. Ankeny (eds.), *Mutating Concepts, Evolving Disciplines: Genetics, Medicine and Society*. Dordrecht: Kluwer Academic Publishers (2002), 215–35.

30 Compare Denis Kenny, Inheritable genetic modification as moral responsibility in a creative universe (Chapter 5, this volume).

Traditional and feminist bioethical perspectives on gene transfer: is inheritable genetic modification really *the* problem?

Rosemarie Tong

9.1 Introduction

Although feminist bioethicists have critiqued the new reproductive and genetic technologies in general,[1] they have written relatively little on the specific topic of gene therapy. To be sure, there are exceptions to this rule. Mary B. Mahowald reflects in depth on genomic alterations and women in her book *Genes, Women, Equality*.[2] In addition, Jackie Leach Scully[3] and Anita Silvers[4] have routinely challenged both the reigning boundaries between somatic cell gene transfer (SCGT) and germ-line gene transfer (GLGT) on the one hand, and the standard definitions for genetic "treatment" and genetic "enhancement" on the other. Some traditional bioethicists, such as Eric Parens, have also challenged these same boundaries.[5] But when they have done so, they have neglected, overlooked, or chosen to ignore the ways in which raising the so-called "woman question"[6] can help *all* bioethicists, feminist or non-feminist, provide better advice about which types of gene transfer should be encouraged and which discouraged.

In the following essay, I first offer a fairly traditional bioethical analysis of gene transfer, with an emphasis on GLGT and other forms of inheritable genetic modification (IGM). I then provide some feminist critiques of this mode of analysis, each of which raises the woman question with respect to gene transfer. Finally, I suggest that if traditional bioethics incorporates feminist understandings about gene transfer into its corpus, it has a better chance of serving the best interests of men and women equally.

9.2 Traditional bioethical approaches to gene transfer

For more than 25 years, most traditional bioethicists have embraced SCGT for treatment purposes, but not for enhancement purposes. In addition, they have virtually closed the door on IGM for any purpose, most especially for purposes of enhancement. However, whether traditional bioethicists will continue to honor the reigning boundaries between SCGT and IGM on the one hand, and the standard definitions for genetic "treatment" and genetic "enhancement" on the other, is unclear. Indeed, there is increasing reason to think they will relax both of these boundaries.[7]

9.2.1 Gene transfer for therapeutic purposes

To date, only one kind of gene transfer has generally been permitted, namely, SCGT for the purposes of treating a severe genetic disease. SCGT has not yet resulted in many patients being cured.[8] Nevertheless, around 900 clinical protocols for SCGT experiments have been submitted and approved worldwide.[9] Progress has been slow, and successes such as the development of a promising treatment for severe combined immunodeficiency disorder or SCID[10] have been offset by unexpected tragedies such as the development of leukemia among some subjects in the SCID trial, and the death of a patient in a University of Pennsylvania study of gene transfer for a metabolic disorder primarily affecting the liver.[11] The latter subject died from a reaction to the vector used to deliver genetically-altered cells to him.[12]

Because of the difficulties associated with SCGT, there has been some pressure to move in the direction of IGM. Many research scientists believe that IGM may potentially be easier to perform than SCGT because pre-embryos to be used for *in vitro* fertilization (IVF) procedures, which are the most likely candidates for IGM, are housed in *petri* dishes where they are easily manipulated. If a pre-embryo tests positively for a genetic disease, scientists could try to correct its defective genes *before* inserting it into a woman's womb. Should the experiment work, not only the baby (as would be the case in SCGT) but also all of his/her descendants would be born without the disease. Significantly, this particular difference between SCGT and IGM has triggered several concerns within the traditional bioethics community.

Opponents of IGM claim, first, that it poses too many unpredictable, unavoidable, and serious long-term risks to the genetically-altered individuals and their offspring to be justified.[13] In their estimation, the risk–benefit ratio is such that apart from circumstances where IGM represents the only option (e.g., diseases transmitted via the germ line), there is no real justification for using IGM to eliminate conditions (such as cystic fibrosis, CF). Like many genetic diseases, CF could be addressed through the far less risky means of carrier screening, prenatal diagnosis followed by abortion, or perhaps SCGT (subsequent to the birth of the afflicted individual) in the future.[14] Second, opponents of IGM insist that it places multiple human generations in the role of research subjects who have not given consent. As they see it, future generations have the right to determine their *own* destinies, in particular because their views about what counts as a favorable human trait may substantially differ from the present generation's views about the same human trait.[15] Third, opponents of IGM claim it violates the right of the individual and his/her descendants to have their own unique, genetic identities. More accurately, IGM substitutes other individuals (at least in terms of genetic identity, and perhaps even in a deeper sense of personal identity) in the place of the individuals who would have been born. At the very least, it substitutes for the individuals who would have been born very different versions of their original selves.[16]

Opponents of IGM also raise two additional objections to it, both of which apply equally to SCGT – namely, that IGM will never be "cost effective" enough to warrant wide-scale use,[17] and that success in using IGM for therapeutic purposes may encourage scientists to use it for enhancement purposes.[18] Because wealthy people may wish to use their ample resources to perfect their children and because people of ordinary means will not be able to afford "fine tuning" their sons and daughters, the chasm between the rich and the poor could grow as the rich add genetic privileges to their other privileges.[19]

However, not all traditional bioethicists are opponents of IGM; some of them are clear advocates for it. Such advocates claim, first, that its risks have been exaggerated. They contend that far from being morally undesirable, IGM is actually morally preferable to SCGT in that it obviates the need to perform equally costly, risky SCGT in multiple generations.[20] Second, advocates of IGM reason that if society entrusts parents to act in the best interests of their children when they decide to procreate with their own unaltered genes, society should also generally trust parents to act in the best interests of their future children and foreseeable (or at least imaginable) descendants when they consent to IGM on their pre-embryos. The fact that this generation can neither acquire the permission of future generations nor know their genetic "needs" and "preferences" is not a sound justification for banning IGM. If it were, says Ray Moseley, it would likewise be "unethical to do anything affecting future generations, including produce them."[21] IGM advocates rebut the third argument outlined above, that IGM will result in a person *different* than the one who would have been born without IGM, with the claim that *no* person whatsoever exists at the pre-embryonic or preimplantation stage. All that exists is a cluster of living human cells that has the potential to differentiate in numerous ways.[22] Therefore, whatever genetic changes are made, they are not made on a *particular* person with an established identity, but merely on a totipotent cell cluster that is utterly devoid of an identity.[23]

With respect to the fourth objection, that IGM will not be cost effective, IGM advocates maintain that "it is too early to know what the relative cost of germ-line intervention will be when the technique is fully developed."[24] Finally, regarding the fifth objection, namely that medically necessary genetic treatments will pave the way for medically unnecessary genetic enhancements, some IGM advocates maintain that the line between permissible treatments or therapies and impermissible enhancements can and will be held.[25] However, other IGM advocates make the more debatable claim that the treatment–enhancement boundary should simply be crossed. As they see it, provided that genetic enhancements are safe, effective, and no more unjust than other practices ordinarily permitted in a free and democratic society – for example, sending one's children to the best schools – they should be permitted.[26]

9.2.2 Gene transfer for enhancement purposes

The argument that triggers the most debate within the traditional bioethics community is the one that supports gene transfer for enhancement purposes. Although some traditional bioethicists classify any and all genetic interventions as "enhancements",[27] I prefer to refer to *health-related* genetic interventions as "treatments" (or "therapies," should they become sufficiently proven), reserving the term "enhancement" for *non-health-related* genetic interventions. According to LeRoy Walters and Julie Palmer, examples of health-related genetic treatments include improving the general functioning of the immune system (a physical treatment); eliminating the genes associated with senile dementia (an intellectual improvement); and eliminating the genes associated with sociopathic tendencies (a moral improvement). In contrast, examples of non-health-related genetic enhancements include helping people sleep fewer hours (a physical improvement); increasing the efficiency of long-term memory (an intellectual improvement); and stimulating capacities for "friendliness" (a moral improvement).[28] Implicit in the distinction between health-related genetic treatments and non-health-related genetic enhancements is, I admit, a fairly narrow conception of health, certainly not the very broad conception of health that the World Health Organization (WHO) espouses. WHO asserts that health is "a state of complete physical, mental, and social well-being and not merely the absence of disease or infirmity."[29] A past advocate of the WHO definition of health, I now regard it unfavorably as destroying one of the distinctions I would most like to maintain – specifically the opposition between a treatment on the one hand and an enhancement on the other. Were the decision up to WHO, virtually everything I categorize as an enhancement would be recategorized as a treatment, a recategorization that would, frankly, destroy my line of argumentation.

The ethical issues and questions raised about health-related genetic treatments, such as risk–benefit, informed consent, fairness, and cost also will apply to non-health-related genetic enhancements.[30] And since even the risks and costs of health-related genetic *treatments* remain very high, it would seem imprudent to consent to non-health-related genetic *enhancements*. It is one thing to take considerable risks to avoid the depths of forgetfulness that Alzheimer disease causes, and quite another to take these same risks in order to memorize the contents of the *Encyclopaedia Britannica* in one night. Of course, the case against genetic enhancement would be considerably weakened were both non-health-related genetic enhancements and health-related genetic treatments to become entirely safe, effective, voluntary (in the sense of not socially coerced and fully consented to by the individuals themselves), and affordable. Proponents of genetic enhancement would then be able to argue effectively that *if* there is nothing intrinsically wrong about parents trying to improve their children's minds through education, their physical appearance through cosmetic dentistry, and their character through self-help programs and spiritual counseling, then there is nothing intrinsically wrong about parents trying to improve their children through genetic enhancements. Indeed, lawyer and bioethicist John A. Robertson has already speculated that " ... prenatal (genetic) enhancement might turn out to be preferable (to postnatal enhancement) because an existing child will not be the immediate object of the effort."[31] Rather than subjecting an existing child to cosmetic surgery to straighten her "ugly" nose, why not instead ensure that the child is born with an appropriately-shaped nose so that she never has to feel badly about her appearance?

Although Robertson's views have certainly not met with universal approval in the traditional bioethics community, resistance seems to be weakening. The more that science promises (and delivers) in the way of treatments for devastating genetic diseases, the less inclined the traditional bioethics community is to eschew IGM. Likewise, the more society emphasizes the values of choice and control, the less able the traditional bioethics community is to mount persuasive arguments against seemingly harmless genetic enhancements. Thus, among the questions feminist bioethicists need to ask is the following one: will moving more rapidly in the direction of both IGM and the further weakening of the distinction between genetic treatment and genetic enhancement serve women's particular interests at this time?[32]

9.3 Feminist bioethical approaches to gene transfer

With respect to the question of whether moving more rapidly in the direction of IGM is likely to serve the best interests of women, the short answer is that it is not likely to do so. Although feminist bioethicists have not, to my knowledge, systematically debated the pros and cons of IGM, it is easy enough to imagine them engaging in such a debate. It is also easy to imagine them concluding that, on balance, IGM is at present too full of question marks to benefit women.

Most feminist bioethicists – say the majority of the feminists who belong to the International Network on Feminist Approaches to Bioethics (FAB) – are likely to stress that whether IGM is used before the embryo is implanted in a woman's womb or during the course of time she gestates the embryo *in utero*, her body will be exposed to risks the genetic father and others involved in the process will escape. Preimplantation genetic interventions require ovulation stimulation, egg retrieval, external fertilization of the egg, and embryo transfer into the womb of the woman, and *in utero* genetic interventions on behalf of the fetus require a woman to subject herself as well as her fetus to the risks of fetal surgery or manipulation. To be sure, chances are that in its beginning phases, IGM will be largely confined to preimplantation embryos simply because it is at present technically easier to manipulate *in vitro* than *in vivo* embryos. Therefore, until postnatal IGM becomes a reliable technique, some women who would have preferred to have their child in the "old-fashioned way" may instead feel obliged to have their (future) child the modern, *in vitro* way in order to guarantee its genetic health. Of course, the women who "choose" to have their child using *in vitro* processes will be exposed to the routine risks, inconveniences, stresses, strains, and expense of the IVF process.[33] But they will also be exposed to additional negative consequences.

In the first place, women will be asked, perhaps together with their partners, to consent to one or more particular genetic interventions for their (future) child.[34] At first, such interventions will be highly experimental; as traditional bioethicists opposed to IGM have stressed, many pre-embryos will be destroyed in the process. In addition, some of the pre-embryos that survive the process of genetic intervention may be worse off rather than better off as a result of the intervention. Should a pre-embryo's imperiled condition become apparent before it is placed in a woman's womb, the woman will be faced with the decision whether to "discard" it. Depending on her moral views about the status of pre-embryos, her decision to discard will be either very easy or quite difficult. A woman who believes that life begins at conception may insist on implantation even though her IVF health care team may be strongly opposed to such an implantation. Much discussion and subsequent regulation will occur about whose responsibility it will be if the child is born in a diminished or perhaps even severely compromised condition.

Questions and decisions similar to these raised above will also present themselves if the pre-embryo is implanted in the woman's womb and its imperiled condition becomes apparent only after the gestational process is well underway. The woman will then be faced with the decision whether to have a termination, perhaps the very decision she had sought to avoid by consenting to the taxing process that IVF coupled with genetic intervention presents. In the event that the woman decides that she must continue the pregnancy, she will probably bear most of the responsibility for caring for a severely compromised child. Child-rearing tends to remain women's work, particularly when the child has serious disabilities.[35]

Over and beyond having to confront potentially difficult discard and abortion questions,[36] the woman who gestates a genetically-altered fetus may share directly in her fetus's fate. Pregnancy blends the physicality of mother and fetus in many ways, according to the physician David Perlman. He comments that:

Fetus and mother are connected via the umbilical cord and exchange blood, nutrients, waste products and antibodies, among other substances. If a retrovirus containing spliced genes is used as the vehicle for delivering genetic changes to early concepti, sperm or ova, as has been proposed and recently attempted, then women may face the danger of having their own genetic material altered by these same retroviruses ...[37]

Although in many countries women are not legally bound to bring a fetus to term that may imperil their own health or life, Perlman and other feminist bioethicists believe that many women will nonetheless feel that they should put themselves at risk for their future child (and in some countries where genetic and reproductive technologies are used, women are not legally protected in this manner). Because women's "goodness" is still measured in terms of how self-sacrificial they are, women who fail to go the "extra mile" on behalf of their (future) child are likely to be viewed as "bad" women, as I have argued elsewhere.[38]

9.3.1 Women's (and men's) parental choices: how "free" are they?

Although traditional bioethicists may not be entirely convinced that the pressure on women to sacrifice themselves for their children is as strong as some feminist bioethicists believe, there is considerable evidence that such pressure exists. Until relatively recently, it was simply assumed that a pregnant woman's interests coincided with those of her fetus, with the obvious qualification that she was not planning on aborting her fetus electively (i.e., for personal reasons unrelated to her fetus's health status or overall life possibilities). Indeed, no sacrifice seems too great for some pregnant women who, in my experience, sometimes impose behavioral restrictions on themselves that their physicians regard as unnecessary, and even submit to experimental medical procedures for the sake of their (future) child's well-being.[39] As feminist bioethicists have observed, it is precisely because most women seem willing to do *more* than necessary for their children that society is leery of women who regard their own lives as no *less* important than those of their children. Women who view themselves as just as valuable, if not more valuable than their pre-embryos, fetuses, or children are, in the estimation of feminist bioethicists, *least* likely to participate in risky genetic experimentation on their (future) child if doing so involves considerable inconveniences or even risks to themselves. They are, also in the estimation of feminist bioethicists, *most* likely to be viewed by society as "bad" women acting against their offspring's best interests.[40]

Feminist bioethicists' speculations that women who refuse to submit their (future) child, and therefore themselves, to inconvenient or even risky genetic experimentation are likely to meet with social disapproval are bolstered by the growing number of cases which challenge the decisions of pregnant women to refuse medical treatments or procedures such as caesarean sections, blood transfusions, or fetal surgeries intended to benefit their (future) children.[41] For instance in the U.S.A., despite Supreme Court rulings that have interpreted an individual's right to self-determination and bodily integrity as including an individual's right to protect his or her body from risk-inducing intrusions, lower courts are still petitioned to order involuntary caesarean sections, blood transfusions, and even fetal surgeries on pregnant women. Thus, feminist bioethicists speculate that it is only a matter of time before women are pressured to consent to gene transfer or manipulation on their IVF pre-embryos or very early implanted embryos, interventions that will put the woman as well as the child at risk.

Among the reasons that society is likely to pressure women to consent to genetic modifications for their (future) child is that many people believe there is a moral distinction between giving birth to a genetically-diseased child because the only other options were either not conceiving it at all or, subsequent to prenatal screening, aborting it,[42] and giving birth to a genetically-diseased child who could have been born genetically healthy.[43] For example, suppose that a pregnant woman wins a similar *legal* case to that won by a man who refused to donate 21 ounces of bone marrow to his dying cousin.[44] Nevertheless, women in the U.S.A. (and elsewhere) are highly unlikely to win the *moral* case (in the court of public opinion, as it were) that a pregnant woman may refuse to consent to interventions that promise to result in some positive contributions to the health of her (future) child. The point undoubtedly will be made that whereas the man's cousin had the possibility of obtaining bone marrow from an unrelated, compatible, and consenting donor, a genetically-altered pre-embryo (or implanted embryo) will never come to be born unless some woman (either the genetic mother or a gestational mother), despite possible extra risks to her own health and life, agrees to carry it to term in her womb. But even though this observation is true, is it fair to women that simply because of women's biology a society puts more pressure on women than on men to expose themselves to health and life risks?[45] Although society may judge a man who refuses to help a dying relative harshly, it will have a far harsher moral reaction to the pregnant woman who refuses to subject herself to extra risks for her (future) child. According to the psychologist Dorothy Dinnerstein, for a variety of "subterranean" reasons buried deep in the collective human psyche, society fears women and mothers who tend to be non-self-sacrificing much more than it fears men and fathers who are not self-sacrificing. Society knows that without women's willing participation as the gestators as well as the co-conceivers of human life, human life will cease. Dinnerstein argues that it is this instinctual fear that partly explains why society so often condemns insufficiently sacrificial women.[46]

9.3.2 The perfect child and the social equality questions

Feminist bioethicists are, as noted above, concerned that some pregnant women will be pressured to be more sacrificial than they actually want to be. But they are equally concerned that other pregnant women – namely, those who may *want* to take risks for the sake of their (future) children's health – will not be able to afford costly genetic interventions for them and through them for all their descendants. When informed that her embryo has a genetic disease, an economically-disadvantaged woman will have to choose either to terminate her pregnancy or to carry it to term. No matter which "choice" she makes, however, she is unlikely to be at peace with it. On the one hand, if she chooses the former course of action and aborts the embryo, she may for religious or personal reasons feel that she has taken a human life, or others may condemn her. On the other hand, if she chooses the latter course of action and carries the genetically-diseased embryo to term, she will probably bear the brunt of caring for a child with serious physically and/or mental disabilities.[47] Or, in the event she chooses to institutionalize the child, she may be condemned as an "irresponsible" woman who not only has chosen to sentence an innocent child to a "miserable" life but also expects society to pay the bills for her child. With regard to this type of issue, lawyer Margery Shaw has previously argued that:

> … parents should be held accountable to their children if they knowingly and willfully choose to transmit deleterious genes or if the mother waives her right to an abortion if, after prenatal testing, a fetus is discovered to be seriously deformed or mentally defective. They have added to the burdens of the other family members, they have incurred a cost to society, and, most importantly, they have caused needless suffering in their child …[48]

Sympathizing with economically-disadvantaged women's limited set of options, feminist bioethicists stress that in contrast to poor women, rich women will not have to choose between no life and a life limited by severe disabilities for their (future) child. Rather, should IGM become safe, effective, and widely available, they will have the option of using it for their future child and through him or her all their descendants. As soon as gene modification is adequately developed, rich women's financial resources will spare them these kinds of agonizing "choices" that poor women may have to make about their future child's destiny.

Yet, despite the fact that feminist bioethicists regard poor women's lack of access to costly genetic interventions as unfair, many do not wish to encourage women to genetically alter their (future) child, let alone abort it, simply because it has some minor imperfections. Adrienne Asch, for example, has expressed the view that if it is wrong to abort a fetus solely because it is female, because doing so sends the message to women and girls that they are not valued as highly as males, then it is also wrong to abort a fetus solely on account of its having Down syndrome, because doing so sends the message that persons with Down syndrome and other intellectual disabilities are not valued as highly as persons without these genetic limitations. Ableism, says Asch, is no less harmful than sexism.[49]

Were genetic manipulation for treatment of serious genetic disease available, Asch (and many other feminist bioethicists sharing her opinion on disability and "ableism") would probably support pregnant women voluntarily using these techniques to spare a (future) child from a serious genetic disease that makes it very difficult, though not impossible, for a person to lead a meaningful human life. Yet her writings also suggest that she would caution women against genetically altering a (future) child who has only a less severe genetic disease. Asch fears that the drive to eliminate genetic disease altogether – to give birth to normal children only – may lead society to ever greater intolerance of people perceived as "Others": as weak, ugly, or dull-witted. Asch also suspects that society probably will want to do more than genetically alter abnormal people. Gradually, it will seek to enhance "normal" people, thereby further increasing its inability to embrace as fully human any person who is less than perfect.

Because many feminist bioethicists agree with Asch that perfectionist ideas are likely to lead society down paths best left untrodden, they maintain that interventions that provide genetic enhancement should not be offered by health care professionals. As they see it, genetic enhancements are likely to increase the size of the gap that already divides the "rich" and "normal" from the "poor" and "abnormal." Moreover, they are also likely to reflect or, even worse, reinforce existing standards for attributing value to humans that typically manifest some of the worst features of our society: racism, sexism, homophobia, ableism, and so on. For example, as Maggie Little has speculated, in a worst case scenario African-American parents might request lighter skin for their prospective children. Little views such requests as morally disturbing because "the norms of appearance at issue are grounded in or get life from a broader system of attitudes and actions that are in fact *unjust.*" For African-Americans who want their children to look more white than black, the issue is probably not "some aesthetic whimsical preference,"[50] in Little's estimation. It is more likely a function of a racist history in which being black is devalued and being white is valorized. Rather than welcoming and encouraging diversity and change, genetic enhancements may drive a society toward homogeneity and the further ossification of the status quo, which is in fact unjust as it stands.

Yet despite the fact that most feminist bioethicists are opposed to using IGM (and for that matter SCGT) for enhancement purposes, this does not mean they are all or always unwilling to make exceptions. For example, feminist bioethicist Jackie Leach Scully has argued that we should not be fixated on the issue of whether a genetic intervention constitutes a treatment or an enhancement. Rather we should focus on whether the genetic intervention, be it a treatment or an enhancement, is something that increases or decreases women's and other disadvantaged groups' social equality and individual freedom.[51]

The example that Scully provides is gene transfer to lessen or cure congenital deafness. Insisting that the lifestyle in the Deaf community is a good one for children – indeed a better one than the lifestyle for children in the non-Deaf community – many members of the Deaf community are adamantly opposed to any and all interventions to "cure" Deafness. Some feminist as well as traditional bioethicists support their position on the grounds that far from being objective, definitions of the "normal" human being are socially constructed and highly subjective. "Normality," like "beauty," is in the mind of the beholder, they say,[52] and curing a (future) child of his/her "Deafness" may diminish him/her significantly as a person. However, other feminist as well as traditional bioethicists maintain that although life in the Deaf community may be good, it is limited. They also typically add the point that, ultimately, there are some limits on what can reasonably count as a "normal" way for a human being to exist. Is it, for example, "normal" for a human being not to be able to see, touch, hear, feel, smell, taste and/or think?[53] How many of these "basics" can a human being lack and still be regarded as a human being?

Although the technical debate about what counts as "normal" interests Scully, for her the real moral issue is deciding whether it is in the best interest of a (future) child to genetically cure (or not cure) its "Deafness." She suggests that our answer to this question depends on how we view the child. On the one hand, if we view the child as some sort of general abstract person, we may conclude that he/she must, by virtue of the power of definition alone, possess certain characteristics to be whole. On the other hand, if we view the child as a particular flesh-and-blood human being embedded in a complex network of human relationships, we may instead conclude that possessing trait x or y or z is not that important after all. In sum, Scully summons us, as many feminist bioethicists do, to view the self as a relational self,[54] and to ask specific questions like "Will *this* child be more socially equal and individually free if he/she is born 'Deaf' or, alternatively, not 'Deaf'?"

9.4   Conclusions

Clearly, feminist bioethicists share many of the concerns that traditional bioethicists have about genetic manipulation, particularly IGM. However, they voice these concerns in a way that focuses the moral spotlight on *women's* interests with respect to IGM. Because women's bodies are, for some time at least, more likely to be involved in reproductive gene transfer experiments than men's, feminist bioethicists view it as justified to stress women's concerns. However, raising the "woman question" is not the only contribution feminist bioethicists make to the general field of bioethics. Having played the role of the other for all too long, feminist bioethicists, like other bioethicists who write from the margins, have developed the ability to look at old bioethical issues in new ways. Their fundamental concerns are, as Scully correctly notes, about social equality and individual freedom. My own view as a feminist bioethicist is that although the jury is still out about how equalizing and liberating genetic interventions are likely to be, there is reason to think that they are unlikely to benefit all social groups equally, let alone all individuals. Thus, with respect to all genetic interventions, but particularly IGM, the most ambitious of all genetic interventions, I favor keeping the future as "open" as possible for those who come after us.

Because women and other systematically disadvantaged groups know the pain and suffering that accompanies living life not on their own terms but on others' terms, I suggest we heed the following, often-quoted admonition of bioethicist and lawyer Dena Davis:

Deliberately creating a child who will be forced irreversibly into the parents' notion of "the good life" violates the Kantian principle of treating each person as an end in herself and never as a means only ... Parental practices which close exits virtually forever are insufficiently attentive to the child as an end in herself. By closing off the child's right to an open future, they deprive the child as an entity who exists to fulfill parental hopes and dreams, not his own.[55]

From the perspective of this feminist bioethicist, there is no pressing reason for either further weakening the distinction between genetic treatments and genetic enhancements on the one hand or adopting a full-court-press approach to IGM. On the contrary, there is a real need to develop an ethics of restraint and resistance, lest we unreflectively create a future world that is even more socially unequal and individually unfree than the world in which we presently dwell.

NOTES

1 For example, see Susan Sherwin, *No Longer Patient: Feminist Ethics and Health Care.* Philadelphia: Temple University Press (1992); Mary Mahowald, *Women and Children in Health Care: An Unequal Majority.* New York: Oxford University Press (1993); Laura M. Purdy (ed.), *Reproducing Persons: Issues in Feminist Bioethics.* Ithaca, NY: Cornell University Press (1996); Susan Wolf (ed.), *Feminism and Bioethics: Beyond Reproduction.* New York: Oxford University Press (1996); and Rosemarie Tong, *Feminist Approaches to Bioethics: Theoretical Reflections and Practical Applications.* Boulder, CO: Westview Press (1997).

2 Mary B. Mahowald, *Genes, Women, Equality.* New York: Oxford University Press (2000), especially Chapter 13.

3 Jackie Leach Scully, Drawing a line: situating moral boundaries in genetic medicine, *Bioethics* 15 (2001), 189–204; and Inheritable Genetic Modification and disability: normality and identity (Chapter 10, this volume).

4 Anita Silvers, A fatal attraction to normalizing: treating disabilities as deviations from "species-typical" functioning. In: Eric Parens (ed.), *Enhancing Human Traits: Ethical and Social Implications.* Washington, DC: Georgetown University Press (1999), 95–123.

5 Parens (ed.), *Enhancing Human Traits*, Introduction.

6 According to Katharine T. Bartlett, a question becomes a method when it is regularly asked; see her Feminist legal methods. In: D. Kelly Weisberg (ed.), *Feminist Legal Theory.* Philadelphia: Temple University Press (1993), 550–70, p. 551. The so-called "woman question" has been regularly asked by feminists ever since Simone de Beauvoir raised it so forcefully in *The Second Sex,* trans. H.M. Parshley. New York: Vintage Books (1952). Why, she asked, is man the Self and women the Other? Why can man think of himself without woman, whereas she cannot think of herself without man? Why is this man's world, not woman's world? Elaborating on de Beauvoir's statement of the woman question, a variety of feminist thinkers have sharpened it into an analytical tool for the purpose of "identify(ing) the gender implications of rules and practices which might otherwise appear to be neutral or objective" (Bartlett, 555).

7 For example see Mark Lappé, Ethical issues in manipulating the human germ line, *The Journal of Medicine and Philosophy* 16 (1991), 621–32; John A. Robertson, *Children of*

Choice: Freedom and the New Reproductive Technologies. Princeton, NJ: Princeton University Press (1994).

8 Donald B. Kohn, Michael Sadelain, and Joseph C. Glorioso, Occurrence of leukaemia following gene therapy of X-linked SCID, *Nature Reviews Cancer* 3 (2003), 477–88.

9 By the end of 2004 there were almost 900 completed, ongoing or pending trials worldwide in clinical gene therapy. See http://www.wiley.co.uk/genetherapy/clinical/.

10 Alain Fischer, Salima Hacein-Bey, and Marina Cavazzana-Calvo, Gene therapy of severe combined immunodeficiencies, *Nature Reviews Immunology* 2 (2002), 615–21.

11 Assessment of adenoviral vector safety and toxicity: Report of the National Institutes of Health Recombinant DNA Advisory Committee, *Human Gene Therapy*, 13 (2002), 3–13. See also: Lynn Smith and Jacqueline F. Byers, Gene therapy in the post-Gelsinger era, *JONA'S Healthcare, Law, Ethics, and Regulation* 4 (2002), 104–10.

12 *Ibid.*

13 Edward M. Berger and Bernard Gert, Genetic disorders and the ethical status of germ-line gene therapy, *The Journal of Medicine and Philosophy* 16 (1991), 667–83.

14 Lappé, Ethical issues in manipulating.

15 Ray Moseley, Commentary: maintaining the somatic/germ-line distinction: some ethical drawbacks, *The Journal of Medicine and Philosophy* 16 (1991), 641–7.

16 Katherine Nolan, Commentary: how do we think about the ethics of human germ-line genetic therapy? *The Journal of Medicine and Philosophy* 16 (1991), 617–8.

17 Burke K. Zimmerman, Human germ-line therapy: the case for its development and use, *The Journal of Medicine and Philosophy* 16 (1991), 596–8.

18 LeRoy Walters and Julie G. Palmer, *The Ethics of Human Gene Therapy*. New York: Oxford University Press (1997).

19 Maxwell J. Mehlman and Jeffrey R. Botkin, *Access to the Genome: The Challenge to Equality*. Washington, D.C.: Georgetown University Press (1998), pp. 679–81.

20 Walters and Palmer, *Ethics of Human Gene Therapy*.

21 Moseley, Commentary, p. 643.

22 Walter Glannon, Genes, embryos, and future people, *Bioethics* 12 (1998), 187–211.

23 See Christoph Rehmann-Sutter, Controlling bodies and creating monsters: popular perceptions of genetic modifications (Chapter 4, this volume).

24 Robertson, *Children of Choice*, p. 85.

25 W. French Anderson, Human gene therapy: why draw a line? *The Journal of Medicine and Philosophy* 14 (1989), 681–93.

26 Robertson, *Children of Choice*.

27 *Ibid.*, p. 83.

28 *Ibid.*, pp. 101–8.

29 Preamble to the Constitution of the World Health Organization. Adopted by the International Health Conference held in New York from 19 June to 22 July 1946, and signed on 22 July 1946 by the representatives of sixty-one states (*Off. Rec. Wld. Hlth. Org. 2*, 100).

30 Robertson, *Children of Choice*, pp. 99–142.

31 *Ibid.*, p. 167.

32 According to many feminist bioethicists, the woman question is better understood as the gender question. They claim that feminist bioethicists need to focus on how one's gender, be it masculine or feminine, affects one's identity and status in a wide variety of contexts. However, it remains debatable within the entire feminist community whether it is advisable to substitute the gender question for the woman question. For example, Christine di Stephano points out that feminists may have something to lose in their embrace of the enriching differences of race, class, sexual preferences, ethnicity, culture, age, religion, and so on: they may lose themselves. Feminism is, after all, about women in a more basic way than it is about men; see her Dilemmas of difference. In: Linda J. Nicholson (ed.), *Feminism/Postmodernism*. New York: Routledge (1990), 63–82, especially p. 75.

33 See Joan A. Scott, Inherited genetic modification: clinical applications and genetic counseling considerations (Chapter 12, this volume).

34 Feminists insist that women are the final arbiters of their embryos' or fetuses' fates. However, many feminists add the point that because women exist in complex relation networks, they often prefer to make important decisions together with their families or friends. Thus it is not surprising that spouses and partners routinely participate in women's reproductive decision-making.

35 David Perlman, The ethics of germ-line gene therapy: challenges to mainstream approaches by a feminist critique, *Trends in Health Care, Law and Ethics* 8 (1993), 35–46, p. 44.

36 To be sure, difficult discard and abortion questions are also faced by women in present day IVF programs; but the women in these IVF programs face *less* unknowns about the likely health status of their future child than the women who initially consent to experimental gene transfer for their children will confront.

37 Perlman, Ethics of germ-line gene therapy, p. 43.

38 Rosemarie Tong, *Feminine and Feminist Ethics*. Belmont, CA: Wadsworth Publishing Co. (1982), especially pp. 80–157, on maternal ethics.

39 L. Neergaard, Tiny camera in women's uterus helps doctors do surgery on fetus, *The Charlotte Observer* 17 February 1994, 18A.

40 Tong, *Feminine and Feminist Ethics*, pp. 135–57.

41 Janet Gallagher, Fetus as patient, In: Sherrill Cohen and Nadine Taub (eds.), *Reproductive Laws for the 1990s*. Clifton, NJ: Humana Press (1988), 185–235.

42 John A. Robertson, Procreative liberty and the control of conception, pregnancy and childbirth, *Virginia Law Review* 69 (1983), 405–64, p. 449.

43 Margery W. Shaw, Conditional prospective rights of the fetus, *The Journal of Legal Medicine* 5 (1984), 63–111.

44 *McFall v. Shimp* (1978), 127 Pitts. Leg. J. (14) (Allegheny PA).

45 The *McFall* case may seem to be non-analogous due to the distance of the relationship; for references to the self-sacrifice by women more generally for children, see Roberta G. Simmons, Susan D. Klein and Richard L. Simmons, *The Gift of Life: The Social and Psychological Impact of Organ Transplantation*. New York: Wiley (1977).

46 Dorothy Dinnerstein, *The Mermaid and the Minotaur: Sexual Arrangements and Human Malaise.* New York: Harper Colophon Books (1977).

47 Eva Feder Kittay, *Love's Labor: Essays on Women, Equality, and Dependency.* New York: Routledge (1999).

48 Shaw, Conditional prospective rights, p. 111.

49 Adrienne Asch, Can aborting "imperfect" children be immoral? In: John D. Arras and Bonnie Steinbok (eds.), *Ethical Issues in Modern Medicine.* Mountain View, CA: Mayfield Publishing Company (1995), 384–8.

50 Margaret O. Little, Cosmetic surgery, suspect norms, and the ethics of complicity. In: Parens (ed.), *Enhancing Human Traits,* 163–76, p. 166.

51 Scully, Drawing a line.

52 Lennard J. Davis, *Enforcing Normalcy: Disability, Deafness, and the Body.* London: Verso (1995), pp. 1–22.

53 Arthur L. Caplan, The concepts of health, illness, and disease. In: Robert M. Veatch (ed.), *Medical Ethics.* Sudbury, MA: Jones and Burlett Publishers (1979), p. 66.

54 See Anne Donchin, Integrating bioethics and human rights: toward a global feminist approach. In: Rosemarie Tong, Anne Donchin and Susan Dodds (eds.), *Linking Visions: Feminist Bioethics, Human Rights, and the Developing World.* Lanham, MD: Rowman & Littlefield (2004).

55 Dena S. Davis, Genetic dilemmas and the child's right to an open future, *Rutgers Law Journal* 28 (1997), 549–92, pp. 569–70.

Inheritable genetic modification and disability: normality and identity

Jackie Leach Scully

10.1 Introduction

The concept of deliberate, targeted genetic intervention into the human genome has been under discussion since the early 1960s,[1] and the attendant ethical problems have been well-rehearsed in the professional and public arenas. Somatic genetic interventions in humans have been shown to be possible and to effect substantial amelioration in at least a few conditions: the first such "cure" by somatic cell gene transfer (SCGT) was announced in 1990. Although progress in the implementation of SCGT has been slower than hoped, the announcement in 2000 of significant improvement in the condition of children with X-linked severe combined immunodeficiency (SCID) treated by SCGT[2] suggested that somatic genetic intervention may yet become part of the everyday medical repertoire.[3]

The situation is rather different for inheritable genetic modification (IGM), even though IGM may actually face fewer technical difficulties in terms of gene delivery and expression than SCGT. Extensive experience of germ-line modification has been gained from the production of transgenic animals, but as far as is known there have been no attempts to use transgenic technology to modify the human genome, although therapeutic modification of the human mitochondrial genome has been successful.[4]

The abstention is primarily for ethical reasons. Since the 1970s, a professional semi-consensus on the ethics of human genetic interventions has developed. This views somatic, therapeutic (as opposed to enhancing) interventions as ethically acceptable, arguing that they involve no more than the introduction of exogenous material (genes) into an individual's body, and as such are no more ethically problematic than any other expensive, experimental therapy.[5] For germ-line or other inheritable genetic interventions, on the other hand, the majority consensus is that they are ethically unacceptable whether for therapy or enhancement. But this consensus was never absolute, and recently the voices of dissent in both the professional literature and popular discourse have become more confident.[6]

One reason for this is simply that IGM is in many ways a very attractive medical option. The ideal intervention is one that prevents a condition from occurring in the first place: direct genetic manipulation offers a way of doing this, by excising or modifying the pathologic entity, that is, the gene.[7] Other chapters in this book describe in detail IGM technologies as well as the diseases or characteristics that have been proposed as suitable candidates for IGM.[8] As LeRoy Walters and Julie Palmer note, the emphasis today is less on the overtly eugenic aim of improving the human gene pool than on specific clinical situations faced by couples making reproductive decisions.[9] It has been suggested, for example, that parents with a genetic disorder who also have moral objections to abortion, or to preimplantation genetic diagnosis (PGD) plus selection of the "right" embryos and discarding of the others, would opt for IGM as a route to having healthy children. IGM could also be contemplated in cases where the prospective parents are both homozygotic for a particular gene mutation and therefore all of the resulting embryos would be affected, or if the disease causes damage to multiple organ systems during development such that no postnatal therapy would be effective.

Unlike SCGT, which only affects the individual (except for a few rare instances in which the therapy inadvertently delivers the exogenous gene to the germ cells of the individual being treated),[10] IGM would target or modify the pathologic gene in the gametes (germ cells) or zygote, so that it would appear neither in the resulting individual nor in any offspring. IGM thus apparently presents a means of eradicating severe genetic disorders from the local or even global gene pool. Assuming that the technical difficulties of efficient and targeted insertion of the exogenous gene into the recipient genome and safe manipulation of gametes and embryos can be overcome, IGM could therefore result in the elimination of many monogenic disorders from the population. Several authors have argued it would in fact be morally negligent not to take up this opportunity.[11]

The general ethical arguments for and against IGM are well characterized, and I do not intend to repeat them here.[12] In this chapter, I consider IGM from the perspective of its anticipated consumers: people whose impairments or chronic illnesses have a genetic component. I do not consider more general ethical issues related to IGM that would have broader impacts likely to affect everyone, including disabled people. For this reason I do not discuss in detail the possible misuse of IGM for overtly eugenic aims: even though any eugenic program would be likely to target genetically-disabled people, they would not be the only ones affected or threatened by such programs. Nor will I attempt to grapple with the very complex question of whether disability is most accurately or comprehensively described by genetic, medical, social, or other explanatory models.[13] Working from the perspective of disabled people, I focus on some assumptions about normality and health, and about human embodiment and its relationship to identity, that underpin the arguments in support of IGM.

10.2   The marginal perspective of disability

Why is considering IGM from the perspective of disabled people of ethical importance? Why not simply stick to what many see as the proper task of bioethics: evaluating medical interventions to see if they adhere to generally accepted moral standards, and formulating the legislation that helps to guarantee they will? Aside from the point that any new perspective on an old field can be informative, there are two key reasons for thinking that a disability perspective on IGM is needed. First, IGM is most likely to be used as a *therapy*: it would be used to treat genetically-linked conditions thought to be associated with illness or impairment. Together with other forms of genetic medicine such as prenatal genetic testing, IGM is therefore of central relevance to people living with illness or impairment. Whether IGM is technically possible, how much it will cost, who will have access to it, and what the social consequences of its implementation will be, are all matters of intimate concern to individuals and families for whom genetic disorders are everyday reality.

The second reason to consider IGM from a disability perspective may be less obvious. Through living in/with their specific embodiment, disabled and chronically ill people have experiences that give them different perspectives on familiar concepts like normality and health – different, that is, from the perspectives of people whose embodiment is considered unproblematic. Viewed from this marginal perspective, some of the ideas about disability and normality that are the cornerstones of the IGM debate do not look quite the same.

10.2.1   Therapy and normality

The concept of normality is used to establish both the need for IGM and the limits to its implementation. Much of the literature on IGM deals with the possible existence of a slippery slope from therapy to enhancement, and then on the moral status of deliberate attempts to improve the human phenotype. This discussion tends to assume that, unlike enhancements, therapeutic IGM is necessarily less problematic *because* it is therapeutic. One of the most powerful arguments in favor of IGM is therefore the intrinsic beneficence of *any* therapeutic intervention. Authors such as Ronald Munson and Lawrence H. Davis argue that "medicine possesses a therapeutic obligation (not just permission) imposed by its own character. That is, basic to medicine as an enterprise is the *prima facie* duty to treat those who are ill in ways that will help them achieve the degree of health of which they are capable."[14] For these authors this extends to the duty to pursue and employ IGM for therapeutic purposes. In this theoretical literature, therapeutic interventions are those that "bring you from a defective state, that is, disease-producing, towards a normal state."[15] The difference I want to emphasize here is that it is not so much the precise degree of suffering or disadvantage experienced, as the fact that these are states that are culturally recognized as defects or illness, which brings the therapeutic obligation into play. It is of course undeniable that suffering and disadvantage are part of what brings a state to be considered a defect in the first place, but other, less obvious factors are also involved.

Knowing where we consider normality to begin and end is therefore crucial, because these boundaries determine which phenotypes call for an intervention to restore them to normality, and in our society that usually means which of them come within the purview of medicine. These concepts decide where, and to whom, the new knowledge of human genetics is applied. And likewise, deciding that a condition requires medical intervention is a way of signaling where the culturally determined boundary between abnormality (as disease or impairment) and normality is to be found.

Nevertheless, terms like "healthy" and "abnormality" remain poorly characterized, occupying an ambivalent position in which the definitions are both vague (at what point does social drinking become alcoholism, or sadness become clinical depression?) and overdetermined: there are numerous explanatory models available to account for the condition identified as alcoholism, or for depression, short stature, menopausal symptoms, hypoglycemia, or hyperactivity. In this confusing landscape, medicine's impressive and growing ability to measure physiologic and biochemical parameters has encouraged an understanding of disease as deviation from a standard measurement: variations in hormonal levels, or in the length of time taken to reach developmental stages, are now readily used as surrogate markers for disease itself. In the twenty-first century, as genetic loci are correlated with particular phenotypes, the presence of alleles and DNA polymorphisms that deviate from a canonical genomic norm are emerging as a new kind of surrogate marker. There is nothing wrong with using an easily discernible marker, like a blood pressure measurement or a gene sequence, as a proxy for the thing you are really interested in, such as a disease, but it is necessary to be clear that it is a *surrogate*, and the strength of the causal connection – if any – between the marker and what it stands for, should be made explicit. It is questionable whether either of these two provisos is given appropriate weight in the current proliferation of genetic markers in medicine.

The difficulty with superimposing deviation and abnormality is that phenotypic variation is the norm for any living population. Since phenotypic diversity provides the raw material for natural selection, variation is a prerequisite for adaptation (on the population rather than the individual level) to changing circumstances. In biologic terms, divergence from a genomic standard can never be equated straightforwardly with disease. At some point, phenotypic diversity crosses a line into impairment or illness – but exactly where this happens will often depend on the environmental circumstances, and in human communities on the social and medical means available to support people who function anomalously, and on cultural understandings of deviance. Labeling a deviation from a genetic norm as a problem, before the degree of disadvantage (if any) has been established, is a judgment that may be more strongly influenced by cultural habitude than the reality of the embodied experience.

10.2.2   Impaired embodiment and identity

I want now to consider in more detail the relationship between embodiment, impairment, and identity, and how IGM might affect it. Under the influence of philosophical and cultural moves that can broadly be described as postmodern, and of twentieth-century psychoanalytic developments in object relations theory, contemporary theories of the self have shifted away from the notion of a presocial, core, or "true" self towards one that sees selfhood as constructed in part or entirely through interactions with others. Recognition of the extent to which a personal self-concept is made possible by, and maintained within, relationships means that individual subjectivity is understood as *inter*subjective and relational. It is also intersectional, developing through multiple networks whose nature is defined by aspects of gender, race, class, age, and physical ability, in addition to the more contingent factors of individual biography.

It is uncontroversial that the cultures in which people grow up and live play a major role in shaping moral perception and evaluation: what counts as a moral issue and how it is handled cognitively. The epistemologic importance of embodiment, that "we think as we do because of the sorts of bodies we have and the sorts of complex relation with reality which this entails,"[16] is less familiar, and raises the possibility that the experience of a particular *embodiment* can distinguish a moral worldview. Over recent decades, feminist theory has been especially instrumental in reconceptualizing views of the moral self, in part alongside the trend already mentioned away from the socially disembedded and disembodied self of the Enlightenment tradition. Feminist theory has paid closer attention to the important contribution of *gender* to subjectivity and the development of the moral selves of women.[17]

I want to argue that the experience of a variant or anomalous embodiment might generate different interpretations of what constitutes normality, and hence differences in moral evaluation. I will consider in detail here one of the most striking examples in the context of genetic medicine: cases where some people considered disabled, notably the culturally Deaf or people with achondroplasia, claim the right to use reproductive technologies to help them to have – rather than to avoid having – children with "their" disability.

In fact, culturally Deaf people often differentiate deafness from other impairments as not being a disability at all.[18] Paddy Ladd and M. John (1991) write, "Labelling us as 'disabled' demonstrates a failure to understand that we are not disabled in any way within our own community … Many disabled people see Deaf people as belonging, with them, outside the mainstream culture. We, on the other hand, see disabled people as 'hearing' people in that they use a different language to us …"[19] The available evidence suggests that, while most culturally Deaf people either express no preference or would opt for children with unimpaired hearing,[20] some do state a clear desire to have deaf children – and may act upon it. In 2002 a case involving a Deaf lesbian couple in the U.S.A. received widespread media attention. Both partners had a congenital hearing impairment and, while they did not reject the idea of having a hearing child, they said that they felt a deaf one would be "a special gift." They therefore decided to increase their chances of having a deaf child by choosing as a sperm donor a male friend with hereditary deafness. As a result the couple now have two children, both hearing impaired.[21]

Many (although by no means all) members of the Deaf community strongly defended the couple's right to (as it was described) choose the kind of child they wanted to have. On the other hand, this reproductive decision seemed morally incomprehensible to most people outside Deaf culture.[22] Even reports that were broadly supportive used terms like "shocking."[23] By contrast, a later report that a deaf Melbourne couple planned to use PGD to ensure (and not, like the couple in the U.S.A., merely to increase their chances) they had a child with normal hearing, prompted almost no ethical debate. The local regulatory body, the Infertility Treatment Authority, was asked to decide on the legitimacy of the request because, "Some people would say deafness is a disease. Others would say that it is an unfortunate condition."[24] But there was no mention in these reports of those who see deafness as neither a disease nor bad luck, but as another way of being.

With deafness placed as a cultural identity rather than a disability, however, the couples' reproductive decision becomes markedly less bizarre. For those Deaf people whose lived experience of their body allows them to think of themselves as not-necessarily-impaired members of a linguistic minority, it is *not* self-evident that "choosing" deafness violates their child's future freedoms, any more than choosing to practice Judaism or sending the child to Eton. It is a cultural choice that, like any choice, closes off some options while opening up others. From this perspective it also becomes clearer that the preference for a hearing impaired child can be understood as expressing care for the individual,[25] if parents believe their Deaf child is more likely to grow up as the self-confident member of their flourishing community, and also care for the continued existence of the Deaf community itself, ensuring that it endures to provide support to its members.

Most of the ethical analyses, whether the conclusion was for or against the choice made, focused on competition between parental versus the child's rights, and as is often the case with rights-based arguments, were discussions of universalizable rights and harms. There was a distinct neglect of the social, and especially the biologic, contexts within which moral decisions like these are made, a lack which becomes particularly odd when we remember that it was a bodily difference that caused the dilemma to be raised in the first place, and particularly crucial if (as I suggest) it is the incompatible bits of bodily experience that make one decision obvious and the other not. In the case of the Deaf couple, most commentators worked from assumptions about the benefits of being able to hear and the problems associated with being hearing impaired. It was symptomatic of this that there was no discussion of any of the sociologic evidence that the life of a hearing child in a deaf family can have its own difficulties. Naturally, whether these difficulties are encountered or not will depend on the family characteristics and on circumstances like external support, and it might be that the disadvantages are nothing like as great as the disadvantages of being deaf. My point is that where the potential difficulties for the deaf child were *always* enumerated, the potential problems of the hearing child never were. It is as if, because a certain form of embodiment is taken as normative, the fact that it is a *specific* form, and therefore not universally unproblematic, slips out of moral sight.

But real moral agents have a biologically-particular embodiment that, combined with social and material influences, generates a specific (non-generalizable) moral terrain with its own peculiarities of meaning and value. It is from within this terrain that moral judgments are made and justified. I am suggesting that, at least in some cases and under some circumstances, the experience of disability contributes to a distinctive moral perspective. Some evidence in support of this has been provided by qualitative empirical research into the ethics of SCGT done in Switzerland.[26] The question we started with was: do those who are professionally involved in providing SCGT (medical professionals, basic research scientists) differ from its potential consumers in terms of how the associated ethical issues are perceived?[27] We interviewed medical or scientific professionals and people with multiple sclerosis (MS), cystic fibrosis (CF), a variety of skeletal dysplasias, or a hearing impairment. We found significant differences in the groups' assessments of the ethics of SCGT, some of which could be interpreted as reflecting their different experiences of disability or chronic illness. The patient groups differed among themselves in their overall attitude towards therapy in general and gene therapy in particular, with MS patients notably the most positive and Deaf or achondroplasic patients the least. Furthermore MS patients were most likely to agree with a predominantly genetic etiology, while achondroplasic and Deaf participants were least likely to see genes as "the" cause of disease. (Note that achondroplasic participants were fully aware of the genetic etiology of their *condition*, but did not consider achondroplasia to be straightforwardly a *disease*.)

But some of the clearest differences were between the medical professionals and the patient groups. For instance, medical professionals used the therapeutic imperative as an overriding positive value in their ethical evaluation (as one clinician said, "I think there is no major concern … as long as we are trying to cure diseases it's fine."). Potential patients showed more variable responses, noting the value of diversity and expressing some skepticism towards the use of the therapeutic imperative: one CF patient stated explicitly, "I think that 'to cure severe disease' is not grounds for doing everything." And when medical professionals mentioned "risk" as an ethical problem associated with gene therapy, they meant the risk of physical side effects resulting from a novel therapy. MS and CF patients also often spoke of risk, but their understanding of the term was broader. It included disruption to the often precarious equilibrium of their daily lives – what treatment might mean in terms of travel commitments, childcare arrangements, tiredness, time off work, and so on.

Particularly relevant to the discussion here is the very different stance towards disability and identity. Unlike any of the medical professionals, several patients expressed a profound sense that, in both its negative and positive aspects, disability could be an irreplaceable part of a person's identity. We have hypothesized that it is precisely this awareness of the part a disabled embodiment plays in generating *who I am*, that lies behind the fact that some patients found SCGT *less* morally acceptable than termination of a pregnancy, on the grounds that "it's the biggest decision you can make, to change a life, even bigger than ending a life."

The fact that disabled experience cannot be reduced to a singular phenomenon was also pointed up by the variations between patient groups here. Some patients, especially those with MS, perceived the condition as a disruption of their "real" identity and always described it as unwanted, negative, and not part of the self. Others saw their condition as something without which they would not *be* themselves. Achondroplasic and Deaf participants were most likely to describe their impairment as part of their identity, and in fact all the Deaf interviewees also said that they saw their deafness as a *positive* part of themselves. For many people with impaired hearing, whether they grew up in the community or came to it later on, identification with a culturally and political strong Deaf community grounds some of the most satisfying aspects of their lives. It is likely that this consciousness contributed to the uniquely high moral priority that our Deaf participants gave to the risk of estrangement from the Deaf community if they were "cured."

This sense of a condition as a component of identity rather than an identity-deforming problem was unfamiliar to the medical professionals interviewed. None suggested it spontaneously, and when asked what they thought about it as a possibility, they generally expressed surprise or skepticism.

10.2.3   IGM and identity

These findings about attitudes to SCGT are significant, because the question of what a genetic intervention does to individual identity has played a major part in the ethical evaluation of IGM. Germ-line or early somatic interventions have been depicted as a morally more acceptable route to "choosing the kind of people we want to have" than prenatal screening (genetic or otherwise) followed by abortion. Among disability activists, selective termination (selection against fetal abnormalities or defects) has long been considered a potential source of discrimination against disabled people.[28] Some (not all) people with disabilities have argued that offering termination of pregnancy after testing or screening is in direct conflict with the fetus' right to life, and that this is a right that should not be compromised purely because the fetus has an identifiable impairment. Essentially, the ethical question in this situation is the following one: if an impairment is detected prenatally, is it better that this individual not exist at all?[29] Many disabled people strongly contest the assumption that the medical conditions for which genetic testing and termination are offered inevitably result in so poor a quality of life that the individual would be better off not living.

At first IGM appears to offer a happy alternative to selective abortion. The individual is not destroyed, but rather some of its constituents are altered. For example, consider a zygote that undergoes highly efficient gene transfer to compensate for, or even by homologous recombination remove, an allele coding for a mutated dystrophin protein. The zygote remains alive, and we generally assume that it remains the same person. In this case the moral problem of abortion disappears: nobody dies, and the right to life of the embryo is no longer a relevant matter.

But does the modified individual really remain the same person? In popular culture, genetic manipulation is often depicted as the cause of disruption to the identity, as in the production of human–animal hybrids with a mixture of characteristics.[30] Some of the philosophical literature, mostly considering hypothetical interventions that result in major and unprecedented phenotypic shifts, discusses the possibility that a genetic intervention *in itself* ends the existence of a particular person.[31] Because the extent of change involved in the repair of monogenic disorders, that is the actual percentage of the total genome that ends up modified, is small and leaves an overwhelming proportion of the genome unchanged, it seems generally to be concluded that issues of identity do not come into play. In other words, if we have Alex (with a mutant CF allele) and Alex (without a mutant CF allele), changing the terms within the parentheses leaves us with the same old Alex.

This argument relies on a model in which identity is essentially a function of genomic content: the genetic change is insignificant, and *therefore* the change to the individual is insignificant as well. Probably few of the people who find this plausible would also argue that an individual's biologic, psychologic, and social self is entirely derived from his or her genetic constitution. Nevertheless, to conclude that monogenic change is not a cause for concern *because* it is too minor to effect profound change in the whole organism entails a belief that genetic change is the one to worry about – otherwise, the number of gene loci altered would be neither here nor there. This premise itself is vulnerable to challenge.

But as was discussed above, there are models of identity that understand selfhood not as an essential, core component of an organism, whether derived from the genome or something else, but as constructed in relationship with and to others. A corollary of this is that identity depends very much on the nature of the relationships open to you, and that this in turn depends on how others perceive you. In effect, who other people *say* that you are has a profound influence on who you end up knowing that you are. So according to these models, a germ-line change to remove or repair a CF gene would indeed produce a different individual, not immediately through the effect of the altered genetic constitution on the phenotypic self, but through the effect of the altered phenotype on the development of selfhood over time. What is produced is a person who is born and grows up, not as Alex with the condition of CF but as Alex *without* the condition of CF. And these two Alexes are different – increasingly so as time goes on. As with selective termination, the consequence of IGM is the erasure of a *particular* potential individual. The difference is that in the case of IGM, the original biologic organism persists.

It might be argued that this actually holds for *any* form of therapeutic intervention (including SCGT). *Any* successful therapy will alter the life of the individual being treated. The lived experience of chronic asthmatics before the invention of bronchodilators was very different from that of asthmatics today. Their lives were so shaped by periodic incapacity, the need to avoid the triggers of asthmatic attacks, developing strategies to survive an attack and so on, that we might say that the end result was a significantly different person. So Monica (plus salbutamol) is not the same as Monica (without salbutamol). If alteration of identity through the alteration of lived experience is a problem, morally or otherwise, then all therapies become ethically worrying, which is contrary to our moral tradition and also to common sense.

However, there are important differences between the consequences of IGM and of other therapies, which are related to time and the experience of a particular body's capacities. Even where a successful postnatal therapy (conventional or SCGT) is instituted, the person concerned will have spent some time in an embodied form undergoing the lived experience of that condition. By contrast, IGM, involving as it does manipulation of the gametes or early embryo, effectively prevents the condition *ever* forming part of that individual's embodied experience. Furthermore, in many – though not all – cases, somatic treatment of a disability or chronic illness is reversible: the individual could stop taking the tablets, discard the inhaler and so on, and return to the ill state. This option has been removed from the set of choices open to the individual whose germ line has been manipulated. It is not possible for her to re-establish her "sick" identity, should she wish to do so.

This argument is not an attempt to say that alleviating a condition is always wrong because it alters an individual's selfhood, nor that we should endeavor to preserve an individual from experiences that might change her self-concept. An interior sense of identity evolves throughout an individual's life, through the multiplicity of experiences and interactions with others that she undergoes. She may consciously choose some experiences – education, marriage, learning a foreign language, going to a rock festival – because she believes that she will not be quite the same person as she would have been without them, and indeed such conscious manipulation of selfhood tends to be applauded in our society as "taking control of one's life." I only suggest here that both SCGT and IGM should be recognized as means of manipulating – to differing degrees – the identity of the individual. Unlike many types of SCGT, the manipulation in IGM is irreversible.

And, since the use of IGM is likely to be restricted to the treatment of severe abnormalities (at least at first), the result of the manipulation is intended to be a very different lived experience – different enough to produce, by this analysis, a different person.

10.2.4   Preserving disabled identity?

But why should this be a problem? IGM will be offered to cure diseases or disabilities. Even if it involves the erasure of Alex with CF in favor of Alex without CF, surely any reasonable person would find no moral difficulty here. Most of us prefer to minimize the amount of suffering in our lives, and conditions like CF unarguably involve significant suffering.

But the empirical data from our study discussed above suggest that *at least some* disabled people consider their impairment to be a strong, and strongly positive, part of their identity. This was particularly true for Deaf participants who identified with both their condition ("Isn't the hearing impairment a part of me, something that constitutes my being too?") and the social group associated with it ("[Eradication of hearing impairment] would be very sad! Deaf culture and sign would disappear, and that would be a real loss"). But it was also noteworthy that not even all the people with CF who we interviewed saw their CF experience as entirely negative ("(Scientists) just want to get rid of suffering and death, and for me that's not right").

From such a perspective, the germ-line erasure of the potential disabled identity (or the somatic modification of a child's or adult's disabled identity) may be judged to be of as much moral consequence as the eradication of the person through prenatal testing and abortion.

These considerations raise the question of the trade-off between the good of diversity and the evil of suffering. Twentieth-century western history can be read as a series of incomplete attempts to come to terms with human diversity, local *and* global; within this narrative, the past and present treatment of disabled people shows that we are generally not very good at accommodating to the diversity of corporeal forms. IGM and other forms of genetic medicine may provide us with a seemingly morally unproblematic – at least when compared with selective termination or PGD – way of controlling, or giving the illusion of controlling, variant embodiment. Clearly, extremes of genetic variation leading to neonatal death, multisystemic abnormality, or profound intellectual impairment indubitably cause suffering or distress; I am not attempting here to redescribe them as neutral phenotypic variations. But less extreme forms of variant embodiment may not entail suffering, or not in the way that non-disabled people might expect. The phenomenology of variant forms – what it is really like to live with them – is severely under-researched and under-theorized. The key point in this context is that, precisely because there is so little genuine accommodation to variant embodiment, we have very little idea of the extent to which people with impairments would be disadvantaged if society were not, in itself, disabling. Knowing as little as we do about the lived experience of variant embodiments, then, we cannot rule out the possibility that there may be aspects of impairment which people or communities might wish not to lose. We are still too ignorant about the meaning of most genetic impairments to push enthusiastically for their germ-line eradication.

10.3   Some consequences of IGM for disability

IGM and other genetic medical interventions allow us to act upon our cultural beliefs about the (dis)value of embodiments that transgress the limits to normality. The practical consequences are likely to impact on disabled people – as pre-eminent sites of variant embodiment – first and perhaps most profoundly. Among the potential consequences are the message delivered by the IGM commitment; the medicalized extension of the category "disabled"; and the reinforcement of normalization, each of which I discuss in turn.

10.3.1   The expressivity of the IGM commitment

A societal commitment to IGM indicates a preference for (a) some phenotypes over others, and (b) the selection of some phenotypes via genetic manipulation. If IGM were to be taken up in by a significant portion of the population, it might have a negative impact on the overall levels of genetic diversity of the population (though this is debated),[32] but it is unlikely to have that much effect on the extent of impairment or disability in society, since most impairments are not genetically-based. Furthermore, as indicated previously, many theorists find the roots of disablement to be social rather than biologic or genetic. Nevertheless, the *attitudinal* impact of a commitment to IGM would be far-reaching. IGM is a highly contentious technology, the potential risks of which have been repeatedly rehearsed in the professional literature and in public debate. The consensus of opinion up to now has been that IGM is ethically unacceptable for the types of cases that have so far been proposed. And so, if (or when) it is eventually permitted in order to change a particular phenotype, the permission in itself sends out a strong message that *that* phenotype is unacceptable – so unacceptable, in fact, that society is willing to face all the ethical risks of safety to the patient, of increased social polarization, or of stepping onto the slippery slope to overt genetic engineering, in order to eradicate it.

I call this an "expressivist" argument by analogy with the claims about the message sent through selective abortion of impaired fetuses. In addition to their direct consequences, human acts have intrinsic meanings that are readable by the individual or the collective, and which can sometimes be of more importance than the obvious causal effects. The disability critique of selective abortion after detecting a prenatal impairment is that this act "sends a message" that a life with this or similar impairments is not worth living.[33] A number of critics from both inside and outside the disability field have reasoned that, for this to happen, the act must communicate an unambiguous message to a recipient audience. They have questioned whether existing models of communication allow a selective abortion to "say" anything at all.[34] It is by no means certain that decisions made on the part of *individual* patients would be generally understood as a "message," and in fact the biggest flaw in the expressivist argument is the lack of empirical evidence to prove that anything of the kind occurs. I have argued elsewhere[35] that the effectiveness of the expressivist argument, in other words the expressivity of an act, depends less on whether there is intent to send out a message, or on whether there is an accepted code for transmitting it, than on the context in which the act is perceived and interpreted.

But supposing that the decision to implement IGM is indeed interpreted in this way, then the consequences might realistically include decreased acceptance of the presence of disabled persons, since they "need not have happened." There is some evidence that mothers are more likely to be blamed for the birth of children with congenital impairments if prenatal genetic screening is available.[36] A similar attitudinal change following IGM could lead to practical reductions in healthcare provision or societal accommodation for what are perceived as avoidable conditions.

10.3.2   Extension of the category

Many recent authors have raised the possibility that genetic interventions could increase socioeconomic stratification, or lead to the development of new subclasses or ultimately of two species. But once we start to question the assumptions behind the definition of disability, another element emerges. If germ-line or somatic interventions aimed at *enhancement* are permitted, the result could be the creation of a new category of disadvantaged people: those who remain unenhanced. One potential consequence would be to enlarge the category of "disabled" to include people who today would be classified as normal or able-bodied. Shifting a large number of people, perhaps even the majority, into some category of disability is likely to be intolerable both economically and psychosocially. For one thing, it is hard to imagine any healthcare system that could cope effectively with such an increased demand. Psychosocially, stigmatizing great swathes of the population as impaired would have far-reaching consequences. It is possible to visualize this situation leading to greater division between impairments (if, for example, the "new disabled" had greater lobbying power); greater exclusion of those at the bottom of the heap as they are left even further behind; and the domination of social discourse about disability by the voices and needs of the "new disabled" – at the cost of those whose impairments are severe enough to make them always the most vulnerable to exclusion.

10.3.3   Reinforcement of (genetic) normalization

As I indicated earlier, therapeutic interventions are generally seen as ethically less problematic than enhancements. But basing the ethical permissibility of a genetic intervention on whether it can be classed as a therapy or an enhancement has some invidious consequences. IGM is likely to be used first for interventions that are clearly therapeutic. Thereafter, its continued use will demand decisions about whether any given intervention is therapeutic or enhancing, and for these judgments to be made there always needs to be a commonly agreed reference point of normality. Once that point is set, therapy can straightforwardly be defined as any intervention that brings an individual from the region of subnormality into the region of normality, while enhancements are interventions that take her into the region of super-normality – increased height or muscle strength, or improved memory.

The heuristic move of superimposing the boundary between morally permissible and impermissible interventions on the normal/abnormal boundary only works if a standard of nonvariant embodiment is taken as the norm. Since genetic medicine, including IGM, prioritizes the genotype as the foundation of health and normality, it is foreseeable that normal embodiment will also become defined in terms of a canonical genome sequence. My point here is not to deny the existence of limitations, but to show that we cannot class some genetic interventions as therapy and others as enhancements without having an objectively defined contour of normality. This tells us which attributes are normal, and so lacking them means we call what you need therapy, but others are not normal and so obtaining them is an enhancement. Reifying a conceptual boundary in this way will substantially reinforce the idea that there are two groups of people, normal and not-normal, and that we can easily tell them apart. A more subtle point is that for people with variant or disabled embodiments, especially when these are congenital or hereditary, it is *their* embodied experience that is normative. An intervention that brings an anomalously short person up into the range of normal height does not make him or her normal; what it gives is a height that is normal for most other people. From the point of view of the short person this might better be characterized as an enhancement (or even a harm, if the alteration turned out to be damaging or intolerable). So one consequence of making the therapy/enhancement boundary do triple-duty as the morally permissible/impermissible *and* as the abnormal/normal one is to necessitate the exclusion of some people's experience of variation.

In concrete terms, as IGM will inevitably be associated with the elaboration of guidelines, regulations, and laws, the boundary line between therapy and enhancement (between legally permissible and impermissible interventions) will then become incorporated into public policy and legislation. As this boundary will also be serving as the line between normal and abnormal embodiment, the end results could be a legal definition of human normality becoming enshrined in the statute books. This would be unprecedented in international law. Even the corresponding laws regulating selective abortion refer to what is abnormal rather than attempting to define normality (and in many cases a substantial amount of leeway is left for subjectively interpreting what "abnormal" might be). In order for a law to regulate therapy and enhancement it must define what its authors take to be normal, because they will be defining what an enhancement of normal would be. Here technical definition takes on a political power by defining whose needs are legitimate and whose should not exist, and the political and social implications of this for disabled people are enormous.[37]

10.4   Conclusions: disability and bioethics

I have argued that the disability perspective is worth taking into account for two major reasons: because disabled and chronically ill people are among those on whom IGM and similar technologies will have the greatest and most immediate impact, and because the novel perspectives of disabled people, with regard to identity and other aspects of human life, offer new insights into (over)familiar bioethical debates. Both of these are good enough reasons for bioethics to take the perspectives of disabled people seriously, to investigate bioethical questions from this currently marginalized standpoint.

A third reason, however, is that it is the right thing to do. The inclusion of disabled people here is a question of justice. It is no longer tenable to imagine that the ethical norms generated from within a few social niches, with their limitations of standpoint, give adequate voice to the interests of all agents in society. Normative morality is generated by a discursive process undertaken in particular contexts; it is therefore necessary to ensure that the ethical evaluations made within different contexts, other than those which are customarily heard, are brought into the discourses that eventually make the rules. For evaluative processes to be just, they need to include the perspectives of disabled people as well. The historical, and present, reality is that the ethical evaluation of all forms of genetic medicine, including IGM, has been undertaken without inviting those most affected to participate. This exclusion ought to be a cause for concern to all bioethicists and policymakers interested in the creation of just societies, and the just use of IGM.

NOTES

1 John C. Fletcher, Evolution of ethical debate about human gene therapy, *Human Gene Therapy* 1 (1990), 55–68.

2 Marina Cavazzana-Calvo, *et al.*, Gene therapy of human severe combined immunodeficiency (SCID)-XI disease, *Science* 288 (2000), 669–72; W. French Anderson, The best of times, the worst of times, *Science* 288 (2000), 627–9.

3 Subsequent problems in this clinical trial, including the development of leukaemia in some of the children, have since raised more question marks about the general clinical feasibility of SCGT. See Charles Marwick, FDA halts gene therapy trials after leukaemia case in France, *British Medical Journal* 326 (2003), 81; European Society of Human Genetics press release, 18 January 2003.

4 See Jason A. Barritt, Carol A. Brenner, Henry E. Malter, *et al.*, Mitochondria in human offspring derived from ooplasmic transplantation: brief communication, *Human Reproduction* 16 (2001), 513–6.

5 This does not make them entirely ethically unproblematic either. As with any other innovative therapeutic intervention, there are substantial ethical issues to do with the risk/benefit balance, the choice of patients, and the allocation of healthcare and research resources; furthermore, somatic interventions to *enhance* human capabilities occupy a more ambiguous moral area than clearly therapeutic ones.

6 See, for example, Robert M. Cook-Deegan, Robert H. Blank, Ruth Chadwick, *et al.*, Symposium: regulating germ-line gene therapy, *Politics and the Life Sciences* 13 (1994), 217–48; Gregory Stock and John Campbell, *Engineering the Human Germline: An Exploration of the Science and Ethics of Altering the Genes We Pass to Our Children.* New York: Oxford University Press (2000).

7 I am ignoring here the questions of how much genetic and non-genetic factors interact with each other, and the extent to which the phenotypic expression of even "classic" monogenic disorders such as cystic fibrosis (CF) are under polygenic and non-genetic influence.

8 For example, John E.J. Rasko and Doug Jolly, The science of inheritable genetic modification (Chapter 2, this volume).

9 LeRoy Walters and Julie G. Palmer, *The Ethics of Human Gene Therapy.* New York: Oxford: Oxford University Press (1997), p. 77.

10 Christoph Rehmann-Sutter, Germ line risks of somatic gene therapy – an ethical issue. In: Stefan Müller, Jürgen W. Simon, and Jan W. Vesting (eds.), *Interdisciplinary Approaches to Gene Therapy: Legal, Ethical and Scientific Aspects.* Heidelberg: Springer Verlag (1997), 259–67.

11 For example, Ronald Munson and Lawrence H. Davis, Germ-line gene therapy and the medical imperative, *Kennedy Institute of Ethics Journal* 2 (1992), 137–58; Walters and Palmer, *The Ethics of Human Gene Therapy.*

12 See, for instance, Walters and Palmer, *The Ethics of Human Gene Therapy;* Eric Parens (ed.), *Enhancing Human Traits: Ethical and Social Implications.* Washington, DC: Georgetown University Press (1998).

13 For discussions of these points, see Mike Oliver, *The Politics of Disablement.* Basingstoke: Macmillan (1990); Mike Oliver, *Understanding Disability: From Theory to Practice.* Basingstoke: Macmillan (1996); Colin Barnes, The social model of disability: a sociological phenomenon ignored by sociologists? In: Tom Shakespeare (ed.), *The Disability Reader: Social Science Perspectives.* London: Cassell (1998), 65–78; Mairian Corker, Differences, conflations and foundations: the limits to "accurate" theoretical representations of disabled peoples' experience? *Disability and Society* 14 (1999), 627–42; Carol Thomas, *Female Forms: Experiencing and Understanding Disability.*

Buckingham: Open University Press (1999); Jackie Leach Scully, A postmodern disorder: moral encounters with molecular models of disability. In: Mairian Corker and Tom Shakespeare (eds.), *Disability/Postmodernity: Embodying Disability Theory.* London: Cassell (2002), 48–61.

14 Munson and Davis, Germ-line gene therapy, p. 155.

15 W. French Anderson, Genetic engineering and our humanness, *Human Gene Therapy* 5 (1994), 755–60, p. 759.

16 Terry Eagleton, *The Ideology of the Aesthetic.* Oxford: Basil Blackwell (1990), 235.

17 See, for example, Eva Feder Kittay and Diana Tietjens Meyers (eds.), *Women and Moral Theory.* Totowa, NY: Rowman and Littlefield (1987); Iris Marion Young, *Throwing Like a Girl and Other Essays in Feminist Philosophy and Social Theory.* Bloomington: Indiana University Press (1990); Susan Bordo, *Unbearable Weight.* Berkeley: University of California Press (1993); Judith Butler, *Bodies that Matter.* New York: Routledge (1993); Diana Tietjens Meyers, *Subjection and Subjectivity.* New York: Routledge (1994); Susan J. Hekman, *Moral Voices, Moral Selves.* University Park: Pennsylvania State University Press (1995); Diana Tietjens Meyers (ed.), *Feminists Rethink the Self.* Boulder, CO: Westview Press (1997).

18 Harlan Lane, *The Mask of Benevolence: Disabling the Deaf Community.* San Diego: DawnSignPress (1999).

19 Paddy Ladd and M. John, Deaf people as a minority group: the political process. In: *Issues in Deafness.* Milton Keynes: Open University Press (1991), 14–5.

20 S.J. Stern, K. Oelrich, K.S. Arnos, *et al.*, The attitudes of deaf and hearing individuals towards genetic testing of hearing loss, *Journal of Medical Genetics* 39 (2002), 449–53; Anna Middleton, Jenny Hewison, and Robert Mueller, Prenatal diagnosis for inherited deafness – what is the potential demand? *Journal of Genetic Counselling* 10 (2001), 121–31.

21 Liza Mundy, A world of their own, *The Washington Post Magazine*, 31 March 2002, W22.

22 See, for example, Dena S. Davis, Genetic dilemmas and the child's right to an open future, *Hastings Center Report* 27 (1997), 7–15.

23 Mundy, A world of their own.

24 Robyn Riley, Pair seeks IVF deaf gene test, *Herald Sun* 30 June 2002, 3.

25 Jackie Leach Scully, Disabled embodiment and an ethic of care. In: *Bioethics – Interdisciplinary Challenges in Cultural Contexts*, C Rehmann-Sutter, Markus Düwell and Dietmar Mieth (eds), Dortmund: Kluwer (2005), 247–261.

26 Jackie Leach Scully, Christine Rippberger, and Christoph Rehmann-Sutter, Additional ethical issues in genetic medicine perceived by the potential patients. In: Bartha Maria Knoppers (ed.), *Populations and Genetics: Legal and Socioethical Perspectives.* Leiden/Boston: Martinus Nijhoff Publishers (2003), 623–38; Jackie Leach Scully, Christine Rippberger, and Christoph Rehmann-Sutter, Non-professionals' evaluations of gene therapy ethics, *Social Science and Medicine* 58 (2004), 1415–25.

27 For other public surveys on related technologies, see Joan A. Scott, Inheritable genetic modification: clinical applications and genetic counseling considerations (Chapter 12, this volume).

28 Eric Parens and Adrienne Asch, *Prenatal Testing and Disability Rights*. Washington, DC: Georgetown University Press (2000).

29 I phrase the question in this way because in the present discussion I want to avoid trying to disentangle whether the question is really about benefit to the individual, or to the mother, family, or society, or a mixture of all of those.

30 See Françoise Baylis and Jason Scott Robert, Radical rupture: exploring biological sequelae of volitional inheritable genetic modification (Chapter 7, this volume); Christoph Rehmann-Sutter, Controlling bodies and creating monsters: popular perceptions of genetic modifications (Chapter 4, this volume).

31 Noam J. Zohar, Prospects for "genetic therapy" – can a person benefit from being altered? *Bioethics* 5 (1991), 275–7; Robert Elliott, Identity and the ethics of gene therapy, *Bioethics* 7 (1993), 27–40.

32 Hans-Jakob Müller, Treatment of human disorders with gene therapy and its consequences for the human gene pool. In: Klaus Wöhrmann and Jürgen Tomiuk (eds.), *Transgenic Organisms*. Basel: Birkhäuser Verlag (1993), 229–44.

33 See Adrienne Asch, Reproductive technology and disability. In: Sherrill Cohen and Nadine Taub (eds.), *Reproductive Laws for the 1990s*. Clifton, NJ: Humana Press (1988), 69–124; Deborah Kaplan, Prenatal screening and its impact on persons with disabilities, *Fetal Diagnosis and Therapy* 8 (1993), 64–9; Nancy Press, Assessing the expressivist character of prenatal testing; the choices made or the choices made available? In: Erik Parens and Adrienne Asch (eds.), *Prenatal Testing and Disability Rights*. Washington, DC: Georgetown University (2000), 214–33.

34 See Eva Feder Kittay with Leo Kittay, On the expressivity and ethics of selective abortion for disability: conversations with my son. In: Erik Parens and Adrienne Asch (eds.), *Prenatal Testing and Disability Rights*. Washington, DC: Georgetown University (2000), 165–95; Allan Buchanan, Choosing who will be disabled: genetic intervention and the morality of inclusion, *Social Philosophy and Policy* 13 (1996), 18–46; James Lindemann Nelson, Prenatal diagnosis, personal identity, and disability, *Kennedy Institute of Ethics Journal* 10 (2000), 213–28; James Lindemann Nelson, The meaning of the act: reflections on the expressivist force of reproductive decision making and policies. In: Erik Parens and Adrienne Asch (eds.), *Prenatal Testing and Disability Rights*. Washington, DC: Georgetown University (2000), 196–213.

35 Jackie Leach Scully, Assisted reproductive technologies and the expressivist argument. In: Manuela Rossini and Elizabeth Zemp (eds.), *Gender Matters/Gender Talks: Gender Studies at the Interface of Biology, Medicine, the Social Sciences and the Humanities*. Basel: Karger (in press).

36 Theresa M. Marteau and Harriet Drake, Attributions for disability: the influence of genetic screening, *Social Science and Medicine* 40 (1995), 1127–32; Rosemarie Tong, Traditional and feminist bioethical perspectives on gene transfer: is inheritable genetic modification really *the* problem? (Chapter 9, this volume).

37 For more detailed discussion, see Jackie Leach Scully and Christoph Rehmann-Sutter, When norms normalize: the case of genetic enhancement, *Human Gene Therapy* 12 (2001), 87–96.

Regulating inheritable genetic modification, or policing the fertile scientific imagination? A feminist legal response

Isabel Karpin and Roxanne Mykitiuk

11.1 Introduction

The past few years have seen an explosion of legislative activity around developments in genetics and assisted reproduction. In this chapter we examine recently passed legislation in Australia and Canada in the area of genetic modification technologies and reproductive genetics. We demonstrate that legislative control in this area has a twofold purpose. Less controversially it is aimed at providing limits to scientific innovation for the purpose of ensuring safe and ethical research and experimentation. More controversially it is concerned with what should be the proper "nature of reproduction," namely, how it happens (sexually), between whom (a man and a woman, both human), in what kinds of relationships (heterosexual), such that progeny, the product of reproduction, inherit the blood/genes (bodily substances) of only two biological progenitors. It is to this latter purpose that we turn our attention in this chapter, analyzing the role of law in limiting, determining, and constituting reproductive possibilities in an age of genetic modification. Our focus is on new and potential technologies that enable inheritable genetic modification (IGM) of humans, but we read these, and their legislative limits, in the context in which they appear medically and legally, namely alongside other assisted reproductive technologies (ARTs) such as reproductive cloning. We ask what is at stake in the new legislative limits, who benefits, who loses, and what kinds of humans are we left with?

11.2 The nature of reproduction

Beginning in the 1970s, it became routine to screen pregnant women in high-risk groups using blood tests, sonograms, and other, more invasive techniques. Amniocentesis and chorionic villus sampling (CVS) are now used to detect fetuses with anomalies, and therapeutic abortions are offered to women whose

fetuses express chromosomal abnormalities. More recently, people have begun
to use *in vitro* fertilization (IVF), coupled with preimplantation genetic diagnosis
(PGD) and selective abortion. Those who are at a serious risk of passing on an
undesired genetic condition have the option of using PGD to identify embryos
without the condition for implantation.

IGM techniques represent the next stage in ARTs. Instead of aborting affected
fetuses or deciding not to implant those embryos identified as carrying a
genetic mutation, it may be possible to prevent the development of an affected
fetus through IGM. While this is only one of the many ways in which IGM
might be utilized, it is clear that any legislation prohibiting or regulating its use
will impact on reproduction. It is no coincidence, therefore, that the only documented instance of human IGM that has occurred so far is in the context
of reproduction, namely IVF. Researchers at the Institute of Reproductive
Medicine and Science of St Barnabas in New Jersey undertook a controversial
procedure known as ooplasmic transplantation. The process, which has led to
30 births, is now known to have resulted in children who have a small quantity
of additional mitochondrial DNA not inherited from either parent.[1] We will
discuss this case in more detail later in the chapter. Legislation in Australia and
Canada has recently made such procedures illegal.[2]

We argue that regulatory discourses around IGM inevitably affect the nature
of reproduction. The most common type of IGM is germ-line modification.
Germ-line modification epitomizes the connection between reproduction and
genetics as it is conventionally understood. It involves the manipulation of
genetic material in the germ cells themselves, that is, the reproductive cells of an
organism, the sperm, and egg cells. Germ-line modification can also include, in
some definitions, the early 8-cell stage embryo which, when genetically altered,
will probably develop with that alteration in all its cells including the germ
cells. It may also refer to the cells of the embryo that will ultimately develop into
the sperm or egg cells. The technique to which germ-line modification is often
ethically, socially, and scientifically compared is somatic cell gene transfer
(SCGT) which, it is argued, affects only the individual being treated.

The view that somatic cells and germ-line cells are not only distinct but have
completely different trajectories is sometimes offered as scientific fact. Somatic
cells, it is said, cannot be passed from one generation to another and therefore
have a finite life. Germ-line cells, on the other hand, have the potential to be
endlessly passed along to future generations. On the basis of this scientific distinction, some ethicists and state regulatory regimes make an ethical distinction between interventions that modify the germ line compared with those
that modify somatic cell lines. SCGT is viewed as less problematic since, it is
argued, only the person who is the subject of the intervention can hope to benefit from it (or be harmed by it) now and in the future. We suggest, however,
that the distinction relies on a particular construction of identity and reproduction that need not be, and should not be, assumed. Take for instance the

example offered by W. French Anderson, an advocate of SCGT. He describes the difference as follows:

Inserting a gene into somatic cells affects only the patient being treated, similar to when a patient undergoes surgery, takes a medication, or receives a limb prosthesis. However, with germ-line gene therapy (GLGT), a gene is inserted into the DNA of an egg or sperm so that children of the patient will have the inserted gene.[3]

Despite the apparent simplicity of the statement that SCGT affects only the patient being targeted, the kind of therapy that Anderson himself proposes belies it. He intends to cure adenosine deaminase (ADA) deficiency by a direct injection of a retroviral vector carrying a normal copy of the human ADA gene into 13–15-week fetuses. Of course there is no way to "directly" inject a 13–15-week fetus. Rather, injection must occur indirectly through the mother's body.

Clearly, then, at least in the case of *in utero* SCGT, it is nonsense to suggest that only the individual who is being treated is affected.[4] It would be easy, of course, to dismiss this as irrelevant because the essential distinction is at the cellular level. However, this distinction relies on a molecularization of human identity that is not appropriate. In the case of a pregnant woman, there is no separate person until the fetus is born. Up until that time, even though there may be the capacity to identify different cellular components, those components are nevertheless inextricably integrated. The relationship has been described by one of us (IK) as "not-one-but-not-two."[5] Somatic individuals then are not always just that.[6] The erasure of the female body and person in both scientific and legal discourse about genetics is something we find very troubling, particularly when the link is made between genetics and reproduction. We will return to this point in our examination of the legislation in Australia and Canada.

Scientific facts then are themselves disputable. The purported factual distinction between SCGT and IGM is itself founded upon assumptions about the "nature of reproduction." For instance, arguments made by John Harris suggest that were we to permit reproductive cloning, the factual distinction between GLGT and SCGT would be undermined by the capacity to turn those very same somatic cells into germ cells:

… inserting the mature nucleus of an adult cell into a de-nucleated egg turns cells thus formed into germ-line cells. This has three important effects. First, it effectively eradicates the firm divide between the germ-line and somatic-line nuclei because each adult cell nucleus is, in principle, "translatable" into a germ-line cell nucleus by transferring its nucleus and creating a clone. Secondly, it permits somatic line modifications to human cells to become germ-line modifications … If you … cloned a permanently genetically modified bone marrow cell … the modified genome would be passed to the clone and become part of his or her genome, transmissible to her offspring indefinitely through the germ-line … The third effect is that it shows the oft asserted moral divide between germ-line and somatic-line therapy to be even more ludicrous than was previously supposed.[7]

In an attempt to overcome the limits of this distinction, scientists and others now refer to IGM rather than using the more limited term "germ-line modification." Mark Frankel states, for instance, that IGM "encompasses modifications both of nuclear and of extra-nuclear genomes, and modifications that are inadvertent side effects of other, deliberate genetic interventions (of, for example SCGT)."[8] The moral divide becomes that between heritability and non-heritability, which in turn becomes the basis of a distinction embedded in recent legislation in Australia and Canada.

The purported ethical or moral distinction that has been erected rests on assumptions about the "nature" of reproduction. As we noted at the outset, legislative impulses are also geared towards ensuring that the old parameters of reproduction, so-called "natural reproduction," continue to be mapped across new technological possibilities and provide appropriate limits. These parameters include the requirement that reproduction is sexual – meaning, between a man and a woman (not cloning) and that the man and the woman are in a heterosexual relationship (some countries and jurisdictions have legislated to limit the use of IVF and related technologies to heterosexual couples) with each other, and that, the product of that technologically-enhanced reproduction, has a blood/genetic line that only traces back to two progenitors.

Kinship relationships and relationships of inheritance are established on the basis of this "truth" about the "nature" of reproduction, such that it becomes impossible to think about kinship being established, or reproduction taking place, in other ways. Changes that come about by so-called "natural" reproduction are not viewed with the same kind of anxiety as those brought about artificially and with direct intervention.

The idea of natural reproduction itself has shifted, however, with the advent of new technologies. New ARTs, such as IVF and artificial insemination (AI), once considered unnatural and interventionist, have become accepted forms of natural reproduction (in part because they mimic sexual reproduction) although many legislatures have been at pains to ensure that only heterosexual couples use them.[9] Human IGM is the latest source of insecurities about the impact of technology in the realm of reproduction. It has become aligned with transgressive reproductive practices and technologies such as cloning, the creation of human/non-human hybrids, and the creation of chimeras. IGM, like other ARTs, challenges us to rethink the normativity of the established relations of conception, gestation, and *in vivo* reproduction, in other words, to question the very "nature" of reproduction.

Genetic and reproductive technologies force us to rethink not only the limits of the possible in reproduction, but also the boundaries of what it is to be human. The anthropologist Sarah Franklin describes how our sensibilities have already shifted significantly when we can view "a cryopreserved embryo suspended in a liquid nitrogen tank (as) a biological relative," as do many couples undergoing IVF. Franklin describes this as "kinship shorn of a sense of natural limit, but (maintaining) surely a sense of relatedness based on shared bodily substances and genetic ties."[10]

The anthropologist David Schneider has suggested that "kinship is whatever the biological relationship is. If science discovers new facts about biogenetic relationships then that is what kinship is and was all along."[11] Implicit in Schneider's understanding of the relationship between biology and kinship is the existence of a pre-discursive nature or biological order that is revealed as our scientific understanding becomes more sophisticated. On this view, then, not only do we, as Franklin describes the position, "embody scientific knowledges" in that "they describe the nature of our very being"[12], but our conceptions of relatedness or kinship also spring into being when scientific knowledge or natural facts are "discovered." Within this framework, kinship is the "social construction of natural facts."[13] While we do not agree with the relationship between kinship and biology described by Schneider, his account certainly characterizes much of the current Euro-American understanding about the relationship between the "facts" of sexual reproduction and the biological kinship relations it produces. As argued elsewhere by one of us (RM):

> by presuming that biological ties and the "facts of life" exist [and are fixed], we have created a strong rationale for foundational arguments which favor the "naturalness" of family and kinship relations. What has been construed within our understanding of kinship as "natural," then, is a normatively essentialist position having direct bearing upon the way we understand gender and sexuality within the reproductive context.[14]

The biological kinship relation, as described above, is thrown into sharp relief, when as Franklin puts it, "science discovers new facts about biogenetic relationship." For instance, when science discovers new facts that allow a human to be crossed genetically with a pig or a mouse, we must ask whether this alters our cultural conception of who we may call kin. And what are we to make of the way that such new relations also challenge our commonly held understandings of "natural" limits? In an ironic twist, as Franklin suggests, "the very ways in which we are today connected and related through biology undoes the very fixity the biological tie used to represent."[15]

When biological science is deployed to disturb the familiar categories of relation and identity, it troubles mainstream understandings of the role of "scientific truth." Underlying all this is a profound discomfort about the connection between relationship and identity. There is a kind of pervasive anxiety that identity can only be secure if relationships are fixed. Up until now this fixity was assured by the belief that biogenetic relationships were "found," revealed in "nature," and not *made*. We suspect this anxiety stems from the latent threat to liberal notions of identity and individuality bound up with explicit recognition of the inevitability and inescapability of relationship. This concept of inevitability is only acceptable when it can be removed from the realm of choice and instead firmly ascribed to a very particular construction of "nature" that favors the liberal subject but yet, in the lexicon of naturalness, is beyond our capacity to influence or change.

From this perspective, as IGM has the potential to create new kinds and forms of biological kinship, it may also encourage us to revise kinship along radically different lines. In our view, we must not recreate the errors of past legal and social reasoning by attempting to "find" kinship on the basis of processes at the cellular or molecular level. Kinship is, and should be, based on social relationships established by embodied persons. The fear that motivates legislative prohibitions of IGM is based on the spurious construction of human kinship on the basis of invisible processes at the sub-cellular level.

Legal developments that prohibit and regulate the panoply of technologies associated with (or dreamed of) as emanating from recent successes in cloning, stem cell research, and embryonic and gene therapy attempt to reinstate the very limits of the human that Franklin describes as no longer present or at least under threat. Our focus is on the appropriateness of this role for law and why it might be utilized to these ends. The legal scholar Derek Morgan sees the role of law in this context as twofold: first, "not just as an autonomous body of knowledge, but as a factor that contributes to – which, indeed, facilitates – the so called public understanding of science." At the same time, law has a role in declaiming "who we are and whom we want to become, giving a moral and symbolic emphasis to law."[16] The aim of the current chapter is to make sense of the current legislative fixation with policing the limits of heritability and coextensively, we argue, with declaring what kind of human (or perhaps post-human) may be reproduced. It will become clearer just what those limits are understood to be when we examine the legislation in detail. In addition, we contend that feminists should look more closely at the way in which science is being deployed to construct law, and probe more carefully what norms of reproduction are being read into law.

It is imperative, for instance, to consider the position of women in the context of these recent regulatory moves. As we shall see, while much of the legislation that has been passed recently or proposed in this area concerns interventions involving embryo implantation and the manipulation of egg cells, there is little or no mention of the female body or female persons within the legislation itself, particularly in the case of Australian legislation. The Canadian legislation is notable for its specific recognition of the role that women play in reproduction. In the Assisted Human Reproduction Act discussed in detail below, a set of principles are articulated.[17] Principle c states: "while all persons are affected by these technologies, women more than men are directly and significantly affected by their application and the health and well-being of women must be protected in the application of these technologies." In both cases what is overtly policed is the fertility of the scientific imagination. As we shall argue, more often than not the body as flesh is unhinged from any self. In this chapter, we offer an alternative feminist legal response that does not reify a specific construct of nature.

The initial and most intriguing question, however, is the following: what is it about technologically-induced IGM that could call an unusual coalition of feminists and conservatives into being and get them to push collaboratively for legislative change?

11.3   What's wrong with artificial inheritable change?

A large cohort of feminists, disability activists, and progressive thinkers are lining up with moral conservatives to argue for the legal prohibition of human IGM and cloning technologies. To the extent that their reasoning derives from concerns that human cloning and IGM may promote unethical experimentation on women and children, and that both are grossly underdeveloped and even dangerous, it is clear the argument is unimpeachable. Feminists are on firm ground opposing unauthorized experimentation on the bodies of women and children in the name of genetic technology and scientific development. But why is a general prohibition favored, rather than a regulatory regime in which practice and research is subject to ethics approval? In both Australia and Canada, medical practice and scientific research are governed by ethical guidelines applied by university, hospital, and other institutional ethics committees. In the case of publicly-funded research, research funding is dependent on requisite approval by the relevant ethics committee and adherence to professional and regulatory guidelines. In the case of IGM, it is clear that even if the research or practice was shown to be safe and developed in accordance with approved ethical guidelines, it would nevertheless be argued that it should be prohibited. In other words, the concern here is not just with safe and ethical conduct of experiments and medical treatment on humans. Instead, IGM is seen in and of itself as a moral wrong.

11.3.1   Designer babies: simply unnatural?

A number of feminist commentators have argued that the use of IGM will alienate women from the reproductive process. It would, they argue, fundamentally undermine maternal autonomy and result in market control of baby design and production.[18] Further, there is a fear that genetic technologies will go beyond "therapeutic" purposes – to prevent the inheritance of lethal genetic diseases in families – and rather be used to "improve," as Frankel writes, "human traits that without intervention would be within the range of what is commonly regarded as normal, or improving them beyond what is needed to maintain or restore good health."[19] Desirable characteristics will be chosen not by governments, as they were in eugenic programs of the past, but by individuals exercising free choice to enhance the life chances of their offspring. The offerings of the marketplace will create the citizen with the best advantage in the global marketplace: the compliant corporate citizen.

Disability activists perceive the idea of "enhancement" as fundamentally flawed in its overvaluation of certain traits and undervaluation of others.[20] They rightly point out that discourses and practices aimed at enhancement reinforce an individualized and medicalized model of disability, rather than locating disability in a network of exclusionary attitudinal, environmental, and economic barriers.[21] Moreover, as the President's Council on Bioethics in the U.S.A. noted: "both enhancement and therapy are bound up with, and absolutely dependent on, the inherently complicated idea of health and the always controversial idea of normality ... The distinction rests on the assumption that there is a natural human "whole" whose healthy functioning is the goal of therapeutic medicine."[22] Kerry Taylor and one of us (RM) have argued that:

"Normalcy" is used to rationalize medical attempts to eradicate our differences, and to render all bodies alike – healthy and interchangeable ... It is conceivable that genetic enhancements of normal human functions, if sufficiently valuable and widespread, might lead us to revise upward our conception of normal species functioning, with the result that where we draw the line between health and disease, and hence between enhancement and treatment, would correspondingly change. If this occurred, we might come to view certain interventions as being required by justice ... if such enhancements became widespread, we might come to regard a person who lacked them as suffering from an adverse departure from normal functioning.[23] The normal is a cultural and biological imperative, which represents the average, both physically and morally. It also is a means to justify and preserve the status quo. The "average man" [sic] was constructed based on the average of all human attributes in a given country.[24] Thus, the average body became the ideal against which all others are measured. All variations within bodies became characterized in terms of variation from the normal state ... It also creates the existence of deviations from that norm – or, when applied to the body as the site of identity, the presence of "abnormal" persons within a population. In addition to being a quantitative marker of human variability, the normal is a powerful normative tool that is used to determine and rationalize the extent to which certain persons fall *outside* the boundaries of moral responsibility.[25]

It is not surprising then that feminists, disability activists, and other progressive thinkers are concerned about the deleterious social and justice impacts of enhancement technologies associated with IGM. However, we need to ask whether there is anything new in the differential distribution and valuation of particular traits. Or, is the difference in the case of IGM one of luck versus design, nature versus artifice? The legitimate concern described above veers into dangerous terrain, when the defense of human rights, especially women's rights, is conflated with the defense of "nature." Typical objections about enhancement seem to fit that bill. This occurs for instance, when feminists including Judith Levine are concerned that "genetic engineering designs in inequality." She argues that genetic engineering "will artificially confer heritable advantages only on those who can afford to buy them",[26] and implies that natural advantages are neutral and have no impact on social justice and equity. Obviously, it needs to be asked how heritable advantages came to be "advantages" in the first place.

In addition to this implicit valorization of the natural, some radical feminist critiques explicitly rely upon it. They critique various forms of reproductive technologies as fundamentally disruptive of the natural and proper link between the woman and her maternal identity.[27] However, the problem with this sort of argument is, as Margrit Shildrick writes, that "it assumes certain fixed modes of female being … it implicitly counterposes natural with techno-logical reproduction … [and] relies on a closure of identity that in fact may inhibit women's interests."[28]

11.3.2 The critique of genetic determinism

Having argued that the problem with genetic enhancement technologies is that they have a differential impact in terms of equity, it should be noted that feminist and progressive thinkers are also critical of the accuracy of this kind of determin-ist genetic discourse. In other words, in the act of formulating a considered response to the claims being made regarding what is scientifically possible, one quickly falls into the trap of accepting the outcome (i.e., genetically-enhanced individuals) as a concrete possibility. Critical pressure must also be brought to bear on this assumption. A focus on genetic enhancement could, as Frankel suggests, "… lead us to devalue various social and environmental factors that influence human development in concert with genes." Further, as he cautions, "a preoccupation with genetic enhancement may place too much emphasis on the genes and ultimately prevent us from solving problems that are really embedded in the structure of our society."[29]

At various times in the history of genetic research, claims have been made about possible indicators, markers or genetic identifiers for things such as alco-holism, homosexuality, violence, criminality, and so on. The effect of these kinds of claims has been to displace or dismiss more speculative, analytical dis-courses such as psychoanalysis, psychology, sociology, and anthropology. We need to remind ourselves that what we understand as "criminal," for example, is indeed academic. It is a concept that only makes sense within the sociologi-cal discourse that produced it. Genetic discourse borrows from the social sci-ences, identifies particular sociological traits as genetic, and then looks for a gene. Traits such as violence, intelligence, and so on, are treated as if they have a kind of scientific actuality without subjecting them to interpretive work. Richard Lewontin reminds us, however, that "science, like other productive activities, like the state, the family, sport, is a social institution completely inte-grated into and influenced by the structure of all our social institutions."[30] Claims about genetic modification and what can be achieved thus must be viewed as contingent, always contestable, and remarkably political.

11.3.3 What is *so* distinctive about IGM?

Responses to IGM must also be read against the technologies that currently exist and are legal. Why does IGM generate more concern than existing technologies that demand what some have termed "responsible" reproduction through selective abortion? Put another way, these arguments, while important, are not distinctive to IGM but are equally applicable to a wider range of practices that affect somatic cells. Nikolas Rose argues, for instance, that "by the start of the twenty-first century, hopes, fears, decisions and life-routines shaped in terms of risks and possibilities in corporeal and biological existence had come to supplant almost all others as organizing principles of a life of prudence, responsibility, and choice."[31] Technologies such as CVS, amniocentesis, and PGD are becoming routine, particularly for pregnant women over the age of 35. Then why does the specter of changing the germ-line animate legislatures to act prohibitively?[32]

One argument for the differential response is offered by Frankel, who claims that:

enhancement by genetics is ... qualitatively different from enhancement by other means. Existing methods of enhancement ... are not biologically intrusive in a manner that will significantly shape our evolutionary course. Inheritable genetic enhancement would have long-term effects on persons yet to be born. Thus we have little, if any, precedent for this way of using IGM. We would be venturing into unknown territory, but without any sense of where the boundaries should lie, much less with an understanding of what it means to cross such boundaries.[33]

But we routinely make decisions that will have long-term consequences on persons yet to be born – we make decisions to procreate and give life to individuals without their consent (the adolescent refrain "I never asked to be born" is evidence enough). We routinely alter environments with irreversible consequences (think of any number of activities – pollution, building high-rises, sending rockets to the moon), and intervene in political activities, but because these are changes to the environment, they are somehow less constitutive of the individual, somehow less integral to identity. Not only are environmental factors significant on their own, but the new genetics itself reveals the extent to which phenotypes result from complex interactions between genes and environment. This should caution us to investigate what resides at the intersection of genes and environment, and not to focus on one over the other. What Frankel's words indicate instead, we suggest, is an alarmist concern with the scrutiny of boundaries and the dangers of boundary transgression. In our view, this anxiety stems from fears about the vulnerability of bounded notions of the liberal self in the face of new genetic combinations. Later in this chapter, we return to this central anxiety which motivates much of the legislation in the area and claims for law the role of policing those boundaries against *unnatural*[34] transgression.

11.3.4 The common heritage pool

Another argument developed (and later discounted) by Mark Frankel and Audrey Chapman in their report assessing the ethical and social implications of human IGM is that future generations have a right to inherit an unmodified gene pool because the gene pool represents their "genetic patrimony" as the "common heritage of our species."[35] The Universal Declaration on the Human Genome and Human Rights seems to accord with that position, for instance when it states in Article 1, that:

The human genome underlies the fundamental unity of all members of the human family, as well as the recognition of their inherent dignity and diversity. In a symbolic sense, it is the heritage of humanity.[36]

Frankel and Chapman also point to the claim made in the resolution adopted by the Parliamentary Assembly of the Council of Europe on genetic engineering, which states that:

… the rights to life and to human dignity protected by Articles 2 and 3 of the European Convention on Human Rights imply the right to inherit a genetic pattern which has not been artificially changed.[37]

In response to this argument, Frankel and Chapman insist that:

The human gene pool is a heuristic abstraction, not a natural object and lacks a material referent in nature. Individuals inherit a specific set of genes derived from their parents. Thus from a biomedical perspective, there is no intergeneration "human germ line" that could serve as an asset to the future.[38]

A single human gene pool is, as Frankel and Chapman suggest, a linguistic artifice. Yet, there is no doubt that the introduction of inheritable genetically-modified genes will impact on future generations even if only in a miniscule way. It is therefore more useful to think about the modifications themselves as comprising a small pool of genetic resources. Viewed in this way, the concern shifts from one of changing or harming the human gene pool, to one about accessing or controlling the reservoir of genetic material that can be drawn upon to make required modifications. Assumptions should not be made, however, about likely preferences for particular types of genetic modifications. It would be easy to take the view that modifications that correct serious illness should be publicly available and distinguished from those which are merely enhancing and socially desirable. Indeed, one can imagine the latter forming part of a new commodity culture.

However, in our view even this broad distinction is fraught with serious ethical concerns. The line between these two criteria will always be determined at the level of context and situated desire. For instance, while some might consider that deafness is an illness that should be corrected, others may view deafness as an enhancement.[39] Consider for instance the case of a deaf lesbian couple in the U.S.A. who deliberately created a deaf child: Sharon Duchesneau and

Candy McCullough used their own sperm donor, a deaf friend with five generations of deafness in his family, to ensure the birth of a deaf child. They argued that deafness was a defining factor in their cultural identity.[40] In light of examples such as this one, it is far more likely that any market in technologies for IGM will be niche-driven rather than a resource for some non-existent entity called "the common humanity." On the contrary, it is likely that corporations will compete to market genetic traits that serve specific groupings of individuals.

11.3.5 Reproductive agency for women

What about the argument that IGM as a new reproductive technology, like those that have gone before it, is a tool for women that offers them greater control and agency in the reproductive process? These women, it is suggested, would otherwise see themselves as subject to their reproductive biological fate. It is clear that "reproductive choice" is another one of those ideas like health, normality, and naturalness, whose meaning shifts with the technology. Some feminists, including Abby Lippman, see the plethora of "choice" as artificially manufacturing needs. She suggests that women will find themselves increasingly subject to external notions of responsibility and risk avoidance.[41] As each new technological advance is seamlessly incorporated into the experiential matrix of the pregnant woman, it becomes internalized and naturalized, and new demands to reproduce *responsibly* follow. Rose argues for instance that:

In advanced liberal democracies, biological identity becomes bound up with more general norms of enterprising, self-actualising, responsible personhood.[42]

Importantly, however, Rose goes on to argue that the new biomedicine is not individualizing to the extent that "'at risk' groups are joining into groups and organisations, not merely demanding public provision and rights but making their own claims on the deployment of biomedical technologies and the direction of biomedical research."[43] He sees a contradiction in the new legal species of human rights based on simple existence, or what he terms "biological citizenship." While such rights suggest each human life is of equal worth, he notes that these rights have to be read against an equally powerful "biological ethics and genetic responsibility." According to Rose:

As biomedical technique has extended choice to the very fabric of vital existence, we are faced with the inescapable task of deliberating about the worth of different human lives ... this politics is not one in which authorities claim – or are given – the power to make such judgments in the name of quality of the population or the health of the gene pool. On the one hand, in the new forms of pastoral power that are taking shape in and around our genetics and our biology, these questions about the value of life itself infuse the everyday judgments, vocabularies, techniques and actions of all those professionals of vitality: doctors, genetic counsellors, research scientists and drug companies among them, and entangle them all in ethics and ethnopolitics. And, on the other hand, the politics of life itself poses these questions to each of us – in our own lives, in those of our families and in the new associations that link us to others with whom we share aspects of our biological identity.[44]

Recent legislative interventions in Australia and Canada do, however, suggest that the authorities are claiming a right to make judgments about the worth of different human lives. Indeed, a new tension is emerging between an ethic of choice where, with our internalized responsibilities, we make decisions about our genetic futures that may or may not have us becoming trans- or post-human, and a human rights of genetics, where governments at the national and international level take control of human futures by determining for us the outer limits of how and with whom we may reproduce. In other words, human rights instruments seem more concerned with *policing* the outer limits of the human than protecting those that are born in excess of those limits.

A vignette, recounted recently in the *Village Voice*, helps to illustrate this point. A story about "supertots and frankenkids" reminds us that while we may be approaching that day when wealthy parents may pay to have genetic "enhancements" to their progeny, the law is currently more concerned about "banning their birth than in protecting their interests."[45] There is no guarantee that prohibiting the creation of specified biological entities will, in fact, prevent the feared experiments from occurring. It is possible, instead, that the legislative ban might have the perverse effect of prejudicing the interests of the persons or entities born of such experimentation, thus denying them the status of humans and depriving them of the enjoyment of any ancillary rights. As the *Village Voice* article points out, this is the future conjured up by the comic strip and movie "X-Men" and is modeled on the treatment meted out today to undocumented aliens, illegal migrants, or, in the past, to women, African slaves, aboriginal peoples, and people of color generally. While science looks forward, law looks backwards.[46] Law is more effective in determining and allocating interests than it is at defining possibilities in the real world. It is better at defining "illegitimate" offspring than in preventing them from coming into the world.[47] Policing natural reproduction ends in policing the persons that result from unnatural (transgressive) reproduction. According to Erik Baard, "the rights of such unusual progeny are being curtailed before the people even exist."[48] Far from drawing actual limits on nature and science then, statutory prohibitions that police the boundaries of the human end up determining who we may call kin.

We want to suggest that legal and regulatory responses to IGM ought to embrace "the exhilarating prospect of getting out of some of the old boxes and opening up new ways of thinking about what being human means."[49] In order to understand why this is important to a feminist legal ethic, we need to recognize that, to date, a legal, liberal conception of the human person has prevailed that applies only to a fraction of the population, namely those who can operate as autonomous selves – who are actualizing beings because they have the financial resources, the power, and the time to enact themselves in such a way.

As we suggested previously, we need to be wary of collusion between science and law in the effort to freeze the meanings of categories and remove them from social contestation. Science is often deployed to place facts beyond dispute, while law is deployed to place disputes under restraints. Both may be deployed to "reproduce" the bounded notions of the liberal self.

While feminist responses are, for the most part, aware and critical of the limits of liberal selfhood, in some instances as noted above they fail to move away from a hidden discourse of the *natural*. In line with feminist legal theorists such as Martha Fineman, we argue that a particular conceptualization of *natural maternity* operates for liberal individuals as a hidden repository of all its dependencies.[50] The truth of liberalism is that no one is a truly autonomous or independent self, but some lay claim to that status by masking or privatizing their dependencies. Most commonly, this is done through supportive family structures. Therefore we are suspicious of moves that seem to be legislating a particular kind of reproduction on the basis that it most closely replicates the "natural" and results in "natural reproduction."

It is interesting in this light to compare the Australian legislation with its Canadian counterpart. The former was introduced under the auspices of one of the most conservative governments in Australia's history. The latter has been developed with significant input from and participation by feminist thinkers and the women's health community. As will become evident in our examination of the legislation, whereas the Canadian legislation appears to place limits on asexual and species-transgressing reproduction (animal/human), the Australian legislation also prohibits any kind of reproduction that cannot be seen to mirror, in some way, heterosexual monogamous reproduction. On the conservative side, then, there seems to be a panic about the loss of the autonomous liberal subject that "natural" reproduction operates to shore up.[51]

11.4   The legal response in Australia

Prior to the recent legislative developments in Australia prohibiting cloning and regulating embryo research, significant energy was put into legislative provisions that would regulate the control, access, and use of genetic information.[52] The primary outcome of several years' debate over specific (and now defunct) legislation, the *Genetic Privacy and Non Discrimination Bill* 1998 (Cth.), was a 400-page report by the Australian Law Reform Commission recommending, in large part, enhancement of the existing federal and state privacy legislation to manage the use of genetic information. Protecting privacy, rather than property, is the preferred approach, which is justified on the ground that commodification of the human body is a moral wrong. Human dignity, it is argued, demands that we do not treat the body as property.

There is no doubt that information about our genetic profile joins us to others. Each person's unique genetic code perversely reveals who else we are – our familiarly distributed network of identity markers – and who else we might become – the myriad future pathologies lurking down the track. In a sense, then, this is the moment when the liberal individual must face his or her interconnected status. Privacy legislation is a knee-jerk response to the necessary vulnerability we feel when we realize that we are all interconnected. Nevertheless, it cannot work. Under a privacy model, each member of a family not only has the right to choose not to reveal information about themselves but also the right to disclose if they so wish. Disclosure will, however, usually reveal something about other genetically-related family members. Therefore, a different kind of response is required that protects against the discrimination to which the revelation might give rise, rather than protecting against the revelation itself. In the same way, recent legislation around IGM appears to be aimed at protecting the liberal individual not by ensuring safe and ethical conduct of ARTs involving gene therapies, but by prohibiting the therapies themselves. How should we understand this prohibitory legislation? We suggest that in Australia, this legislation is primarily aimed at preserving what has come to be imagined as a kind of "natural maternity," which acts ideologically to preserve the supportive sexual unit for the usually male liberal individual, namely, the heterosexual, monogamous, nuclear family unit.

The new comprehensive Australian federal and state legislation passed over the course of 2002–2004 consists of two primary Acts: the Prohibition of Human Cloning Act (Cth.) and the Research Involving Human Embryos Act (Cth.). Each of the state Acts is a reiteration of the federal legislation.[53] The state legislation is necessary to overcome possible Constitutional limits on the power of the federal government to regulate in this area, and ensure national uniformity. It should be noted at the outset that both Acts provide for a review of their operation as soon as possible after the second anniversary of the day on which the Act received the Royal Assent. A review committee was appointed on 17 June 2005. The committee must present their report to Parliament by 19 December 2005. The review of both Acts must be undertaken concurrently and by the same persons.[54]

The Commonwealth Acts should be read together with the National Health and Medical Research Council (NHMRC) *National Statement on Ethical Conduct in Research Involving Humans*, specifically the notes on the human fetus and the use of human fetal tissue (Supplementary Note 5) and the guidelines for the ethical review of human SCGT and related therapies (Supplementary Note 7). The NHMRC established by the NHMRC Act 1992 (Cth.) is charged with setting down ethical guidelines for research and requires all institutions or organizations that receive funding from it to do research to establish human research ethics committees (HRECs) and to subject all research involving humans – whether relating to health or not and whether funded by the NHMRC or not – to ethical review by HRECs using the statement and supplementary notes as the standard.

While these ethical guidelines are just that – guidelines – the new Common-wealth Acts make certain prohibited acts and offences punishable by imprison-ment. Turning then to the Prohibition of Human Cloning Act 2002 (Cth.), section three sets out the object of the Act:

to address concerns, including ethical concerns, about scientific developments in rela-tion *to human reproduction* and the utilisation of human embryos by prohibiting certain practices. (italics added)

It is within this Act that we find the most comprehensive prohibitions in rela-tion to IGM. While the general prohibition against cloning falls at the margins of what we might describe as IGM, other prohibited practices in the Act are more clearly aimed at IGM. At first blush, one might view these provisions as intended to curtail the production of a radically-modified human being – a hybrid or chimera or trans-human. However, a more considered look suggests that there is also a concern with what might be viewed as deviant reproduction. As stated earlier this seems to be tied to what we would argue is a mistaken cor-relation between human kinship relationships and how they are worked out at the sub-cellular level.

We should be wary of the mystification of social relations based on the invisi-ble realm of molecular biology. The critique – or embrace – of post-humanism can only be done from the standpoint of embodied persons and the relationships they develop in the social world. It is by foregrounding these relationships when interpreting the Australian Prohibition of Human Cloning Act 2002 (Cth.), for example, that we are able to reveal what may even be unconscious assumptions about the nature or naturalness of reproduction. Those assumptions catch us in a questionable feedback loop where what is viewed as unnatural is already prede-termined by particular views about the way reproduction should proceed, namely, sexually between one man and one woman. Consider Section 13:

A person commits an offence if the person intentionally creates a human embryo by a process other than the fertilsation of a human egg by a human sperm, or intentionally develops a human embryo so created.

It is clear that some kind of interpretive work needs to be done to assess what the words "a process other than" are alluding to. By foregrounding the relation-ships or embodied identities that must be involved in any process aimed at the creation or development of an embryo, we can see that a requirement for male to female reproduction is being legislated. One of the ways in which the legisla-tion masks this objective is by disembodying the human gametes that are being regulated. The legislation reads as if it had been written from the perspective of a fiber-optic telescope or a laparoscope. If we were to insist upon a perspective that embodies the gametes, the legislation might read quite differently.

This is further reinforced by the fact that the provision starts by referring to the creation of a *human* embryo whereas *hybrid* embryos are specifically dealt with elsewhere (Section 20). Further, a *human embryo* is defined in the Act as "a live embryo that has a *human genome* or an *altered human genome* and that has been developing for less than 8 weeks since the appearance of two pro-nuclei or the initiation of its development by other means" (italics added). A hybrid embryo, on the other hand, is defined as an embryo created by the fertilization of a human egg by animal sperm, or vice versa, and various other possible chimerical combinations. Clearly, then, what is specifically being policed in this section are deviant forms of human reproduction: non-heterosexual reproduction that transfers genetic heritage. Interestingly, the Canadian legislation does not do this. In other words, it does not mandate a particular kind of reproduction. On its face, the Canadian Assisted Human Reproduction Act, does not appear to contain a provision similar to Section 13.

This conclusion is particularly interesting in light of a recent book by Bryan Sykes, Professor of Genetics at Oxford University, entitled *Adam's Curse*.[55] He predicts the extinction of men unless we can create a designer male gene. He suggests that because of the weakness and singularity of the Y chromosome and the capacity of the two X chromosomes to "pair up and swap genes to minimize bad mutations," the solution might be to fuse genetic material from two women: "the DNA could be extracted from the nucleus of one woman's egg, and made to fuse with the DNA inside another woman's egg."[56] For him, it is a matter of survival of the species, but for now, in Australia at least, such homosexual reproduction is not allowed.

Section 15 of the Prohibition of Human Cloning Act 2002 (Cth.) takes a further step in policing deviant reproduction. It states "a person commits an offence if the person intentionally creates or develops a human embryo containing genetic material provided by more than two persons." Not only is homosexual reproduction banned, but reproduction must continue to be monogamous even at the genetic level. While we know that there may be dangers to any procedure that involves introducing genetic material into a cell, it is not the safety or ethical application of the procedure that is being policed here. Section 15 is a blanket prohibition against use of genetic material from more than two people in any circumstances. As noted at the beginning of this chapter, this is the one area where IGM has already occurred. Micro-implantation techniques already in use make it possible to compensate for mitochondrial genetic diseases either through inserting segments of healthy mitochondria (ooplasmic transplantation) or placing the nucleus of the egg of a woman suffering from the disease into a substitute egg (*in vitro* ovum nuclear transplantation). It is still unclear whether this technology is safe, as there has not been adequate testing. Therefore it would be unethical and premature to allow these techniques to be used on humans as therapeutic procedures, despite the use of this technology to produce 30 babies in 1997, which was reported by research scientists from Saint Barnabas in 2001. The report describes the process and indicates that the babies that have resulted have indeed inherited the mitochondrial DNA from the donor cytoplasm, and will likely produce offspring who will also inherit those genes.[57] These babies have genetic material from three rather than two people. In the context of the Australian legislation, one has to ask again why this particular kind of procedure has been singled out and separately prohibited.[58]

Interestingly, there is no legislation in Australia prohibiting a baby from having three biological progenitors, as opposed to three genetic progenitors. A woman who gestates a baby created from a donor egg makes no genetic contribution to that baby, but nevertheless has a significant biological input through gestation. She nourishes the baby with nutrients produced through her own circulatory system, she carries the baby inside her womb, and the baby is subject to the same environmental changes, positive or negative, to which the woman herself is subjected. Yet the law does not prohibit these exchanges, provided they are not predicated on monetary exchange.[59] In light of the Prohibition of Human Cloning Act 2002 (Cth.), and Section 15 described above, if all three people had instead wished to contribute genetic material to the baby, the law would prohibit the exchange.

Another important section in the Prohibition of Human Cloning Act 2002 (Cth.) reads as follows:

A person commits an offence if:

(a) the person alters the genome of a human cell in such a way that the alteration is heritable by descendants of the human whose cell was altered; and
(b) in altering the genome, the person intended the alteration to be heritable by descendants of the human whose cell was altered.

… in this section: *human cell* includes a human embryonal cell, a human fetal cell, human sperm, or a human egg. (Section 18)

This section specifically targets IGM, but what is particularly interesting is that only *intentional* IGM is prohibited. The legislation is drafted in a way that is clearly concerned not to prohibit SCGT which, some might argue, runs a very small risk of altering the germ line.[60] What it does do, however, is countenance the possibility of heritable change occurring through chance. Change by design is not allowed, but change by accident is. Perhaps this would satisfy those who perceive the problem as related to certain people being allowed to "design in" advantage. If instead the only way in which IGM could occur is if it occurs by accident, then the advantages accrued would be limited to those that have the natural advantage of being the one (in however many thousands) whose germ cells were affected by the modification.

At the same time as the passing of the Prohibition of Human Cloning Act 2002 (Cth.), the Federal government also passed the Research Involving Human Embryos Act 2002 (Cth.). This Act basically sets down rules about how and when an embryo can be used for research purposes. In summary, it limits research only to those embryos created for reproductive purposes that are in excess of what is required by the reproducing progenitors. Licenses that author-ize damage or destruction of an embryo so created are allowed under strict conditions and only with respect to embryos created before 5 April 2002. This time limited provision is, however, repealed as of 5 April 2005. The NHMRC also plays a crucial role under the legislation of approving and monitoring the licensing of the use of excess embryos.

Like its counterpart, the Research Involving Human Embryos Act 2002 (Cth.) also defines a human embryo as "a live embryo that has a human genome or an altered human genome and that has been developing for less than 8 weeks since the appearance of two pro-nuclei or the initiation of its development by other means." We presume that the inclusion in both Acts of an embryo with an altered human genome within the definition of human embryo aims to cover those embryos that may have been genetically altered in their somatic cell lines through *in utero* processes. It also may be directed at covering non-intentional IGM as countenanced in Section 18(1)(b) of the Prohibition of Human Cloning Act 2002 (Cth.). Given that any other kind of alteration is prohibited, it is unlikely that what is being imagined here is an embryo with an intentionally-altered germ line. However, it is reassuring that were such an embryo to be pro-duced and developed, it would be legally considered to have the status of "human embryo," despite its non-legal creation.

As mentioned above, alongside the prohibitory legislation, and operating in tandem therewith, are research guidelines set down by the NHMRC. The NHMRC has recently issued guidelines which mirror the federal legislation. The *Ethical Guidelines on the Use of Reproductive Technology in Clinical Practice and Research* (the *Guidelines)* are intended to provide comprehensive rules govern-ing activities relating to reproductive technology in clinical practice; research aimed at improving outcomes in clinical practice; and other research involving the use of human gametes, embryos, embryonic stem cells, fetuses, and fetal cells.[61]

It is interesting to note that the *Guidelines* do note the desirability of IGM where it precludes passing on a genetic disorder. It is suggested as a goal of con-temporary reproductive technologies that couples avoid passing on a heritable genetic disorder. However, PGD rather than IGM is considered appropriate where a serious genetic condition or disease (including serious chromosome abnormalities not associated with a known condition or disease) is in question. A single thread that is woven throughout the *Guidelines* is the right of a person to know the identities of their genetic parents. This point is presented as an assumption, and is raised in every context where donation of gametes or embryos is examined. Given that one of the possible results of IGM in some contexts is the opportunity for more than two genetic progenitors, it is worth asking how law and social discourse would manage this multiplicity of parental possibili-ties. Perhaps this is another reason why, so far it, has been directly excluded as a possibility in the Australian legislation.

11.5   The legal response in Canada

In response to growing public concerns about new reproductive and genetic technologies, the Government of Canada appointed the Royal Commission on New Reproductive Technologies in October 1989. In November 1993, under an "ethic of care" framework,[62] the Royal Commission made public 293 recommendations, concluding that "decisive, timely, and comprehensive national action is required with respect to the regulation of new reproductive technologies."[63] In particular, the Royal Commission called for legislation to set clear boundaries around acceptable and non-acceptable uses of ARTs and genetic technologies, and to regulate and monitor the use of acceptable practices and developments in this field. To achieve this goal, the Royal Commission stated that the federal government should use its power under the *Criminal Code* to prohibit practices that "because of their unsafe or unethical character (are) considered unacceptable under any circumstances."[64] In addition, the Royal Commission recommended the establishment of a national regulatory commission charged with the responsibility of setting and enforcing standards for those practices deemed acceptable.

The Canadian government's final response to the Royal Commission is An Act Respecting Assisted Human Reproduction and Related Research (AHR Act) which was given royal assent on 29 March 2004.[65] In 1996, Bill C-47, An Act Respecting Human Reproductive Technologies and Commercial Transactions Relating to Human Reproduction, was proposed.[66] Bill C-47 contained a list of prohibited activities which included, amongst others, implanting animal embryos into humans or vice versa; fusing human and animal zygotes or embryos; maintaining human embryos outside the human body (beyond the 14-day limit); germ-line alterations; fertilizing animals with human sperm, or vice versa; and retrieving the ovum or sperm from a fetus or cadaver with the intention of maturing it. Under the various pressures of an upcoming federal election, the proposed regime failed to materialize, and Bill C-47 died on the order paper in 1997.

Unlike Bill C-47 which was exclusively prohibitory in nature, the AHR Act combines both criminal prohibitions with a regulatory framework. Since the original Bill C-47 died, and the introduction of the AHR Act, significant changes have occurred in the development of reproductive and genetic technologies. Notable among these changes is the growing interest in stem cell research and the increased use of IVF-related technologies. These changes, as well as a shift in attitude towards these technologies, are reflected in the AHR Act. Where the preamble of Bill C-47 began with an expression of grave concern "about the significant threat to human dignity, the risks to human health and safety, both known and unknown, and other serious social and ethical issues posed by certain reproductive and genetic technologies," the declaration of principles in the AHR Act provides that:

the benefits of assisted human reproductive technologies and related research for individuals, families and for society in general can be most effectively secured by taking appropriate measures for the protection and promotion of human health, safety, dignity and rights in the use of these technologies and in related research.

Another difference between Bill C-47 and the AHR Act is that the former contained a set of legislative objectives. Although the AHR Act is silent about the objectives of the legislation, information published by Health Canada at the time that precursor draft legislation was introduced states that it has two primary objectives: first, to "ensure that Canadians using assisted human reproduction techniques do so without compromising their health and safety," and second, to "ensure that promising research involving human reproductive materials takes place within a regulated environment."[67] This second purpose, while not overtly expressed in the text of the draft legislation, appears to inform many of the activities that would be controlled through license under the Bill.

Rather than a statement of objectives, the AHR Act contains a declaration of principles that informs the Act and guides lawmakers in interpreting and implementing the legislation. Notable principles set out in the Bill include:

The Parliament of Canada recognizes and declares that:

(a) the health and well-being of children born through the application of assisted human reproductive technologies must be given priority in all decisions respecting their use ...

(c) while all persons are affected by these technologies, women more than men are directly and significantly affected by their application and the health and well-being of women must be protected in the application of these technologies ...

(e) persons who seek to undergo assisted reproduction procedures must not be discriminated against, including on the basis of their sexual orientation or marital status ...

(g) human individuality and diversity, and the integrity of the human genome, must be preserved and protected.

Because these principles are enshrined in a statutory declaration, they have greater legal force than if they were set out in a preamble to the legislation. As stated earlier, principle c is significant and noteworthy in its deliberate recognition of the unique position that women occupy in relation to the application of reproductive and genetic technologies. As far as we can determine, Canada is unique among nations in signaling that women, more than men, are impacted by the development and use of reproductive and genetic technologies. How this principle will be interpreted, and therefore the direct effect that it will have on decisions about applications of the technologies, remains to be seen. However, its inclusion as a statutory principle means that courts interpreting this legislation will be called upon to take seriously and account for the embodied and social situatedness of women in relation to the use of such technologies in both the reproductive and research context.

Principle e of the AHR Act, which provides that "persons who seek to undergo assisted reproduction procedures must not be discriminated against, including on the basis of their sexual orientation or marital status," is noteworthy in light of the comments made above in relation to the Australian legislation. Whereas one of the unstated, but nonetheless we argue animating, concerns in Australia is the regulation, indeed prohibition, of homosexual reproduction, it is important to ask whether similar procedures, if performed in Canada, would or could escape prohibition where they conflict with this principle. This is not to suggest that procedures that would facilitate homosexual reproduction and that might be rightfully regulated due to health and safety concerns would be forced to be on offer. But one could argue that where the safety of such procedures had been demonstrated, their use could not be prohibited solely because they facilitated homosexual reproduction.

Finally, the inclusion of principle g in the AHR Act, which provides that "human individuality and diversity, and the integrity of the human genome, must be preserved and protected" highlights the individual as worthy of protection and objectifies the human genome as worthy of the same. While at first blush this principle looks to be reinforcing a liberal humanist conception of the bounded individual while simultaneously clinging to the fiction of the human genome, one could argue that this principle reflects a healthy ambivalence and tension about both entities and concepts. The Canadian legislation draws attention to the issue of diversity which may be important in developing an interpretation in line with the feminist arguments developed in this chapter. At best, diversity, as set out in this principle, is of equal importance to human individuality and the integrity of the human genome. Arguably then, novel forms are also worthy of protection when they contribute to diversity. According to more conventional interpretations, interests of diversity such as sexual preference, disability, race, and color are also to be protected in the application of the reproductive and genetic technologies regulated by the legislation.

As stated earlier, the AHR Act identifies both prohibited and controlled activities. Those activities prohibited under the legislation include creating a human clone or transplanting a human clone into a human being; creating *in vitro* embryos for any purposes other than creating a human being; improving or providing instruction in assisted human reproductive procedures, germ-line genetic alteration of a cell of a human being, or *in vitro* embryo such that the alteration is capable of being transmitted to descendants; transplanting a sperm, ovum, embryo, or fetus of a non-human into a human being; for the purpose of creating a human, using any human reproductive material or any *in vitro* embryo that is or was transplanted into a non-human; creating hybrids for the purpose of reproduction; or transplanting a hybrid into a human or non-human. While most of these prohibitions cover the same procedures banned in the Australian context and are motivated by a similar aim – to curtail the production of a radically-modified human being, a hybrid, or a chimera – there are several notable differences. On its face, the AHR Act does not appear to contain a provision similar to that section in the Australian Prohibition of Human Cloning Act 2002 (Cth.) which prohibits the intentional creation of a human embryo by a process other than the fertilization of a human egg by a human sperm, or the intentional development of a human embryo so created. Thus, while the Canadian legislation is animated by a fear of species transgression and a concern about cloning (asexual production), it is less concerned about homosexual reproduction.

For purposes of the AHR Act, chimera means "(a) an embryo into which a cell of any non-human life form has been introduced or (b) an embryo that consists of cells of more than one embryo, fetus or human being." While hybrid is defined as a human ovum that has been fertilized by a sperm of a non-human life form, or into which the nucleus of a cell of a non-human life form has been introduced, it also includes an ovum of a non-human life form that has been fertilized by a human sperm, or into which the nucleus of a human cell has been introduced. Finally, the definition of hybrid in the AHR Act also includes a human ovum or an ovum of a non-human life form that otherwise contains haploid sets of chromosomes from both a human being and a non-human life form. Accordingly, the AHR Act's prohibition on the creation of hybrids is very strong.

The same is not true of the prohibition on the creation of chimeras. As Jason Scott Robert notes: "the definition of 'chimera' in the AHR Act does not capture the insertion of human cells into non-human embryos, or the implantation of a creature so created in a human or non-human life form." He goes on to explain that "according to the AHR Act, it is prohibited to insert non-human cells into human embryos or to insert human cells into human embryos, while it is not prohibited to insert human cells into non-humans."[68] Unless this omission is an oversight, the most likely explanation for this kind of transgenesis is the creation of human-to-animal chimeras to be used to conduct research on human biology, as Robert argues. What is striking about the AHR Act, therefore, is that while the creation of human-to-human chimeras is prohibited, the coming into being of novel beings, provided they involve the insertion of human cells into non-human embryos, is not. While at first glance, what appears to motivate most of the prohibitions in the AHR Act is a desire to protect the sexual conjugation of human gametes with the result being genetic recombination with its unpredictability of a new phenotype, what is also permitted is the limited exercise of the scientific imagination provided it protects the boundaries of the liberal legal subject.

11.6 New genetic futures: a postmodern feminist legal ethics

In the new genetic future then, so-called "natural maternity" is increasingly undermined by moves toward deviant reproduction, be it homosexual, asexual, monosexual, or clinical. Bart Simon describes the postmodern subject as "an unstable, impure mixture without discernable origins; a hybrid, a cyborg."[69] It is this same subject that conservatives fear we will become if reproduction is "de-naturalized." For instance Joan Didur argues, "[g]enetic engineering in the lab ... is represented as a violent assault on nature and a form of contamination invading the otherwise pure and untainted boundaries of the body of the liberal subject."[70] Liberal subjectivity depends on the exclusion of the other and the capacity to insist upon an autonomous, individuated "I." This kind of "I," however, cannot be sustained by many of us when we are pregnant or live with a disability, for example. Rather, in these contexts subjecthood has to accommodate the other. This, we argue, is not a bad thing. On the contrary, dependency and connection are inevitable relations for us all. If our conception of selfhood was not limited to untainted bounded bodies but instead incorporated dependency and transgression, we suggest we would have a more just society.[71] It is precisely those people whose embodiment transgresses the liberal norm who are the most disempowered in our society. Katherine Hayles argues for instance that "what is lethal is not the post-human as such but the grafting of the post-human onto a liberal humanist view of the self."[72] It is this very liberal humanist view of the self that permeates legal thinking.

Against this liberal view of selfhood, Shildrick argues "the postmodernist approach necessitates an ethic of openness and responsibility towards differences where none is given prior privilege ... acknowledgement of difference deconstructs any reliance on subject/object distinctions, and uncovers the assumption of the subjective autonomy as a mechanism to police boundaries." Shildrick confronts the inviolability of the liberal self with "the leakiness between one's self and others."[73] While critics of the unstable subject of postmodern theory charge postmodern feminism with an ethics of arbitrariness not far removed from nihilism, we argue to the contrary that postmodern feminism is not lacking in ethics, but instead has an ethics radically at odds with the ethic of liberal individualism or humanism. We affirm (with Shildrick) the basis for a more appropriate ethic is a "responsibility towards differences not as the disembodied site of diverse claims, but as an awareness of the irreducible but fluid bodily investments which ground our own provisional being in the world and our interaction with others."[74]

The same concerns are echoed by Marilyn Strathern, and Margaret Davies and Ngaire Naffine. Franklin describes Strathern, for instance, as interested in the way that Western knowledge practices operate to rework the inevitable interconnections of bodies and identities through forms of possessive individualism.[75] This is similar to the analysis that Davies and Naffine offer of legal understandings of identity. As they write: "our jurisprudential understanding of the person is that of a proprietor of self and of the external world. In modern Western law, to own is to be. We are quintessentially possessive individuals."[76] Interestingly, however, this does not translate into a property right over the self. Indeed, as Davies and Naffine argue, the "dogmatic legal position is that persons are *not* property."[77] To be constituted as property raises the possibility of becoming the property of another, and that would not accord with autonomous liberal selfhood.

It is one of those disturbing paradoxes of liberal identity, therefore, that in order to retain one's subjecthood, identified by Davies and Naffine as the person as mind, there must be individual control of one's object body. It is the boundaries of our bodies therefore that must be relentlessly and vigilantly policed. But this view of the self as a unitary, bounded, self-possessing autonomous individual fails to account for myriad relations of dependency and interconnection. Davies and Naffine argue that:

the person does not have to be viewed as a unitary, bounded, self possessing autonomous individual, always in command of his own being and always able to exclude others. The relationship of the pregnant woman to her foetus reveals just some of the failings of this view. So too does the relationship of persons in the acts of sexual intercourse.[78]

With the development of IGM we are challenging liberal selfhood in its very production. There is something fundamentally disruptive for liberal selfhood in the congruence of boundary transgression through reproduction that the manipulation of genetic identity brings about. While some have described this transgressivity as giving rise to the post-human, we want to make a clear distinction between critical post-humanism – a variant of postmodernism hinted at in our discussion of Hayles above – and extropianism, the completion of the enlightenment project and the perfection of the liberal self. This latter post-humanist project is susceptible to an apocalyptic outcome. Liberal selfhood and transgressive or hybrid selfhood can only go together to the detriment of those who cannot transcend their interconnected subjectivity. Indeed the likely outcome of the liberal self-grafted onto the transhuman is the feminist nightmare of reproduction co-opted to the needs of global capital, producing genetically-engineered hybrids that are compliant corporate citizens. However, as Simon asks, are "revulsion, rejection and exclusion the only viable modes of resistance to corporate technoscientific practice"?[79]

Any post-humanist future worthy of embrace needs to be carefully distinguished from one that simply attempts to actualize the liberal humanist fantasy of the self. That self typically aims to transcend its material limits. Critical post-humanism, on the other hand, emphasizes that being human means being embodied. It offers the possibility of breaking out of the constraints that liberal humanism has placed on being human. IGM also offers emancipatory potential in its refusal to close the parenthesis of relationship and kinship. The resulting transgressive kinship can become a step towards the recognition of a plurality of relationships and forms of kinship. What needs to be critiqued more fully is the impulse to limit legal and social recognition to kinship ties of a restrictive type.

NOTES

1 Jason A. Barritt, Carol A. Brenner, Henry E. Malter, *et al.*, Mitochondria in human offspring derived from ooplasmic transplantation, *Human Reproduction* 16 (2001), 513–6.
2 For Australia see the Prohibition of Human Cloning Act 2002 (Cth.) at http://www7.health.gov.au/nhmrc/embryo/; and for Canada see Bill C-6, An Act Respecting Assisted Human Reproduction and Related Research 2004 at http://www.parl.gc.ca/LEGISINFO/index.asp?Lang=E&Chamber=C&StartList=2&EndList=200&Session=12&Type=0&Scope=I&query=4096&List=toc (last accessed 31 March 2005).
3 W. French Anderson, A new front in the battle against disease. In: Gregory B. Stock and John Campbell (eds.), *Engineering the Human Germ-Line*. Oxford: Oxford University Press (2000), 43–8, p. 43.
4 In addition, Anderson notes that there is a small chance that a low level of inadvertent gene transfer into germ-line cells may occur. See also John M. Kaplan and Ina Roy, Accidental germ-line modification through somatic cell gene therapies: some ethical considerations, *The American Journal of Bioethics* 1 (2003), 1–6, who argue that the risk of accidental germ-line modification is not significant enough to preclude further somatic therapies.
5 Isabel Karpin, Legislating the female body: reproductive technology and the reconstructed woman, *Columbia Journal of Gender and Law* 3 (1992), 325–49; Reimagining maternal selfhood: transgressing body boundaries and the law, *Australian Feminist Law Journal* 2 (1994), 36–62.
6 Carlos Novas and Nikolas Rose, Genetic risk and the birth of the somatic individual, *Economy and Society* 29 (2000), 485–513.
7 John Harris, Goodbye Dolly? The ethics of human cloning. In: Hugh LaFollette (ed.), *Ethics in Practice: An Anthology*, 2nd edn, Oxford: Blackwell (2002), 199–208, p. 205.
8 Mark S. Frankel, Inheritable genetic modification and a brave new world: did Huxley have it wrong? *Hastings Center Report* 33 (2003), 31–6, p. 32.
9 See for example Section 8(1) of the Infertility Treatment Act 1995 (Vic.) which provided: "A woman who undergoes a treatment procedure must – (a) be married and living with her husband on a genuine domestic basis; or (b) be living with a man in a *de facto* relationship." This was successfully challenged, however, in *McBain v. State of Victoria* [2000] FCA 1009 (28 July 2000) as contravening *The Sex Discrimination Act 1984* (Cth.).
10 Sarah Franklin, Biologization revisited: kinship theory in the context of the new biologies, 2001, http://www.comp.lancs.ac.uk/sociology/papers/franklin-bioligization.pdf (last accessed 1 April 2005).
11 D. Schneider, *American Kinship: A Cultural Account*. Chicago: University of Chicago Press (1980), p. 23, quoted in Franklin, Biologization revisited, p. 3.
12 Franklin, Biologization revisited, p. 3.
13 Marilyn Strathern, *Reproducing the Future: Essays on Anthropology, Kinship and the New Reproductive Technologies*. New York: Routledge (1992), p. 17.

14 Roxanne Mykitiuk, Beyond conception: legal determinations of filiation and the new reproductive and genetic technologies, *Osgoode Hall Law Journal* 39 (2002), 771–815, p. 774.

15 Franklin, Biologization revisited, p. 8.

16 Derek Morgan, Science, medicine and ethical change. In: Andrew Bainham, Shelly D. Sclater and Martin Richards (eds.), *Body Lore and Laws*. Oxford: Hart Publishing (2002), p. 331.

17 Bill C-6, An Act Respecting Assisted Human Reproduction and Related Research, date of Royal Assent: 29 March 2004.

18 Marcy Darnovsky, Human germline manipulation and cloning as women's issues. In: *Our Bodies Ourselves: Inspiring a Movement of Women's Health around the World*, 20 November 2000, http://www.ourbodiesourselves.org/clone2.htm (last accessed 30 March 2005).

19 Frankel, Inheritable genetic modification, p. 33.

20 Gregor Wolbring, *Science and the Disadvantaged*, Occasional Papers of The Edmonds Institute, 2000, www.edmonds-institute.org/wolbring.html (last accessed 29 March 2005).

21 See also Rosemarie Tong, Traditional and feminist bioethical perspectives on gene transfer: is inheritable genetic modification really *the* problem? (Chapter 9, this volume), and Jackie Leach Scully, Inheritable genetic modification and disability: normality and identity (Chapter 10, this volume).

22 The President's Council on Bioethics, *Beyond Therapy: Biotechnology and the Pursuit of Happiness*, October 2003, http://bioethicsprint.bioethics.gov/reports/beyondtherapy, pp. 8–9 (last accessed 29 March 2005).

23 Allan D. Buchanan, Dan W. Brock, Norman Daniels, *et al.*, *From Chance to Choice: Genetics and Justice*. Cambridge: Cambridge University Press (2000), pp. 98–9.

24 Lennard J. Davis, *Enforcing Normalcy: Disability, Deafness and the Body*. New York: Verso (1995), p. 26.

25 Kerry Taylor and Roxanne Mykitiuk, Genetics, normalcy and disability, *Isuma* 2 (2001), 65–71, p. 66.

26 Judith Levine, What human genetic modification means for women, *World Watch* July/August 2002, p. 28.

27 Gena Corea and Renate D. Klein (eds.), *Man-Made Women: How New Reproductive Technologies Affect Women*. London: Hutchinson (1985); Robyn Rowland, *Living Laboratories: Women and Reproductive Technologies*. Bloomington: Indiana University Press (1992).

28 Margrit Shildrick, *Leaky Bodies and Boundaries: Feminism, Postmodernism and (Bio)ethics*. London: Routledge (1997), p. 199.

29 Frankel, Inheritable genetic modification, p. 33.

30 Richard Lewontin, *Biology as Ideology: The Doctrine of DNA*. New York: Harper Perennial (1991), p. 3.

31 Nikolas Rose, The politics of life itself, *Theory, Culture and Society* 18 (2001), 1–30, p. 18.

32 In Australia to date, each of the states has taken a different approach. In NSW, for instance, there has been no specific regulation of reproductive technology. In Victoria, on the other hand, there has been regulation but it has been aimed at controlling rather than prohibiting the work of fertility clinics, Infertility Treatment Act 1995 (Vic.); see also Reproductive Technology (Code of Ethical Research Practice) Regulations 1995 (SA) and Human Reproductive Technology Act 1991 (WA).

33 Frankel, Inheritable genetic modification, p. 34.

34 Here we are using "unnatural" to refer to non-normative reproduction.

35 Mark S. Frankel and Audrey Chapman (for the American Association of the Advancement of Science), *Human Inheritable Genetic Modifications: Assessing Scientific, Ethical, Religious and Policy Issues*, 2000, http://www.aaas.org/spp/sfrl/projects/germline/report.pdf, p. 33 (last accessed 29 March 2005).

36 United Nations, *The Universal Declaration on the Human Genome and Human Rights*, 11 November 1997, http://www.portal.unesco.org/shs/en/ev.php-URL_ID=1881& URL_DO=DO_TOPIC&URL_SECTION=201.html (last accessed 29 March 2005).

37 The Council of Europe Convention for the Protection of Human Rights and Dignity of the Human Being with Regard to the Application of Biology and Medicine. Parliamentary Assembly of the Council of Europe, Recommendation 934 on Genetic Engineering. Adopted 26 January 1982 in *Texts Adopted by the Assembly 33rd Ordinary Session, Third Part* (Strasbourg: The Council, 1982), recommendation 934, Article 4(i). The Convention on Human Rights and Biomedicine is slightly less specific in outlawing interference with the germ line but not indicating why this kind of interference should be prohibited; Article 13 states: "An intervention seeking to modify the human genome may only be undertaken for preventive, diagnostic or therapeutic purposes and only if its aim is not to introduce any modification in the genome of any descendants," see "Convention on Human Rights and Biomedicine," 1997, http://conventions.coe.int/treaty/en/Treaties/html/164.htm (last accessed 31 March 2005).

38 Frankel and Chapman, Human inheritable genetic modifications, p. 34.

39 Jackie Leach Scully, Drawing a line: situating moral boundaries in genetic medicine, *Bioethics* 15 (2001), 189–204.

40 Julian Savulescu, Deaf lesbians, "designer disability" and the future of medicine, *British Medical Journal* 325 (2002), 771–3.

41 Abby Lippman, The politics of health: geneticization versus health promotion. In: Susan Sherwin (ed.), *The Politics of Women's Health: Exploring Agency and Autonomy.* Philadelphia: Temple University Press (1998), p. 64.

42 Rose, The politics of life itself, p. 18.

43 *Ibid.*, p. 19.

44 *Ibid.*, p. 22.

45 Erik Baard, Supertots and Frankenkids: on the rights of those not yet designed, *Village Voice*, 23–29 April 2003, http://www.villagevoice.com/issues/0317/baard.php (last accessed 29 March 2005).

46 Roxanne Mykitiuk, Fragmenting the body, *Australian Feminist Law Journal* 2 (1994), 63–98, p. 69.

47 Mykitiuk, Beyond conception.
48 Baard, Supertots and Frankenkids, p. 3.
49 N. Katherine Hayles, *How We Became Posthuman: Virtual Bodies in Cybernetics, Literature, and Informatics.* Chicago: University of Chicago Press (1999), p. 285.
50 Martha A. Fineman, *The Neutered Mother, the Sexual Family, and Other Twentieth Century Tragedies.* New York: Routledge (1995).
51 Fineman, The neutered mother.
52 For a comprehensive analysis and critique of the bill, see Isabel Karpin, The genetic connection: owning our "genetic heritage," *Journal of Law and Medicine* 7 (2000), 376–89.
53 Health Legislation (Research Involving Human Embryos and Prohibition of Human Cloning) Act 2003 (Vic.); Prohibition of Human Cloning Act 2003 (SA); Research Involving Human Embryos and Prohibition of Cloning Act 2003 (Qld.); Human Cloning and Other Prohibited Practices Act 2003 (NSW); Human Cloning and Other Prohibited Practices Act 2003 (Tas.); Human Embryonic Research Regulation Act 2003 (Tas.); Human Cloning and Embryo Research Act 2004 (ACT); and Human Reproductive Technology Amendment Bill 2003 (WA). The Northern Territory is in the process of drafting legislation.
54 See Section 25, Prohibition of Human Cloning Act 2002 (Cth.) and Section 47 of the Research Involving Human Embryos Act 2002 (Cth.). A six-person review committee chaired by the Hon John Lockhart AO QC was announced on 17 June 2005. An issues paper was released on 4 August 2005 and is available at http://www.lockhartreview.com.au (last accessed 19 August 2005). The timetable for the review includes submissions to be made by 9 September 2005 and a final report by 19 December 2005. Notably the review is aimed at "assessing the scope and operation of the existing regulatory framework. It is not the purpose of the review to revisit underpinning community debate and rationale for the legislation." (issues paper).
55 Bryan Sykes, *Adam's Curse: A Future without Men.* New York: W.W. Norton (2003).
56 Richard Pendlebury, Men are doomed! *Daily Mail* 18 August 2003.
57 Barritt, Brenner, Malter, *et al.*, Mitochondria in human offspring.
58 It is possible that the intent was simply to prohibit the procedure while its safety was unproven. Given that both Acts were drafted in light of their mandatory review 2 years later, it is also possible that words qualifying the prohibition and tying it to technological advances were seen as unnecessary. Both Acts specify that the review must consider developments in technology in relation to ARTs and developments in medical and scientific research.
59 In Australia, eggs cannot be sold but they can be donated, as can sperm; see Prohibition of Human Cloning Act 2002 (Cth.), Section 23 (see also the various State counterparts).
60 Kaplan and Roy, Accidental germ-line modification.
61 NHMRC, *Ethical Guidelines on the Use of Reproductive Technology in Clinical Practice and Research,* 2004, http://www7.health.gov.au/nhmrc/publications/synopses/e56syn.htm (last accessed 29 March 2005). These guidelines replace existing *Ethical Guidelines on Assisted Reproductive Technology* (1996); Supplementary Note 5 – *The Human Fetus and*

the *Use of Human Fetal Tissue* (1992), and Supplementary Note 5 of the *National Statement on Ethical Conduct in Research Involving Humans.*

62 The Royal Commission on New Reproductive Technologies (RCNRT) says that "[t]he ethic of care means that a large part of ethical deliberation is concerned with how to build relationships and prevent conflict, rather than being concerned only with resolving conflicts that have already occurred," see RCNRT, *Proceed With Care: Final Report of the Royal Commission on New Reproductive Technologies.* Ottawa: Minister of Government Services, Canada (1993), p. 53. The interests of individuals and communities thus may be considered interdependent.

63 RCNRT, *Proceed With Care*, p. 107.

64 *Ibid.*, p. 108.

65 In October 2003, the Bill was passed by the House of Commons; however it died on the order paper (after its second reading in the Senate) on 13 November 2003, when Parliament was prorogued in the wake of a leadership change precipitated by Prime Minister Jean Chretien's retirement. The House of Commons reinstated the Bill, renumbered as Bill C-6, at the same state as it had been when the previous session was prorogued.

66 Bill C-47 *Human Reproductive and Genetic Technologies Act*, 2nd Sess., 35th Parl., 1996.

67 Health Canada, *Assisted Human Reproduction – Frequently Asked Questions*, http://www.hc-sc.gc.ca/english/media/releases/2001/2001_44ebk3.htm, May 2001 (last accessed 29 March 2005).

68 Jason Scott Robert, Regulating the creation of novel human beings, *Health Law Review* 11 (2002), 9–19, p. 15.

69 Bart Simon, Introduction: toward a critique of posthuman futures, *Cultural Critique* 53 (2003), 1–9, p. 4.

70 Joan Didur, Re-embodying technoscientific fantasies: posthumanism, genetically modified foods, and the colonization of life, *Cultural Critique* 53 (2003), 98–115, p. 108.

71 See also Karpin, "Reimagining maternal selfhood," and "Peeking through the eyes of the body: regulating the bodies of women with disabilities." In: Melinda Jones and Lee Ann Basser Marks (eds.), *Disability, Divers-ability and Legal Change.* London: Martinus Nijhoff (1999), 283–300.

72 Hayles, *How We Became Posthuman*, pp. 286–7.

73 Shildrick, *Leaky Bodies and Boundaries*, p. 179.

74 *Ibid.*, p. 180.

75 Franklin, Biologization revisited, p. 3.

76 Margaret Davies and Ngaire Naffine, *Are Persons Property? Legal Debates about Property and Personality.* Aldershot: Ashgate (2001), p. 98.

77 Davies and Naffine, *Are Persons Property?* p. 181.

78 *Ibid.*, p. 185; see also Karpin, "Reimagining maternal selfhood," and "Peeking through the eyes of the body."

79 Simon, Introduction, p. 8.

12

Inheritable genetic modification: clinical applications and genetic counseling considerations

Joan A. Scott

It is entirely speculative at this point whether technologies to alter the human germ line will develop to the point where they are deemed safe and effective enough to be made available to prospective parents, much less considered ethically acceptable. But even the possibility that such profound technologies might be used has prompted intense debate. The scientific, ethical, moral, and social issues raised by these technologies have been debated in this volume and elsewhere. Missing in the discussion thus far, however, have been the perspectives of the couples or individuals who might consider the use of such technologies, consideration of the clinical or research setting in which these technologies might be offered, and the impact of that setting on couples, or the perspectives and concerns of the health professionals and researchers who may be in the position of counseling the families and providing the services. Additionally, the public has not yet been invited into the discussion in any meaningful way. In the interest of extending the debate, this discussion will try to anticipate some of the patient, genetic counseling, and application aspects of technologies developed to alter the human germ line and articulate the need to include many more voices and perspectives in the debate. Some may consider this discussion premature, perhaps even inappropriate at this point in time, but given the speed with which scientific progress is made, it seems prudent to at least introduce these issues into the debate.

12.1 The application of inheritable genetic modification technologies to humans

When will bench and animal research have progressed to the point that human clinical trials of inheritable genetic modification (IGM) might be considered ethically justifiable, at least from the technical standpoint? Some believe that there will never be enough data to feel confident of the safety of IGM in humans. In the 2000 report of the American Association for the

Advancement of Science on IGM, the working group made the following recommendation:

Human trials of inheritable genetic changes should not be initiated until techniques are developed that meet agreed upon standards for safety and efficacy. In the case of the addition of foreign genetic material, the precise molecular change or the changes in the altered genome should be proven with molecular certainty, probably at the sequence level, to ascertain that no other changes have occurred. Furthermore, the functional effects of the designed alteration should be characterized over multiple generations to preclude slowly-developing genetic damage and the emergence of an iatrogenic genetic defect. In the case in which attempts at IGM involve precise correction of the mutant sequence and no addition of foreign material, human trials should not begin before it can be proven at the full genome sequence level that only the intended genetic change, limited to only the intended site, has occurred. If it is shown at the full genome sequence level that the sequence of a functionally normal genome has been restored, there will likely be no need for multigenerational evaluation. [1]

For the purpose of this discussion, let us assume that we are at some time in the future and that these technical issues have been addressed – techniques have advanced to the point where animal studies demonstrate that one gene can cleanly replace another, without leaving any footprint behind, and that the introduced gene is under appropriate control so that it is expressed in the right tissues at the right time. Additionally, the techniques of adding genes have developed to the point that in animal studies the added genes can be demonstrated to be stable over multiple generations. The rest of this chapter will examine issues related to offering the first IGM trials in humans – who might be candidates for such technologies; in what setting and under what circumstances IGM might be made available and by whom; the comparable risks and benefits that would need to be weighed by the individual or couple considering IGM versus alternative options; what the counseling issues might be that are specific to this situation; and why an individual or family might consider the use of such powerful technologies.

12.2   Candidates for IGM

There is considerable debate about who will be the first candidates for IGM. Some believe that the first clinical applications for IGM will be for couples at risk for having a child with a serious genetic condition. One of the strongest arguments against IGM in these circumstances, however, is that there are relatively few genetic situations for which IGM would be the *only* technology available for such a couple and that other, less risky reproductive options would be more appropriate.

12.2.1   Alternatives to IGM

Depending on the mode of inheritance of the particular disorder in question, some of the reproductive alternatives available for at risk couples to prevent the birth of a child with a genetic condition include adoption, conceiving using donor egg or sperm, prenatal diagnosis followed by termination of an affected pregnancy, or *in vitro* fertilization (IVF) followed by preimplantation genetic diagnosis (PGD).

Opponents argue that the availability of these alternatives make it unethical, or at least inappropriate, to offer IGM with its potentially greater risks and unknowns and ethical dilemmas. However, while it may be true that these alternatives do exist, it would be a disservice to the families faced with these decisions to minimize or trivialize the physical or psychologic burden each poses, or the difficulty couples may have in deciding which option is best for them. Adoption can be a lengthy and stressful process as can conception using donor gametes. Prenatal diagnosis involves invasive procedures that carry risks of miscarriage. Additionally, if the purpose is expressly to prevent having an affected child, prenatal diagnosis implies that the couple would at least entertain the possibility of terminating an affected pregnancy. Pregnancy termination poses a significant psychologic burden and many find it to be a morally unacceptable option.

PGD is the method most cited as the obvious alternative to IGM. In this procedure, eggs retrieved from a woman who has undergone hormonal hyperstimulation are fertilized using well-established IVF techniques. At the 6- to 8-cell stage, one cell is removed from each of the embryos that are produced and tested for the gene in question. Only those embryos that demonstrate the desired genetic characteristic are selected for transfer. By testing and selecting only "normal" embryos for transfer, a couple can initiate a pregnancy knowing they would not be faced with the difficult decision to terminate. However, PGD is also not without its moral dilemmas, technical difficulties, and risks. PGD requires the creation of many embryos. Only those with the desired characteristics are selected for transfer. Some find the notion of "picking and choosing" offspring by whatever selection criteria, even to prevent a serious genetic disease, problematic, as well as the fate of the unselected embryos, whether they are not selected because they do not have the right genotype or because they are "surplus," normal embryos. Because of the technical difficulties in performing genetic analysis on a single cell, there is also the risk of misdiagnosis and implanting an affected embryo. Finally, there is some question as to whether the techniques of IVF and PGD themselves carry an increased risk for producing birth defects or congenital abnormalities.[2]

12.2.2   Genetic situations for IGM

However problematic these options may be, they are available and thus there are relatively few genetic situations that have been put forward where IGM would be the *only* option for a couple of having an unaffected child that is genetically related to them. David Resnik *et al.*, propose several situations:

1. both parents homozygous for an autosomal recessive gene,
2. one parent homozygous for an autosomal dominant mutation or the mother homozygous for an X-linked dominant mutation,

3. father carries an X-linked dominant mutation,
4. parents heterozygous for multiple alleles.[3]

In the first scenario, both parents would be affected with an autosomal recessive condition and therefore have only the recessive gene to pass on to their offspring. One hundred percent of their children would be affected – like both of the parents. Having both parents affected with an autosomal recessive condition is certainly a rare situation and one could rightly question whether the investment in research for such an uncommon situation is justifiable, but as treatments for genetic conditions improve and more individuals survive to reproductive age, it is perhaps a plausible scenario. The example that is frequently used is cystic fibrosis (CF). Better therapies make the life expectancy of CF such that this scenario is not inconceivable.

The second scenario is similarly quite rare. In this case, the affected parent has only the dominant allele to give to his or her children, so again 100% of his or her children would be affected.

If we approach IGM with the presumption that it is, at least initially, offered only to individuals who have no other options of having an unaffected child that is genetically related, the third situation would not be an appropriate application of IGM. As Resnik correctly states, all of the female offspring of a man who carries an X-linked dominant gene would inherit his X-chromosome and the abnormal gene. However, all of his sons would inherit his Y-chromosome and be unaffected. This couple would have the alternative option of PGD or prenatal diagnosis and of selecting only male embryos and fetuses.

In the fourth scenario it is suggested that PGD is not a practical option because the parents produce various combinations of unaffected embryos, embryos that carry one or more of the recessive mutated genes like the parent, and embryos affected with one or more of the recessive genetic conditions, making it unlikely to get the right combination of genes in an embryo. For example, consider a situation in which both parents are carriers of mutations causing CF and Tay-Sachs disease. IVF followed by PGD and embryo selection would be available; however, Resnik argues that statistically only 1 of 16 embryos would be homozygous normal for both conditions and available for transfer. Given the large numbers of embryos that would have to be produced to get the right combination of genes and the low success rate of IVF and PGD, he suggests that PGD as an approach to prevent the birth of a child carrying either mutation becomes unlikely. However, if the intent is to prevent having a child affected with Tay-Sachs, CF, or both, then transferring heterozygous embryos is certainly appropriate. Over half of the embryos produced would be homozygous normal or carriers for one or both abnormal alleles. Since everyone in the population carries an estimated 6 to 8 lethal, recessive alleles, these embryos would not carry a genetic burden that exceeds populational norms.

The above situations assume that the reason for considering IGM is to prevent a serious condition in an offspring. Because the genetic situations described are so exceedingly rare, however, many believe that it will be parents seeking enhanced characteristics for their offspring that will ultimately drive the development and utilization of IGM. The enhancements sought could be for health-related reasons, for example parents seeking to add genes that will boost immunity in their offspring. Or they may be for purely aesthetic or performance reasons – genes to enhance physical characteristics or increase musical talent, for example.[4] Although in some respects the counseling issues will be the same regardless of the intent of the IGM – discussion of safety and risks, for example – the motivational factors, not to mention the broader societal implications, will be entirely different. This chapter focuses primarily on IGM in the context of genetic disease conditions.

12.3 Setting and oversight mechanisms for IGM studies in humans

The first use of IGM, assuming agreed upon medical safety and efficacy standards have been met, will likely occur in a research setting. Although the intent of this chapter is not to review the regulatory climate for IGM, the setting and oversight mechanisms will pose additional challenges for couples who might avail themselves of this technology as well as confound the counseling issues; thus some discussion is warranted.

The specifics of the oversight mechanism will vary from country to country, but in the U.S.A., the Food and Drug Administration's (FDA's) Center for Biologics Evaluation and Research (CBER) has authority over gene transfer technologies and regulates both the gene and the vector used to deliver the gene.[5] Any investigator wishing to test a gene transfer product, therefore, must first submit an Investigational New Drug (IND) application, which includes the scientific and animal data justifying its use in humans and documents that an Institutional Review Board (IRB)-approved protocol, discussed in more detail below, is in place. The FDA can also step in and stop a trial if adverse events are reported that indicate unacceptable risks.

The Recombinant DNA Committee (RAC) of the National Institute of Health (NIH) Office of Biotechnology Activities (OBA) also provides some oversight of gene therapy trials in the U.S.A. The RAC reviews all federally-funded somatic cell gene transfer (SCGT) trials or trials taking place at federally-funded institutions. Only protocols that raise novel issues are required to go through full public RAC review. Novel issues identified that could warrant a public review include:

1. a new vector/new gene delivery system,
2. a new clinical application,
3. a unique application of gene transfer,
4. other issues considered requiring further discussion.[6]

Although the RAC is not a regulatory body and cannot ultimately approve or reject protocols, local Institutional Biosafety Committees (IBCs) cannot give final approval of a protocol until the RAC has reviewed the protocol or determined that the protocol raises no new issues and full RAC review is not needed. The advantage of RAC reviews are that they are public, so new issues can be brought to a public forum for discussion. The RAC has stated:

> Public discussion of human gene transfer experiments (and access to relevant information) shall serve to inform the public about the technical aspects of the proposals, meaning and significance of the research, and significant safety, social, and ethical implications of the research. RAC discussion is intended to ensure safe and ethical conduct of gene transfer experiments and facilitate public understanding of the novel area of biomedical research.[7]

The local IRB, which must approve all federally-funded research involving humans and protocols submitted with IND applications to the FDA, also plays a role in oversight. Federal requirements stipulate that the informed consent documents approved by the IRB contain information about the purpose of the study, a description of what is involved by participating in the trial, the potential risks, potential benefits and alternatives to participating in the research, a statement about the confidentiality of records, a statement about compensation for injury, a contact person to whom questions can be directed, and a statement that participation is voluntary.[8]

The oversight of SCGT studies in the U.S.A. has not been without controversy.[9] The tragic death of Jesse Gelsinger in 1999 led to renewed scrutiny of regulatory procedures and uncovered significant gaps in the current oversight system[10] and steps were taken to rectify deficiencies in the system. Although some complain about duplication of effort and sometimes confusing instructions from both agencies, there are some advantages to the oversight by both the FDA and the RAC. The FDA, regardless of funding source, must review and approve all gene transfer trials. However, FDA reviews are not public. The RAC's reviews are all public; however, privately-funded protocols are not required to be submitted to the RAC.

With regard to IGM specifically, the RAC has stated that they will not entertain protocols involving germ line gene transfer (GLGT) at this time.[11] And although the FDA has not explicitly made the same statement, it stopped fertility clinics in the U.S.A. from performing ooplasm transfer as a method of treating infertility in 2001, citing safety concerns. In this procedure, ooplasm from a normal donor egg is injected into the egg of a woman who had previous failed *in vitro* attempts due to poor embryo development. The theory behind the procedure is that the ooplasm from the donor introduces some unknown beneficial components into the recipient's oocytes. As a result of this procedure, the embryo has three genetic parents – the nuclear DNA from the two parents (as is normal), and the mitochondrial DNA from the mother and the donor of the ooplasm. The authors of the major research paper on the technique cited this as "the first case of human germ line genetic modification resulting in normal children."[12] The FDA sent a letter to all fertility clinics in the U.S.A. stating that the FDA has jurisdiction over "the use of human cells that have received transferred genetic materials by means other than the union of gamete nuclei."[13] Additionally, the FDA stated that:

The FDA feels further public discussion is necessary to: 1) evaluate the potential risks of this procedure, 2) recommend how safety should be monitored, 3) assess how efficacy might best be determined, and 4) determine what further non-clinical data will be needed to support additional human clinical trials.

Thus both agencies have acknowledged the need for public discourse regarding gene transfer studies. What would constitute adequate background research such that the FDA or the RAC would consider a human IGM trial is not clear at this point since neither group has issued any guidance. But the assumption is that, at least in the U.S.A., clinical trials of IGM could not occur without prior approval of at least the FDA (and the RAC if federally funded), and an IRB-approved informed consent process in place, and some public discourse. It is worth noting that IRBs will likely vary considerably regarding their expertise and knowledge about IGM, calling into question the robustness of the informed consent process. Julie G. Palmer has developed a draft consent form for a hypothetical IGM trial illustrating how complex the information and consenting process could be.[14] Thus it will be important for an individual or couple considering IGM to understand that they are participating in a research protocol with all that involves. There will likely be a team of health care professionals, researchers, and scientists with whom the couple will interact. There may be follow-up studies that are required to monitor outcomes or psychologic impact.

Who will provide the information needed by a couple to make an informed decision about proceeding with IGM? The principal investigator in a research protocol is ultimately responsible for the conduct of a clinical trial; however, most researchers are not trained in the skilled communication processes that counseling for IGM will likely require, as discussed more fully below. Additionally, the relationship between researcher and subjects in any clinical trial can be complex and sometimes conflicting. Whereas the researcher has a vested interest in the research itself and in furthering scientific and medical information, the subject is motivated by an entirely different set of factors and expectations. A health care professional not directly involved in the research project who can provide complex technical and risk information in a context that is meaningful, and who has the counseling and communication skills necessary to provide support throughout the decision-making process would be more helpful to the couple or individual.

12.4   Counseling issues in IGM

Individuals or couples who might consider the use of IGM will need extensive information and counseling in order to make an informed decision about participating in an IGM trial. There will be a great deal of factual information that will need to be understood and numerous personal issues resolved. First, an at-risk couple will need to fully understand their genetic situation and their risks of having an affected child. Given the risks of their particular situation they will need to know all of the alternative reproductive options available to them including adoption, conceiving using donor gametes, prenatal diagnosis, and PGD. The relative risks, benefits, burdens, merits, and limitations, both physical and psychologic, of each option will need to be weighed against IGM. The couple will need to weigh the possibility of future treatments for the disorder they are trying to prevent, including the possibility of SCGT for their child, against intervening or trying to prevent the disorder in the first place. If the individual or couple considers IGM as a viable alternative, they should understand the ethical and moral dilemmas that have been raised. Even if they do not adhere to any one position or find a particular option morally objectionable, as potential early adopters of a controversial experimental procedure they should be aware of what the public perceptions are and what the public discourse has been. They also must clearly understand that they are participating in research rather than receiving a proven therapeutic technique.

Additionally, before participating in an IGM trial, the individual or couple must have full disclosure of the risks and benefits of the procedures they are considering. Theoretically, there are several ways one could introduce a gene into the germ line and the relative risks, benefits, and limitations that a couple will need to consider will depend on which approach is being proposed, as well as the supporting technologies that might be employed. For example, IVF, PGD, or follow-up prenatal diagnosis could be recommended depending on the technique in question; the risks involved with those procedures also must be factored in.

Clearly this is a great deal of information to impart and for a couple to digest and process. These discussions are likely to require multiple sessions that may extend over a long period of time, depending on how much knowledge and previous experience the couple has at the beginning of this process.

12.4.1   Techniques involving embryo manipulation

Some feel the most straightforward approach technically to altering the human germ line will be to introduce the gene into egg or sperm cells, a fertilized egg, or preimplantation embryo. For example, one way this might be approached is that eggs retrieved from a woman who has undergone hyperstimulation could be fertilized using standard IVF procedures. The new genetic material could be injected directly into the fertilized egg or at very early stages of cell division. Alternatively, the embryos might be grown in culture until they reach the blastocyst stage, at which point embryonic stem (ES) cells are removed and the gene introduced. The modified ES cells could then be induced to differentiate into gametes used for fertilization or the nucleus of a modified ES cell could be inserted back into an egg cell with its own nucleus removed and the resulting embryo transferred into a woman's uterus to initiate a pregnancy.[15]

Regardless of the specific approach, most advocate that IGM should not be considered until techniques to replace one gene cleanly with another, without leaving any trace behind, are developed. By cleanly replacing one gene for another, the introduced gene will, presumably, insert into the genome at the place where it will be under appropriate regulatory control, resulting in normal gene expression. How accurately and consistently this can be accomplished, however, is uncertain.

Other approaches envision adding one or more genes into the embryo via an artificial chromosome.[16] It has even been suggested that these could be engineered with regulatory features that would enable the recipient child to decide at a later time whether to activate the added genes or not, thus avoiding some of the criticism of IGM regarding the lack of informed consent of the recipient.

IGM techniques that involve manipulation of gametes or embryos allow some opportunity to test for unanticipated outcomes. Follow-up testing of an embryo using PGD could prevent an embryo from being transferred that had not incorporated the new gene or chromosome correctly. Prenatal diagnosis and monitoring the pregnancy with ultrasound might provide additional opportunities to look for obvious problems. However, PGD and prenatal diagnostic techniques are limited in their ability to detect genetic abnormalities, and ultrasound can detect only the most obvious structural fetal defects. Thus, an error introduced by IGM may very well not be detected until its effect made itself known, which is potentially not for some time. In addition to the risks of IGM are the risks of the supporting assisted reproductive technologies including IVF, embryo cryopreservation, intracytoplasmic sperm injection (if it is performed), and PGD.

12.4.2   SCGT approaches

Theoretically, a gene could be delivered to the reproductive tissue of the parent using the same techniques that are currently being employed to deliver genes to other tissues in SCGT trials. The major problem with this approach is that it is subject to all of the technical difficulties and risks inherent in SCGT – selecting and designing a vehicle that delivers the gene and its regulatory elements to the targeted tissue, without widespread dissemination to other tissues, but with a high enough efficiency that most of the reproductive tissue incorporates the gene, and achieving stable gene expression and maintenance. Many feel that the technical challenges and risks of the SCGT approach will be difficult to overcome. However, some who may want to consider IGM, but object to the approaches outlined above because they involve manipulating embryos, may be more amenable to SCGT.

In summary, all of the techniques proposed for IGM are fraught with significant technical difficulties and risks, and many require supporting technologies that in and of themselves have inherent risks. Whether IGM involves gene replacement or gene addition, the potential risks and unknowns are considerable. An error in gene replacement could result in an undetected mutation whose effect may not be apparent until the child that resulted from that procedure becomes an adult, or perhaps not even until a later generation. Techniques that involve adding genes, whether they insert into the resident genome or reside in artificial chromosomes, involve additional risks due to the difficulty of ensuring the appropriate gene regulation and stability across generations. Although this discussion began with the assumption that IGM technology had advanced to the point in animal studies where clinical trials in humans could be ethically offered, animal studies can never completely predict risk in humans. Any individual or couple considering IGM would have to be willing to accept the risks of the IGM procedure, as well as all of the supporting and follow-up technologies. How well-known those risks are or whether they can be quantified in any reasonable or helpful way is questionable. Thus, the couple or individual will also need to be able to accept a considerable level of uncertainty.

12.4.3   Decision-making and IGM

How will individuals or couples weigh their options? They will come to this decision with diverse psychologic and moral frameworks and rich personal histories. Understanding these frameworks will be critical in helping individuals and couples work through decision-making in choosing between reproductive alternatives. Decision-making around *any* pregnancy, childbirth, and parenthood is laden with biologic, psychologic, and social significance,[17] even without the additional burden of being at risk of having a child affected with a severe disorder or of making decisions about complex and controversial technologies. Reproductive decision-making in the context of a risk for an abnormality is influenced by an individual's view of self, previous experience, family and social environments, experience with the disorder, ethnic and cultural background, the value and meaning placed on parenthood and family, coping strategies, problem-solving abilities, and religious and moral beliefs. It is a complex process that occurs over time and is made even more difficult when all of the outcomes of the available options are not knowable or foreseeable, as in the case of IGM.

Do we have any experience in reproductive decision-making in other arenas that provide some guidance as to how couples faced with the decision to undergo IGM may respond? An extensive body of literature has developed over the 30 years that prenatal diagnosis has been available which documents the complexity of the issues related to reproductive decision-making. Various studies have shown that direct experience with a disorder, the magnitude of the perceived risk, the perceived severity of a disorder, the desire to have more children, the availability of prenatal diagnosis, and the acceptance of termination as an option all influence reproductive decisions and the acceptance of prenatal diagnosis.[18] Once a decision has been made the couple may experience additional anxiety or distress. For example, P.G. Frets *et al.*, found that the availability of prenatal diagnosis influenced the decision to have children for at-risk couples.[19] However, of significance is that those couples for whom prenatal diagnosis was available reported their decision-making as being more burdensome than those couples without this option. Thus, prenatal diagnosis did not provide an "easy way out."

PGD is the technique most similar to proposed IGM techniques. However information about decision-making for PGD is scant. PGD is not a simple procedure; it involves hormonal stimulation to retrieve multiple eggs, complex analysis of the embryos, and cryopreservation of excess embryos, yet results in a low "take home" baby rate. Even in the best hands, the probability of achieving a live birth from a combined IVF/PGD attempt is only about 20%. Undertaking IVF and PGD therefore requires considerable dedication and resources on the part of the family and the team of clinicians and scientists providing the services. A very small study of clients who had undergone PGD, half of whom had prenatal diagnosis in a previous pregnancy and 36% of whom had a previous pregnancy termination, found that PGD was an acceptable alternative to prenatal diagnosis, but it was by no mean an easy solution. In fact, 35% of clients who had had both prenatal diagnosis and PGD found PGD *more* stressful than prenatal diagnosis.[20] In 2003, the Genetics and Public Policy Center at Johns Hopkins University conducted interviews with selected key informants about the development and use of reproductive technologies, including IGM. Included were 10 women who had had PGD for a single gene disorder. Although very supportive of the technology, these women expressed surprise at the low success rate of IVF – they had assumed that because they were fertile, they would have greater success in achieving a pregnancy – as well as dismay at the failure rate of being able to make a diagnosis based on a single cell. Once a pregnancy was achieved, these women expressed significant reluctance in putting the pregnancy at additional risk by doing confirmatory prenatal diagnosis.[21]

People's perceptions of their own risk will influence their reproductive choices.[22] How an individual views her risks and the value and weight given to alternatives solutions is not at all straightforward. Risk perception is not just an understanding of objective, numeric information, but a more qualitative process of how that number is internalized and understood.[23] Factors that can influence risk perception include previous experience, how readily possible outcomes can be brought to mind, the implications of those outcomes, and how optimistic or pessimistic a person is, to name a few. For example, 35 is the commonly accepted age to offer prenatal diagnosis because it is at that age that the risk of miscarriage from the procedure begins to equal the risk that a woman will have a live birth with a chromosome abnormality. These guidelines assume, however, that women value these two adverse outcomes equally. In fact, some studies have shown that when women consider just these two outcomes, on average, women considering prenatal diagnosis view chromosome abnormalities as 22% worse than miscarriage[24] and that when other possible outcomes are added, the value that women place on information outweighs all other risks,[25] thus calling into question the rationale for age 35 as the cut-off for offering prenatal diagnosis.

Personal experience with a disorder can also significantly influence an individual's views of reproductive options. In the hypothetical genetic situation that we have been considering – a couple both of whom are affected with an autosomal recessive condition or one parent homozygous for a dominant gene – the couple will come to this situation with a lifetime of complex experiences related to their own conditions, including whether they even consider it to be something that needs "preventing." This will significantly impact their perceptions of the risk of having a child with a condition similar to theirs, balanced against future medical options for that child. Studies evaluating the attitudes of affected patient populations toward reproductive technologies have found conflicting results. In 2001, Lidewij Henneman et al., found that adults with CF and parents of affected children considered prenatal diagnosis an acceptable reproductive option in general, but would have found it difficult to make a personal decision to abort.[26] Similarly, Diane Beeson and Theresa Doksum reported on interviews with families with an individual affected with either CF or sickle cell anemia. When addressing the availability of carrier testing and prenatal diagnosis, they described what they call "experiential resistance":

Family members become unwilling to equate the meaning of the life of a person with a genetic disorder to their disease, or even the suffering that may accompany it. They are unable to avoid seeing many other fulfilling dimensions of the life of an affected person.[27]

Another important aspect of their research was that this resistance was not fully articulated until some probing by the interviewer; thus simple surveys of the population or even cursory genetic counseling will miss the "essential elements of rational thought, moral concerns, and lived experience upon which counselees' resistance is based."[28]

These and other studies have been limited to examining carrier testing, prenatal diagnosis, or PGD, not specifically the use of IGM. There has been little research into how at-risk families would view such technologies. Among the informants in the 2003 study conducted by the Genetics and Public Policy Center were adults affected with a genetic condition and parents of affected children.[29] One woman with achondroplasia said about the hypothetical use of IGM to prevent having a similarly affected child:

I would not be for that. Nothing wrong with being a dwarf. It goes along the same lines of having these limbs lengthened. A dwarf is a dwarf ... It's going to wipe out a lot of things. I mean, there's no such thing as the perfect world, but it sounds like these scientists are trying to make it a perfect world. There's no such thing as a perfect human being.

But a man with achondroplasia was more accepting of IGM:

I would say that would be a decision based on personal belief. Would I do that? No. But I would find it acceptable if somebody else did it … You know, you never know what battles people have internally, and you never know what it is like. So although I may disagree personally with some decisions, it's not my responsibility to put that on somebody else.

And from a woman with a teenage daughter with CF, regarding IGM to prevent CF:

I think it's fine; it's wonderful … If they could do something to fix the CF gene, it would just be remarkable the way it would just change the lives of 30,000 people we have living here in the United States, some of whom are truly suffering and not only they are, the families are.

A man with Marfan's who has affected children said about IGM for Marfan syndrome:

… I think that this could be something wonderful. If we could eliminate the genetic loci from any future generations, that would just be absolutely amazing. It would be truly beyond words.

How common are these sentiments? We really do not know. These individuals represented a small group of patients who self-selected to participate in this study. Additionally, a full discussion about the risks and limitations of IGM technologies was not provided as part of the interview. So although *conceptually* there was general support of the idea of eliminating destructive genes from the population, the question of *at what cost* was not fully explored in this study. Much more needs to be done to determine how these technologies are viewed in the patient population and how likely they are to avail themselves of them. It is also important to remember that what people *say* they will do when questioned, and what they will *actually* do when faced with the situation and full disclosure of the risks, can be two very different things. Before the gene for Huntington disease was identified, for example, studies showed a high interest in presymptomatic testing. However, the uptake of testing since the gene has been identified has, in fact, been low.

12.4.4 Counseling approaches

How does one approach counseling individuals or couples in this situation? Historically, there have been two basic approaches to providing genetic counseling in the reproductive context. One has been the teaching approach, which holds that the client is there for information only and the counselor's role is to educate. It assumes that decisions are made on the basis of a rational understanding of the information and that the client is able to make a decision if the information is presented in a factual and neutral way.[30] The second is the counseling or psychologic approach, in which it is believed that decisions are based

on complex interactions between the information and the subjective meaning
of that information. Here the role of the counselor is to help the client work
toward understanding the information in a meaningful way and as such the
counselor is an active participant in the counseling session.[31] This approach
provides a better opportunity for informed decision-making. Given the complexities of IGM and the many issues that an individual or couple would need
to consider, it seems a better model to consider.

The central ethos of the counseling approach has been that the counselor is
non-directive. This concept has been misunderstood as meaning that the counseling is value-neutral or that the counselor is prohibited from giving advice or
being directive. A broader, and more correct interpretation, however, is that
non-directive counseling is an approach that promotes client autonomy, and
that counselors actively participate in the counseling session by utilizing various counseling models and techniques appropriate to the situation to foster
decision-making. The key tenets of non-directive counseling – respect for the
client, providing a safe and supportive environment, addressing emotional and
psychologic issues, and utilizing interventions that support the client's
autonomous decision-making skills – are certainly relevant in the context of
providing counseling for IGM.[32]

Again, the clinical and counseling situations we have been considering presume that the reason for the IGM is to prevent a serious genetic defect in a
child. In this situation the couple or individual faced with the decision will
most likely be very familiar with the disorder and have had a lifetime of experience with the health care system. If IGM were being considered for enhancement purposes, however, it is clear that the experiences and motivations of
candidate couples would be completely different. Trying to anticipate and
develop an understanding of the experiential and psychologic framework that
would motivate a couple to consider the use of such powerful technology for
these reasons is more difficult, and providing appropriate guidance and counseling would be potentially infinitely more complicated.

12.4.5 Attitudes of researchers and health care professionals about IGM

How do the health care professionals caring for these families or who would
provide the services feel about IGM? Isaac Rabino surveyed members of the
American Society of Human Genetics on their attitudes about gene therapy.
Although there was less support than for somatic cell therapy (64% as compared to 96% support for somatic cell therapies), the majority of respondents
supported the use of IGM – with the caveat that it was proven safe and effective,
and used to prevent serious disease but not for enhancement purposes.[33]

This was similar to findings in the 2003 interviews conducted by the
Genetics and Public Policy Center that included PGD providers.[34] Among this

small group, there was general support for IGM although the need for a safe procedure was repeatedly emphasized. As one provider stated:

… I would not do it if the technique is not safe. It has to be super, super safe. But once it's safe, no, I wouldn't draw a line. I think it's up to the couple what they want to do with their babies, provided, obviously, that the baby's going to be accepted by society … [When discussing the future of IGM] Again, I don't know where society is going to be 10 years from now. I think 20 years ago people would not have been as accepting of sex selection as they are now. Society changes, and our feelings towards things change. And I think as science changes those boundaries, people tend to open up … I think people get comfortable with technology.

12.4.6   Attitudes of the general public about IGM

In addition to the key informant interviews, the Genetics and Public Policy Center conducted 21 focus groups in five locations around the U.S.A. in 2003 about what the public thinks, knows, and feels about reproductive genetic technologies, including IGM.[35] In contrast to the health care providers and even some of the patients interviewed and quoted above, a more cautionary tone was notable. Although support for the idea of eradicating serious diseases was frequently voiced, the potential downsides were well-recognized and articulated. One woman said about the possibility of correcting the gene for sickle cell anemia:

… treat the child so that they don't have sickle cell and their kids don't have sickle cell. … I think that is a good thing. I think I would recommend it.

But another woman discussing CF stated:

I like the idea of this one thing [CF], and maybe a few other life threatening, horrible disease kinds of things, but I know it would never stop.

This concern about a technology and its practitioners careening out of control was raised by many; for example:

It's all or nothing. If you've gone down this road at all, you've gone down completely. You can talk about matters of degree, but you're playing God. … if we can actually do it, I think that's great. But there is a lot of downside that goes with it. We're talking about the best intentions of medicine, and assuming that this is all going to be for good. But how many movies have we seen [with] so many nightmare scenarios of people manipulating this. So opening that door at all means its open, regardless of the degree.

The issue of social inequities was raised repeatedly:

I mean, obviously this is not going to be available to everybody, regardless of whether it's subsidized by insurance or whatever. There are going to be some people that are able to have super kids, or improved kids, and a lot that aren't.

And finally the larger question of how we view ourselves and our place in the world was expressed:

People get caught up in making the perfect child. You are trying to create the perfect life and making the perfect child, and that is not synonymous.

We are not meant to have a planet of complete, perfect individuals that are going to live to 100 years old.

When evaluating reproductive genetic technologies, including IGM, participants considered 6 key factors in determining the appropriateness of the technology:

1. whether embryos would be destroyed,
2. the nature of the disease or trait being avoided or sought,
3. technologic control over "natural" reproduction,
4. the value of suffering, disability, and differences,
5. the importance of having genetically-related children, and
6. the kind of future people desire.

That the public is deeply ambivalent about these technologies and concerned about the wider societal impact was also demonstrated in a survey done by the Genetics and Public Policy Center in 2004 of 4834 members of the general public.[36] Americans were much less approving of IGM than PGD or prenatal diagnosis to prevent the birth of a child with fatal disease and very few supported its use to have children with selected traits. Participants also expressed a high level of concern for some societal implications of all of these technologies.

12.5   Summary

This chapter began by acknowledging the hypothetical nature of the scenarios discussed. Indeed, there are those who would argue that the risks involved with IGM are such that even if technical issues are satisfactorily addressed (and that is a major qualifier in some people's minds), the larger ethical issues would preclude any use of IGM. Undoubtedly, IGM in humans will bring with it numerous questions, not the least of which is "for what purpose is it permissible?". This chapter does not address the very complex issues of parents seeking IGM for enhancement purposes. There are also large gaps in our knowledge of where stakeholder groups and the general public stand on the issues that IGM raises. More studies and public dialogue is needed to fully explore attitudes about IGM and the values that shape those attitudes.

If the debate about the use of IGM is to be meaningful, it should be grounded in real applications, not speculation. As the science moves forward, we should foster discussion about who might be a potential recipient of IGM, for what purpose and under what circumstances, in what setting, and at what cost. This debate should be conducted in a public arena that includes not just scientists and ethicists, but the families who may be impacted, the health professionals who care for these families, policymakers who must address the many policy implications, and the general public.

Acknowledgment

The author would like to thank the Genetics and Public Policy Center at Johns Hopkins University and The Pew Charitable Trusts for the data on public attitudes.

NOTES

1 Mark S. Frankel and Audrey R. Chapman, *Human Inheritable Genetic Modifications: Assessing Scientific, Ethical, Religious, and Policy Issues,* prepared by the American Association for the Advancement of Science, Washington, DC, September 2000, http://www.aaas.org/spp/sfrl/projects/germline/report.pdf (last accessed 29 March 2005).

2 Christine Gicquel, Veronique Gaston, Jacqueline Mandelbaum, *et al., In vitro* fertilization may increase the risk of Beckwith-Wiedemann syndrome related to the abnormal imprinting of the KCN1OT gene, *American Journal of Human Genetics* 72 (2003), 1338–41; Roger Gosden, Jacquetta Trasler, Diana Lucifero, *et al.,* Rare congenital disorders, imprinted genes, and assisted reproductive technology, *Lancet* 361 (2003), 1975–7.

3 David B. Resnik, Holly B. Steinkraus and Pamela J. Langer, *Human Germline Gene Therapy: Scientific, Moral and Political Issues.* Austin, TX: R.G. Landes Company (1999); David B. Resnik and Pamela J. Langer, Human germline gene therapy reconsidered, *Human Gene Therapy* 12 (2001), 1449–58.

4 Genetics and Public Policy Center, Johns Hopkins University, *Human germline genetic modification:* issues and options for policymakers, 2005, http://www.dnapolicy.org (last accessed 31 March 2005).

5 U.S. Food and Drug Administration, Human gene therapy and the role of the Food and Drug Administration, September 2000, http://www.fda.gov/cber/infosheets/genezn.htm (last accessed 29 March 2005).

6 National Institutes of Health (NIH), Guidelines for research involving recombinant DNA molecules, April 2002, http://www.od.nih.gov/oba/rac/guidelines/guidelines.html, (last accessed 29 March 2005).

7 NIH, Guidelines for research involving recombinant DNA molecules.

8 Kennith Cornetta and Franklin O. Smith, Regulatory issues for clinical gene therapy trials, *Human Gene Therapy* 13 (2002), 1143–9.

9 LeRoy Walters, The oversight of human gene transfer research, *Kennedy Institute of Ethics Journal* 10 (2000), 171–4.

10 Cornetta and Smith, Regulatory issues for clinical gene therapy trials; Lynn Smith and Jacquelione F. Byers, Gene therapy in the post-Gelsinger era, *JONAS Healthcare, Law, Ethics, and Regulation* 4 (2002), 104–10.

11 NIH, Guidelines for research involving recombinant DNA molecules.

12 Jason A. Barritt, Carol A. Brenner, Henry E. Malter, *et al.*, Mitochondria in human offspring derived from ooplasmic transplantation, *Human Reproduction* 16 (2001), 513–16.

13 U.S. Food and Drug Administration, Biological Response Modifiers Advisory Committee (BRMAC), Ooplasm transfer as method to treat female infertility, Briefing Document for Day 1, 9 May 2002, http://www.fda.gov/OHRMS/DOCKETS/ac/02/briefing/3855B1_01.pdf (last accessed 29 March 2005).

14 Julie Gage Palmer, Appendix A. Consent form for participating in a study of inheritable germline modification. In: Audrey R. Chapman and Mark S. Frankel (eds.), *Designing our Descendants: The Promise and Perils of Genetic Modifications*. Baltimore, MD: Johns Hopkins University Press (2003).

15 LeRoy Walters and Julie G. Palmer, *The Ethics of Human Gene Therapy*. New York: Oxford University Press (1997); Resnik, Steinkraus, and Langer, *Human Germline Gene Therapy*; Frankel and Chapman, *Human Inheritable Genetic Modifications*; Resnik and Langer, Human germline gene therapy reconsidered.

16 Gregory Stock and John Campbell (eds.), *Engineering the Human Germline*. New York: Oxford University Press (2000).

17 Jon Weil, *Psychosocial Genetic Counseling*. New York: Oxford University Press (2000).

18 E.E. Ekwo, J.O. Kim and C.A. Gosselink, Parental perceptions of the burden of genetic disease, *American Journal of Medical Genetics* 28 (1987), 955–63; P.G. Frets, H.J. Duivenvoorden, F. Verhage, *et al.*, Model identifying the reproductive decision after genetic counseling, *American Journal of Medical Genetics* 35 (1990), 503–9; P.G. Frets, H.J. Duivenvoorden, F. Verhage, *et al.*, Factors influencing the reproductive decision after genetic counseling, *American Journal of Medical Genetics* 35 (1990), 496–502; Weil, Psychosocial genetic counseling; Kenneth P. Tercyak, Suzanne B. Johnson, Shearon F. Roberts, *et al.*, Psychological response to prenatal genetic counseling and amniocentesis, *Patient Education and Counseling* 43 (2001), 73–84.

19 P.G. Frets, H.J. Duivenvoorden, F. Verhage, *et al.*, Analysis of problems in making the reproductive decision after genetic counseling, *Journal of Medical Genetics* 28 (1991), 194–200.

20 S.A. Lavery, R. Aurell, C. Turner, *et al.*, Preimplantation genetic diagnosis: patients' experiences and attitudes, *Human Reproduction* 17 (2002), 2464–7.

21 A. Kalfoglou, J. Scott, and K. Hudson, PGD patients' and providers' attitudes about the use and regulation of PGD, *Reproductive BioMedicine Online* 11 (2005), in press.

22 Bonnie S. LeRoy and A. Walker, Genetic counseling: history, risk assessment, strategies, and ethical considerations. In: Richard A. King, Jerome I. Rotter, and Arno G. Motulsky (eds.), *The Genetic Basis of Common Diseases*. New York: Oxford University Press (2002), 87–102; see also Rosemarie Tong, Traditional and feminist bioethical

perspectives on gene transfer: is inheritable genetic modification really *the* problem? (Chapter 9, this volume), and Jackie Leach Scully, Inheritable genetic modification and disability: normality and identity (Chapter 10, this volume).

23 Weil, Psychosocial genetic counseling.

24 Ryan A. Harris, A. Eugene Washington, David Feeny, *et al.*, Decision analysis of prenatal testing for chromosomal disorders: what do the preferences of pregnant women tell us? *Genetic Testing* 5 (2001), 23–32.

25 Miriam Kuppermann, David Feeny, Elena Gates, *et al.*, Preferences of women facing a prenatal diagnostic choice: long-term outcomes matter most, *Prenatal Diagnosis* 19 (1999), 711–6; Miriam Kuppermann, Robert F. Nease, Lee A. Learman, *et al.*, Procedure-related miscarriages and Down syndrome-affected births: implications for prenatal testing based on women's preferences, *Obstetrics and Gynecology* 96 (2000), 511–6; Harris, Washington, Feeny, *et al.*, Decision analysis of prenatal testing for chromosomal disorders.

26 L. Henneman, I. Bramsen, T.A. Van Os, *et al.*, Attitudes towards reproductive issues and carrier testing among adult patients and parents of children with cystic fibrosis (CF), *Prenatal Diagnosis* 21 (2001), 1–9.

27 Diane Beeson and Theresa Doksum, Family values and resistance to genetic testing. In: Barry C. Hoffmaster (ed.), *Bioethics in Social Context.* Philadelphia: Temple University Press (2001), 153–79.

28 Beeson and Doksum, Family values and resistance.

29 Unpublished data; see also Genetics and Public Policy Center, Johns Hopkins University, Human germline genetic modification: issues and options for policymakers.

30 Patrcia McCarthy Veach, Bonnie S. LeRoy and Dianne M. Bartels, *Facilitating the Genetic Counseling Process: A Practice Manual.* New York: Springer (2003).

31 McCarthy Veach, LeRoy and Bartels, *Facilitating the genetic counseling process.*

32 J. Weil, Psychosocial genetic counseling in the post-nondirective era: a point of view, *Journal of Genetic Counseling* 12 (2003), 199–211; McCarthy Veach, LeRoy and Bartels, *Facilitating the genetic counseling process.*

33 Issac Rabino, Gene therapy: ethical issues, *Theoretical Medicine* 24 (2003), 31–58.

34 Unpublished data; see also Genetics and Public Policy Center, Johns Hopkins University, Human germline genetic modification: Issues and options for policymakers.

35 A.L. Kalfoglou, T. Doksum, B. Berhardt, *et al.*, Opinions about new reproductive genetic technologies: Hopes and fears for our genetic future, *Fertility and Sterility* 83 (2005), 1612–21.

36 Genetics and Public Policy Center, Johns Hopkins University, Human germline genetic modification: issues and options for policymakers.

Can bioethics speak to politics about the prospect of inheritable genetic modification? If so, what might it say?

Roberta M. Berry

13.1 Bioethics, inheritable genetic modification, and politics: informing the policy-making craft

New genetic knowledge and technique continue to generate a torrent of possibilities and associated worries. We hope we might be diagnosed more effectively, treated with pharmaceuticals tailored to our genomes for improved efficacy and diminished side effects, or cured by new somatic cell gene transfer (SCGT) technologies. But we also fear that we might be shunned from the workplace if our employers learn of the vulnerabilities foretold by our genomes, denied health insurance on the basis of genetic test results though we are currently asymptomatic, or misled regarding the prospects of success and the risks of harm while serving as subjects of experimental gene-based research. The possibilities and worries surrounding inheritable genetic modification (IGM), in particular, are remarkable in their variety, nuance, and difficulty.

The focus of these possibilities and worries will vary according to the roles and responsibilities of those who may soon face choices about IGM. First, for parents, there is the hope that future children might enjoy lives free of genetic contributions to burdensome or deadly disease and disability, but also the fear that parents might choose badly – whether due to an overabundance of daring or caution, concern or neglect, perfectionism or ennui, piety or irreverence. If parents do engineer their children, will they be volunteering them as subjects in a grand research project, with risks that are unknowable and, potentially, equally grand? If parents forbear from engineering, will they render their children vulnerable to health risks and to discrimination by social institutions on account of their vulnerability? Would choices to proceed or refrain vindicate or dishonor their commitments to the communities – religious, disability, or ethnic – which partially constitute their social identities?

Second, bioscience and biotechnology researchers, and physicians and other health care professionals also face concerns distinctive to their roles and responsibilities. Would IGM constitute the latest breakthrough in promoting individual well-being and public health, or a revival of old eugenic programs dressed in new garb? Would devoting resources to the development of this technology constitute a justified allocation of resources to meet evolving reproductive health care needs, or an unwarranted devotion of scarce resources to satisfy the demand for "extreme" reproductive care of the well-to-do procreative avant-garde?

Third, members of many kinds of communities – families, research and health care professional groups, religious and secular affinity groups, ethnic and racial identity groups – will encounter issues associated with IGM as they impact their lives in communities. Spouses, for example, may hold differing religious or ethical beliefs about IGM that they must reconcile if they are to engage in the joint practice of procreation and parenting. Research and health care professional groups also are engaged in a joint enterprise, bound together by practical considerations as well as goals, aspirations, and professional norms that are constitutive of their practice; they too will be called on to engage and cope with issues associated with IGM as members of their communities. Leaders of religious communities may be called on to counsel community members about choices on IGM in ways that locate this technology within the tenets of their faith. Disability communities may struggle to decide whether IGM that targets the genetic contribution to a disability can be reconciled with embracing those with the disability; they may also struggle with the implications of IGM for the continuing existence of their communities. And when genetic conditions appear disproportionately among particular racial and ethnic groups, group members may ponder whether scarce research dollars should be devoted to research on IGM that might benefit future generations, to the development of effective and affordable treatments for the living, or to some combination of these.

Finally, the prospect of IGM will command the attention of political communities, the civic societies within which individuals and these diverse private communities conduct their affairs. If we accept the premise that the mission of modern pluralistic democratic political communities includes advancing individual flourishing and the common good – acknowledging that though the premise is uncontroversial, conceptions of what constitute individual flourishing and the common good are not – then the reasons why IGM will command the attention of these communities are evident. Personal well-being, procreation, and parenting are widely recognized as important components of individual flourishing, and public health is widely recognized as an important component of the common good. IGM implicates all of these components of individual flourishing and the common good. Yet it is not obvious how the political community could best vindicate its mission given the perplexing array of questions posed for individuals and private communities, as surveyed above.

These questions arise at the three-way intersection of bioscientific and biotechnological innovation with the complexity of human life systems and with the morally fraught practice of procreation – the locus of other especially difficult questions in politics, including fetal tissue research, stem cell research, and human reproductive cloning. If questions that arise at this locus, including those surrounding IGM, are particularly likely to challenge the ability of the political community to vindicate its mission, can it expect to find help from the discipline of bioethics, which devotes much of its effort to problems that arise at this three-way intersection?

Bioethics, as a branch of ethics that concerns itself with normative questions associated with interventions in human life systems, routinely takes on novel questions generated by bioscientific and biotechnological advances applied to a complex subject matter with implications for morally fraught human experiences, from procreation to death and dying. To answer these questions, bioethics must consider the implications of interventions for the whole person: the biological being, the psychological or "intentional" being, and the social being – a being in part constituted by her membership in a web of private communities. The biological being is itself vastly complex, consisting of multiple, interactive levels from the molecular to the cellular to tissues and organs and organ systems. Alternative accounts of the intentional and social being, and the relationships among these and the biological being, are legion, and variously anchored in theology, social science, the literary imagination, neurobiology, behavioral genetics, sociobiology, and artificial intelligence studies, to name a few.[1] Bioethics, ambitiously, aims to penetrate this vast complexity to shed light on and facilitate practical decision-making about contemplated interventions, often at the leading edge of innovation, in the biological being – including those related to human practices that tap into deeply held moral beliefs anchored in diverse worldviews shared by members of private communities.

I will assume here, without attempting to support the claim, that bioethics succeeds reasonably well in this ambition: the combined efforts of bioethics scholars and clinical bioethicists have yielded insight and helped people make better informed, more reflective practical choices. Policy-makers face different sorts of choices, though. They are called on not to make particular choices at the bedside or in the genetic counselor's office, but to craft rules of general application that will influence the choices of members of the political community – by prohibiting or restricting some choices perhaps, and permitting or encouraging others. If bioethics can help individuals understand and cope with the choices they face, can it also help policy-makers cope with the questions posed by IGM for their mission?

My thesis is that bioethics can speak helpfully to politics about IGM by explicating both the past and an imagined future. In the balance of this chapter, I will attempt to support this thesis by illustrating how historical analysis can illuminate the competing understandings of individual flourishing and the common good that will complicate the task of IGM policy-makers and by illustrating how future imaginings can cast IGM policy issues in concrete, contextualized terms that help sharpen the issues and thereby facilitate practical reasoning and decision-making. I conclude that a bioethically informed politics can cope with the novel, complex, and potentially divisive problems posed by IGM technologies by an ongoing, incremental, iterative process of policy-making: a "navigational approach" that continually listens to soundings of the past and future, and revises its course accordingly.

13.2   History as prelude

Novel bioscience and biotechnologies force us to work through their normative significance without the aid of centuries of deliberation and reflection by our progenitors and the resulting rich and nuanced understandings of practical problems that might be passed along by parents, incorporated in homilies, or codified in professional codes and laws. A time-honored strategy for coping with the novel is to search for its familiar aspects, to which old knowledge can be brought to bear. To suggest a body of the familiar that might help to illuminate the problems that policy-makers will face in IGM policy-making, I sketch three histories that engage the intersection of bioscientific and biotechnological advance with the complexity of human life systems and with the morally fraught practice of procreation, the locus where IGM issues will arise: (1) genetic medicine; (2) eugenics; and (3) reproductive medicine and counseling.

13.2.1   Genetic medicine

Modern bioscientific research began to flower in the nineteenth century and advanced rapidly in the twentieth. In the nineteenth century, Claude Bernard pioneered experimental method in medicine[2] and Louis Pasteur and Robert Koch pursued an association between microorganisms and diseases.[3] Justus von Liebig, Carl Ludwig, and Rudolf Virchow investigated life systems in ways foundational to modern research programs in organic chemistry, physiology, cell biology, and, eventually, molecular biology.[4] These advances in bioscience eventually infused clinical practice, yielding vast new powers to cure and ameliorate disease.[5] New knowledge of the connection between microorganisms and disease supported new protocols and, eventually, new treatments: operations were conducted under antiseptic conditions, and sulfa drugs and antibiotics were developed to cure infectious diseases.

Bioscience research programs in evolutionary science and genetics also were begun in the nineteenth century. The Darwinian theory of evolution and Mendelian "laws" regarding the transmission of characters from generation to generation initiated research programs that examined life from social-evolutionary and organismal-hereditary perspectives. These two perspectives were integrated in an early-twentieth-century "synthesis" that supplied support for the role of natural selection as a mechanism in the "received view" of evolution developed by Charles Darwin and subsequent researchers in evolutionary theory; dissident theories challenged certain aspects of the "received view," and contemporary research programs in evolutionary biology, evolutionary psychology, and sociobiology have emerged from the ensuing debate.[6]

Beginning in the twentieth century, researchers also pursued an understanding of Mendelian genetics at the molecular level, bringing the field of biochemistry to bear in the realm of genetics. This work led to fresh insights and techniques, and a burgeoning biotechnology enterprise built upon them. A cascade of innovations followed upon James Watson and Francis Crick's announcement of the structure of DNA in 1953 and subsequent work showing how Mendelian characters were related to underlying molecular structures. In 1973, Stanley Cohen and Herbert Boyer invented a recombinant DNA technique allowing a fragment of DNA to be snipped from one organism and inserted into the DNA of another[7] and by 1978, an early biotechnology enterprise had inserted human DNA into bacteria, commandeering them to produce human insulin.[8] The production of transgenic animals, animals with DNA inserted from other organisms to render them useful for various industrial applications or as models for the study of disease, took off after the U.S. Supreme Court affirmed the right to patent these life forms in a 1980 decision involving genetically engineered bacteria used in the dissipation of oil spills.[9] In 1988, the first multicellular animal was patented, the "Harvard oncomouse," engineered to be a model for the study of cancer. Many hundreds of transgenic animals have been created and patented since.[10]

In the second half of the twentieth century, human and clinical genetics advanced rapidly, pursuing population studies to better understand patterns of inheritance and bringing knowledge of genetics to bear in clinical medical settings. In the field of human genetics, James Neel drew on his doctorate in fruit fly genetics, his training as a medical doctor, and his studies in statistical methods in pursuing pioneering work on the effects of radiation exposure on residents of Hiroshima and Nagasaki and their descendants.[11] Neel also undertook the study of several hereditary diseases; he detected a pattern of recessive inheritance in sickle cell anemia – only children who inherited recessive genes from both parents suffered the disease – matching the conclusions reached through study of the underlying molecular processes by Linus Pauling and others, an early integration of results in the developing fields of human genetics and molecular biology.

The first clinical genetics department was established by Victor McKusick at Johns Hopkins University in 1957, and rapidly developed an extensive research program – with ties to Neel's program in human genetics – investigating genetically influenced disorders. With the discovery of the cause of Down syndrome and other chromosomal disorders, physicians increasingly referred patients with these disorders in their family histories to clinical geneticists for counseling.

While the programs of Neel and McKusick were especially prominent, there were many other centers of research in human genetics and clinical genetics in the U.S.A. by the end of the 1950s. By 1971, almost 900 disorders caused by a single gene had been identified, and over the course of the 1960s and 1970s, these subjects moved from research frontier to institutionalization in the curricula of most American medical schools.

Advances across these fronts of human and clinical genetics, molecular genetics, and genetic technologies supplied the incentive – the search for clinical benefits – and the bioscientific and biotechnological foundations for a new research program in genomics. In the last decade of the twentieth century, the massive effort to map and sequence the human genome – a taxpayer-supported project extending across academia, industry, and government – was underway, with wide synergistic effects across the frontiers of genomic research and development.[12] Winning Congressional approval for the Human Genome Project (HGP) was testimony to the persuasive power of the promise of clinical benefits across a range of diseases: "[The HGP] was created not by citizens concerned about cancer or heart disease or even genetic disorders, but rather by scientists who argued that a concerted research program was an expeditious way to improve research on all diseases."[13]

To this point, the opportunities for clinical medical benefits flowing from the HGP (or, more broadly, from the confluence of human genetics, clinical genetics, and the new genomic knowledge and know-how) have been limited. Human SCGT experimentation was underway by the 1990s and, by the turn of the twenty-first century, over 400 clinical trials had been conducted, with mixed results.[14] The death of an 18-year-old volunteer in an SCGT experiment in 1999 cast a pall over the research program and prompted a number of investigative studies, Congressional hearings, and regulatory reform proposals.[15] But hopes remain high both for eventual success with SCGT and for improved conventional therapies thanks to new understanding of the mechanisms of disease processes.[16]

13.2.2   Eugenics

Modern eugenics programs, launched by the "founder of the faith" Francis Galton in the late nineteenth century, constituted a significant social movement by the early twentieth, encompassing adherents from across the political spectrum who were united by a shared commitment to improving the human race by measures focusing on heritable characteristics.[17] Eugenicists generally believed that human characteristics were significantly influenced by heredity and that it was important, feasible, and morally right to exert influence over the inheritance of these characteristics to improve the race. Eugenicists variously favored "negative" eugenic measures, including involuntary sterilization of the "unfit" or voluntary abstention from procreation by those likely to pass along disease or disability, and "positive" eugenic measures, including encouraging procreation by those with desirable characteristics.[18]

In one widely-cited instance of American judicial encounter with the early-twentieth-century eugenic project, Justice Oliver Wendell Holmes conferred the approval of the U.S. Supreme Court on eugenic sterilization in his 1927 opinion in *Buck v. Bell*. That case tested the constitutionality of a Virginia involuntary sterilization law pursuant to which Ms Carrie Buck, a young woman who had been determined (incorrectly, we now know[19]) to be mentally disabled. In upholding the statute and permitting the sterilization to proceed, Holmes invoked a public health analogy, and opined both that the welfare of all required individual sacrifice and that the sacrifice after all might not be so great when those doing the sacrificing were "imbeciles":

We have seen more than once that the public welfare may call upon the best citizens for their lives. It would be strange if it could not call upon those who already sap the strength of the State for these lesser sacrifices, often not felt to be such by those concerned, in order to prevent our being swamped with incompetence. It is better for all the world, if instead of waiting to execute degenerate offspring for crime, or to let them starve for their imbecility, society can prevent those who are manifestly unfit from continuing their kind. The principle that sustains compulsory vaccination is broad enough to cover cutting the Fallopian tubes ... Three generations of imbeciles are enough.[20]

A theme evident in Justice Holmes's private correspondence about his opinion in *Buck v. Bell* – and that runs throughout his private and public writings and court opinions – is a deep faith in the guidance that could be found for all realms of life, including public policy, from science.[21] He was a committed social Darwinian, and believed that eugenic policies reflected scientifically sound reform principles that aligned public policy with the laws of nature: "In Holmes's jurisprudence, law was an exercise in social scientific mastery over the conduct of human social affairs, and eugenics was an exercise in scientific and surgical mastery over the conduct of human reproductive affairs, all for the purpose of advancing human welfare along the path of evolution."[22] Accordingly, Holmes wrote to his friend Harold Laski, a British socialist and eugenicist, of his satisfaction in writing the opinion upholding the involuntary sterilization law: "I wrote and delivered a decision upholding the constitutionality of a state law for sterilizing imbeciles the other day – and felt that I was getting near to the first principle of real reform. I say merely getting near. I don't mean that the surgeon's knife is the ultimate symbol."[23]

The decision in *Buck v. Bell* eliminated doubts about the constitutionality of involuntary sterilization regimes in the U.S.A. By the 1930s, most states had enacted involuntary sterilization statutes, and many tens of thousands of Americans, determined by the eugenic science of the day to be "unfit," were sterilized involuntarily over the next few decades until the repeal of these statutes in the 1960s.[24] The U.S.A. was a leader in developing and implementing these policies; in 1933, the German Nazi regime drew on the American approach in enacting its first involuntary sterilization law.[25] The Nazi statute, as the historian

Daniel Kevles recounts, cast a very wide net in identifying those characteristics that would justify sterilization, including "feeblemindedness, schizophrenia, epilepsy, blindness, severe drug or alcohol addiction, and physical deformities that seriously interfered with locomotion or were grossly offensive ... Within three years, German authorities had sterilized some 225,000 people ... About half were reported to be feebleminded."[26]

Pre-World War II eugenicists included "mainline" and "reform" eugenicists; the reformers disavowed the mainline program as unscientific and reflecting race and class prejudice: genetic influences yielding undesirable features, such as low intelligence and "anti-social character," and desirable features, such as high intelligence and high "levels of activity," were distributed evenly, they thought, rather than clustered by race or class as the mainliners assumed. The disproportionate representation of undesirable features among certain groups was caused by unjust social conditions, not by heredity. Some reform eugenicists also conceived of eugenics as a new source of meaning in human life: a cause that could unite humankind in striving for improvement of the race in a post-Darwinian world in which other sources of meaning were no longer plausible.[27]

There was religious and secular opposition to the mainline eugenics program from non-eugenicists as well, citing its violations of human dignity by coercive sterilization, its biological reductionism, its obsession with bodily perfection to the exclusion of other values, and its racism and classism. Most reform eugenicists also rejected the mainliners' advocacy of involuntary sterilization, as opposed to voluntary measures, to achieve eugenic goals.[28] Reform eugenicists, including British scientists J.B.S. Haldane and Julian Huxley, and Americans Hermann Muller and Theodosius Dobzhansky, aimed to distance eugenics from the mainline program and to connect it instead with the emerging fields of human and clinical genetics and with social reforms aimed at eliminating the social causes of apparent disparities in fitness between races and classes.[29]

Connections with human and clinical genetics were forged in a variety of ways. Eugenicists authored books on human genetics and patterns of inheritance of disease that were aimed at general practice physicians, with the goal of encouraging physicians to counsel their patients whose children might be at risk. They worked in cooperation with leading physicians such as Lionel Penrose, whose focus was in finding cures for genetically-influenced conditions but who was willing to work with reform eugenicists to advance and disseminate knowledge about genetically influenced diseases.[30]

Reform eugenicists attempted to forge other connections at the intersection of human genetics, clinical genetics, and procreative practices. Haldane articulated a utopian vision of a future world in which reproduction was conducted according to eugenic science and was separated from sexual bonding; his 1924 novel, *Daedalus*, served as inspiration for Aldous Huxley's *Brave New World*.[31] Muller gathered the signatures of 22 British and American scientists for his

1939 "Geneticists' Manifesto" advocating the substitution of science for super-stition in procreation, declaring it "an honor and a privilege, if not a duty, for a mother, married or unmarried, or for a couple, to have the best children possi-ble, both in respect of their upbringing and of their genetic endowment."[32]

While mainline eugenics was utterly discredited by its association with the programs of the Nazi regime,[33] the reform eugenics program continued to attract support in the post-World War II period.[34] Reform eugenicists were well aware of the need to distance themselves from the Nazi horrors if they were to advance their cause, and they worked hard to do so and to strengthen ties with the rapidly growing fields of human genetics and clinical genetics. The American Society of Human Genetics was founded in 1948, and five of its first six presidents were directors of the American Eugenics Society.[35] Muller, awarded the Nobel Prize in 1946 for his work showing genetic mutations in fruit flies caused by X-rays,[36] founded the *American Journal of Human Genetics* and wrote in the preface to its first issue, in September 1949, of the importance of connecting the science of human genetics with clinical practice, and of the role of the new journal in fostering ties between the two:

an unfortunate compartmentalism has for many years hindered persons in medicine and in the other specifically human disciplines from attaining the necessary knowledge of genetics and, *mutatis mutandis*, has hindered geneticists from mastering the more special human subjects. Although this situation has prevailed for over a generation, we believe that the time is now ripe for a fertile liaison, and it is for the purpose of the pres-ent society and journal to subserve it.[37]

Muller stressed in his preface the importance of bringing sound science and progressive social policies to the program of postwar reform eugenics and stressed the difference between this program and the eugenics program of the Nazi regime:

There remains, not least, the question of the guidance of reproduction away from geneti-cally less favorable and in the direction of more favorable paths, in other words, the ques-tion of eugenics. As we have pointed out above, this whole subject has fallen into disrepute because it has been so perverted by unscientific propagandists and cranks, with hastily conceived remedies which they desired to foist upon the community as substitutes for social measures with which they did not agree. We do not wish this kind of eugenics …

At the same time, we must be careful not to be panicked into throwing away the wheat with the chaff. It is the present writer's considered opinion that eugenics, in the better sense of the term, 'the social direction of human evolution,' is a most profound and important subject and that it will in due time be worked on seriously, not in a spirit of ill-considered partisanship and prejudice, but in one of scientific objectivity combined with social consciousness.[38]

The program of postwar reform eugenics, pursued by Muller and others, aimed at educating the public and influencing procreative choices. Muller warned in 1949 that people with genetic mutations that in an earlier age would have killed them were now, due to improved living conditions and medical care, surviving to reproduce, with a resulting increase in the "genetic load," a problem aggravated by the effects of man-made radiation in the new nuclear age.[39] He urged voluntary measures to persuade those who were healthy to reproduce, and those with high "genetic loads" to refrain from reproduction to avert a future in which increasing numbers of "invalids" required increasing levels of support to compensate for their disabilities.[40]

Muller also revived the idea, first articulated in his 1939 "Geneticists' Manifesto," of a more scientific approach to procreation for superior characteristics. In 1959, he began to advocate and gather support for "germinal choice," a program of eugenic artificial insemination made feasible by new technology for freezing sperm. He gathered support from prominent scientists including Ernst Mayr of Harvard University, James F. Crow of the University of Wisconsin, and Crick, co-discoverer of the structure of DNA. Muller and his collaborators could not agree, however, on the characteristics that should determine who would be invited to deposit sperm, and critics of the program cited shifts in Muller's own opinions about the selection criteria.[41]

As the fields of human and clinical genetics, fueled by the work of Neel and McKusick and others, advanced rapidly in the postwar period, support for reform eugenics programs faded. Opponents of the postwar reform eugenics program, like those of the prewar mainline eugenics program, criticized it for its reductionism and excessive focus on bodily perfection; there were also objections questioning the legal and ethical implications for procreation and parenting of biotechnologies such as artificial insemination and *in vitro* fertilization (IVF).[42] In addition, Kevles observes that the scientific complexity emerging from genetic research was inconsistent with the foundational assumptions of the reform eugenics program about the desirability and feasibility of guiding human inheritance: "Human genetic research may have been spurred in part by reform eugenic goals, but the more that was revealed about the complexity of heredity in human beings, the less did eugenics (even much of the reform variety) appear defensible in principle, or even scientifically within reach."[43]

13.2.3 Reproductive medicine and counseling

In the last half of the twentieth century, new genetic knowledge and new techniques enabled prospective parents to learn more than any previous generation of parents about the health prospects of their future children – both *in utero* and before conception. New knowledge about conception and the early product of the union of egg and sperm and new techniques also enabled prospective parents to exercise far more control over the reproductive process and the genetic make-up of their future children.

Beginning in the 1950s, medical geneticists could provide parents of a child affected by a genetically influenced condition with some information about the likelihood that a subsequent child would suffer the same condition.[44] By the 1970s, genetic screening tests were used extensively to detect carrier status in high-risk groups for diseases including sickle cell anemia, Tay-Sachs, cystic fibrosis (CF), and muscular dystrophy.[45] With this new knowledge, potential parents could choose to refrain from procreation, adopt, or attempt artificial insemination with sperm from a donor who was not a carrier in cases where this eliminated the risk of the genetic condition. And in those states in which it was permitted, abortion was an option for those who found it morally acceptable and who wished to avoid the birth of a child with a possible or near-certain risk of suffering from a genetic condition. By the 1960s, amniocentesis could determine fetal sex and thus reveal the risk of Duchenne muscular dystrophy in a male child; by the 1970s, Down syndrome and X-linked conditions could be detected. The 1973 U.S. Supreme Court decision in *Roe v. Wade*[46] established a constitutional right to abortion under most circumstances in all American states. Thereafter, the development and use of prenatal screening tests expanded rapidly, and "therapeutic" abortions were available as an option for those who, preconception, were unaware of their risk as well as those who, knowing of the risk, "lost" the genetic lottery.[47]

The first "test tube" baby, Louise Brown, was born in 1978, and thereafter IVF followed by transfer of pre-embryos to a woman's uterus allowed those who were aware of their risk, as well as single parents, homosexual couples, and couples with fertility problems, to select both the ova and sperm that would be brought together in fertilization attempts *in vitro*. By the 1990s, pre-implantation genetic diagnosis (PGD) became available for use in conjunction with an IVF procedure. This allowed future parents to test for certain conditions in the pre-embryos created *in vitro* and selectively transfer to the woman's uterus only those that were not affected by a detected condition.[48]

The option of curing those future children or newborns who test positive for genetically influenced disease has proved far more difficult to develop. By 1974 a newborn screening and treatment program for phenylketonuria (PKU) was shown to be effective; newborns who tested positive could be placed on a childhood diet free of phenylalanine, thereby averting severe mental disability and premature death.[49] But effective treatments for other genetically influenced diseases, at the turn of the twenty-first century and for the foreseeable future, remain elusive. Opportunities for effective cure continue to lag behind our ability to predict and diagnose,[50] leaving patients and their doctors with hard choices about prevention by forbearing from serving as a genetic parent, discarding affected embryos created for use in an IVF procedure, or aborting an affected fetus.

During this period of rapid growth in reproductive knowledge and technique, genetic counseling expanded rapidly as well. On historian Diane Paul's account, genetic counselors from the 1940s through the 1960s subscribed to the view that "the heredity of the population should be a matter of public concern."[51] And, in the 1970s, the U.S. Department of Health, Education, and Welfare explicitly embraced the goal of reducing the incidence of disability through prenatal testing and abortion.[52] This approach was abandoned in the course of just a few years in the 1970s. The new ethos of genetic counseling was client centered: to respect and safeguard client autonomy.[53] On this approach, clients should receive information and support in making their reproductive choices, but should not be advised of any public interest in the choices they made for themselves and their children.[54]

Some argue that the old ethos prevails under the thin veil of the new, and that public health, or "eugenic," choices continue to be encouraged.[55] Paul explicates the argument in support of this claim, beginning with policy-makers' assumption that the "right" choices are those that reduce the incidence of genetically influenced and other conditions in the population:

> Policy makers generally assume that individual and social interests are congruent, that families will act 'rationally.' (Thus policy analyses of screening programs usually assume that all fetuses identified as abnormal will be aborted.) ... [T]he assumption that normal people will do what they can to avoid the birth of children with disabilities has a long history ... By the 1960s, it seemed politic to drop the old label for this program. As Frederick Osborn wrote in 1968, 'Eugenic goals are most likely to be attained under a name other than eugenics.' Of course eugenics and reproductive choice are congruent only if families ordinarily make the 'right' decisions.[56]

Paul concludes that complaints of current-day "eugenic" reproductive medicine are founded in observations of the constellation of pressures on future parents to avoid bringing an affected fetus to term:

> Subtle pressures to make the 'right' choice are what many people have in mind when they characterize contemporary genetic medicine as a form of eugenics. Of course many women welcome the opportunities to learn more about their fetus and to act on the results. But some women also feel that they have no realistic alternatives to the decision to be tested or to abort a genetically imperfect fetus. Of course they are under no legal coercion. But they may nevertheless feel pressured to be tested and avoid having children with disabilities – by their doctors, who fear being sued if the child is born with a genetic disorder, by anxiety over the potential loss of health or life insurance, by their inability to bear the enormous financial costs of caring for a severely disabled child, or by the lack of social services (even with national health insurance) for handicapped children.[57]

Even if this argument is correct, subtle pressures are different from enforced policies of coercive eugenics. As Kevles argues, a return to the eugenics of the past, even with the advent of new reproductive technologies, is highly unlikely. The public, including those who formerly were targeted for eugenic measures, would not countenance such intrusions. And the constitutional protection of reproductive rights, established in *Roe v. Wade* and related cases over the last part of the twentieth century, serves as an additional bulwark against new efforts to enforce any sort of coercive eugenic plan.[58]

13.3   The future imagined

Novel technologies challenge us not only because we have no history of deliberation and reflection to draw on, but also because we have no present, concrete, contextualized experience with their implications. This compromises our capacity to engage in practical decision-making, including personal ethical decision-making and policy-making. For example, most of us have, on some occasion, opined about the choices of others and later discovered, when faced with similar choices in our own lives, that the considerations were far more complex, nuanced, and difficult than we had realized – and that our choices in context are different from those we envisioned from a distance. Courts refuse to decide issues posed in the abstract or that involve hypothetical rather than genuine conflicts, in part because they recognize that good practical decision-making requires assessment of the complex particulars presented forcefully by parties locked in genuine conflict.[59]

Given the intense public scrutiny and concern aroused by manipulations of DNA in any living organisms and by interventions of any sort in the products of human conception, it seems likely that policy-makers will engage in prospective regulation of IGM rather than waiting until research and experimentation are far advanced. They will not have the benefit of addressing issues fully formed and presented in their complex particulars by advocates who can recount the details of their experience with IGM and the contested issues that have arisen from this experience. Clinical and scholarly bioethics, however, often involves contemplation of imagined future states of affairs in ways that aim to make as vivid and "real" as possible the future implications of present choices. I will sketch here a few examples of the ways in which bioethics might speak to politics about a future involving IGM, drawing on imagined examples of IGM for:

1. prevention of disease: Huntington disease (HD);
2. prevention of physical disability: deafness; and
3. prevention of behavioral disability: extreme shyness.

13.3.1   Prevention of disease: HD

HD is an incurable, invariably fatal, degenerative disease whose symptoms (involuntary movements, personality changes, and progressive dementia) begin in middle age and worsen over several years until death.[60] HD is an autosomal dominant disease: those who inherit one "HD gene" from a parent will suffer the disease.[61] As symptoms of the disease do not manifest until well into the reproductive years, an asymptomatic parent may procreate while unaware that she will suffer the disease, and that there is a 50 percent chance she will pass the disease on to her child.[62] In an imagined future in which IGM might ensure both that the child and the child's descendants would not suffer the condition, the gains in personal well-being to each child and descendant rescued from this fate would be enormous, by the lights of any worldview. The experiences of procreation and parenting would be transformed as well. Generations of future parents would be spared the experience of unwittingly passing along a gene that would doom their children to suffering and premature death or, if not afflicted themselves, of experiencing first the loss of their afflicted spouses, then their adult children.

If only a few parents engaged in IGM, however, relatively few children would realize the gains in personal well-being and relatively few parents would be spared the impact on their experience of procreation and parenting. And the public health benefits (including reduced incidence of the disease and accompanying reallocation of research and palliative resources to advancing other individual or community interests) would be relatively limited as well. The numbers of persons afflicted might not even be reduced if those engaging in IGM (presumably, those aware of their risk) otherwise would have adopted, procreated by use of donor gamete or gametes, or refrained from procreation and parenting altogether.

For broader impact on personal well-being, procreation and parenting, and public health, policy-makers likely would need to implement policies that would expand the use of IGM significantly. A screening test, perhaps subsidized, and perhaps mandated for those seeking a marriage license, might expand awareness of risk, yielding greater use of IGM. For those previously unaware of their risk, the tests might bring unwanted knowledge that diminished their quality of life. But this might be considered a modest price to be paid for the sake of future lives saved. And some parents would welcome the knowledge, which would allow them time to arrange their affairs and make choices for themselves and their loved ones in anticipation of a shortened life span.

But subsidizing or mandating testing also might not be sufficient to achieve significant public health gains. Subsidies might be necessary to make the services available to all. And a mandate with penalties attached might be required to persuade those who were carriers to guard against careless procreation the old-fashioned way; analogies could be drawn to quarantines imposed on those with potentially deadly infectious disease and mandatory tracing of the sexual partners of those with potentially deadly sexually transmitted disease. Penalties for defiance of a mandate to procreate by IVF with IGM rather than copulation would surely be problematic for many members of the political community, however. Other modes of procreation and parenting – adoption, PGD and discarding of affected embryos, or abortion of affected fetuses – might be offered as acceptable alternatives to those subject to the mandate. But mandating any of these, even in the alternative, would be controversial as well. There would be no obvious, easy path to achieving far-reaching public health benefits in connection with an IGM cure for HD.

13.3.2   Prevention of physical disability: deafness

It is hard to imagine that any religious or secular worldview would count the suffering and early mortality associated with HD as good or desirable. But in the case of hereditary deafness, policy-makers will face an additional complicating factor: the condition will be viewed as good and desirable by some, but not by others.[63] There will be disagreement about the content of "personal well-being," which will be attributable, in part, to the different social circumstances of those who are members of the Deaf community and those who are not. Prospective parents who are deaf may value highly their membership in the Deaf community, which includes participation in a rich and nuanced language community, and may wish to pass on that membership to their children in the same way that members of religious communities wish to pass on that membership to their children. Deaf parents also might worry that a hearing child would be torn between the Deaf community of her parents and the hearing world in the same way that members of religious communities worry that an education that satisfies the curricular requirements established by secular authorities may pull their children away from the family and religious community. As deaf persons may associate primarily with members of the Deaf community, assortative mating will make it more likely that their children will be congenitally deaf: "If both partners carry the same type of recessive gene for deafness, all their children will be deaf."[64]

So, in addition to the range of concerns that policy-makers might consider in the case of IGM for HD, they might, in the case of IGM for deafness, consider whether the content of personal well-being and the experience of procreation and parenting might be dependent on the nature of the private communities into which a prospective child would be born. They might also consider whether a policy promoting IGM for deafness might disparage deaf people and the Deaf community, and reduce the willingness of the hearing community to accommodate difference, rather than advance public health.

If IGM could "correct" hereditary deafness, what stance should policy-makers take toward parental choices about that IGM? At present, if a hearing child were born to parents who viewed deafness as good and desirable and if the parents engaged in some procedure to render their child deaf, this surely would constitute criminal child abuse. But if instead these parents were knowingly to bring a child who was deaf into the world rather than discarding affected pre-embryos or aborting an affected fetus, we would not view this as child abuse, but as the exercise of procreative and parenting choice. If safe and effective IGM were available to correct congenital deafness, and deaf parents refused to employ it, would this constitute criminal child abuse or an exercise of procreative and parenting choice?

13.3.3 Prevention of behavioral disability: extreme shyness

It now seems likely that the range of behavioral characteristics that extends from comfort in social situations to extreme shyness is genetically influenced. If current-day investigators are correct that "extreme shyness can be a precursor for serious disorders, such as social phobias and depression,"[65] and if IGM that would reduce the likelihood of a future child being extremely shy could be developed, should its use be permitted or encouraged, and would it constitute "therapy" as opposed to "enhancement"? While deafness is readily acknowledged as a deviation from species-typical functionality – even if there may be disagreement about whether, in social context, this reflects a diminution in the experience of "personal well-being" – extreme shyness might be viewed as a point in the distribution of temperaments, a "disorder" only if we employ a definition of disorder that captures any attribute that varies significantly from the mean. But perhaps extreme shyness should be considered a disorder because persons whose temperaments lie closer to the mean, as well as those whose temperaments fall at the opposite extreme of gregariousness, do not suffer for it, while extreme shyness places a child at risk for recognized illnesses such as social phobias and depression.

As with deaf parents, extremely shy parents might embrace this behavioral disposition in themselves and their future children simply because it is their own and they see nothing wrong with relating to the social world in way that is different from the way of the "gregarious majority." They would not welcome an intervention aimed at making their child more like the majority, potentially pulling their child away from them and undermining their experience of parenting and family. But if most of those who experience the condition, to the contrary, view it as adversely affecting their personal well-being, then this might lead policy-makers to assess IGM for extreme shyness in a way more like their assessment of IGM for HD.

But they might also consider an additional set of concerns. If the reason why extremely shy persons are at risk for phobias and depression is because of the way they see themselves reflected in the attitudes of others toward them or because of the fact that modern culture demands that they interact with strangers in schools and workplaces, should policy-makers aim to revise the genomes of the extremely shy or, instead, to revise the attitudes, institutions, and practices of the gregarious majority? If, as seems likely, it would be a more cost-effective "cure" to revise the genomes of a small minority than to revise the attitudes, institutions, and practices of the majority, and if this is taken as sufficient justification for engaging in the former strategy as an approach to advancing personal well-being and public health, perplexing questions about the "social" nature of personal well-being and public health are posed.

There are a wide range of minority characteristics, some specific to cultures, some universal at least to contemporary social experience, that might be viewed by most potential parents as adversely affecting the well-being of their future children and their own experience of procreation and parenting. These minority characteristics might include, for example, short stature, distinctive facial features, and early-onset baldness. Presumably, the majority culture would welcome revision of these characteristics and view this as an improvement in public health, broadly conceived, since the public square would now be filled with an increased percentage of those who present pleasing and agreeable features.

If, in these cases and more, however, our regulatory policy permitted engineering the characteristics of the minority to bring them closer to the norm, our conception of therapeutic IGM would threaten to swallow much of what we commonly refer to as genetic enhancement. And it might also raise an alarm: would this not constitute a return to the eugenics programs of the past, or, more precisely, to the evils reflected in eugenics programs of the past? But if the science and technique were sound rather than spurious, and if policy-makers enforced a regime of complete neutrality toward IGM for these conditions rather than imposing a subtle or not-so-subtle coercion, perhaps this would constitute an extension of IGM into a realm analogous to contemporary reconstructive and cosmetic surgery and pharmaceutical correction of conditions that diminish the experience of personal well-being.

13.4   Bioethically informed deliberation: past and future brought to bear on IGM policy issues

I next consider how IGM policy-makers can draw on the past and future to understand better the individual and collective interests at stake, and the points of disagreement about these. If our political community is to cope well with the novel, complex, and potentially divisive questions that IGM will pose, policy-makers will need to bring bioethically informed understanding to bear.

13.4.1   Looking backward

The history of genetic medicine is a story of rapid and highly effective success in advancing the scientific frontier and, in fairly short order, bringing these advances to clinical practice; while the full range of hoped-for advances in clinical genetic medicine are not yet here, there is good reason to expect that they will come. Over the course of this relatively short history, much of the content of personal health, procreation and parenting, and public health has not been very controversial: reducing infectious disease by means of antibiotics and inoculations was uncontroversially good for all of these. Under these circumstances, national and local policy-makers could be quite confident that measures designed to limit the spread of disease, increase the rate of childhood inoculations, and promote biomedical science and technology that might contribute to future breakthroughs in conquering disease (through funded programs such as the HGP) were apt and right.

The histories of eugenics and reproductive medicine and counseling reveal far more controversy about the content of individual flourishing and the common good. State and national policy-makers embraced involuntary sterilization in the prewar period and therapeutic abortions in the postwar period as public health measures that would advance the common good and as congruent with individual flourishing. By the last few decades of the twentieth century, however, these measures were widely renounced for one or more reasons: coercive intervention was inconsistent with procreation and parenting as a component of individual flourishing; measures founded on unsound eugenic science could not in any event contribute to personal health, procreation and parenting, or public health; eugenic notions of "fitness" were simplistic and narrow in their reductionism and their emphasis on bodily perfection as central to conceptions of personal health, procreation and parenting, and public health.

While the eugenic programs of the day were renounced, we have by no means renounced the use of coercion in some form in pursuit of important public health goals – from quarantine to mandatory tracing of sexual partners in cases of sexually transmitted disease – and "subtle coercion" or persuasion surely is a backdrop to some of our current reproductive medicine and counseling. Nor have we crossed a threshold from a dark age of unsound science to a bright new age of sound science: today's sound science is always turning into tomorrow's unsound science; we are continually engaged in risk—benefit assessments about whether to proceed with a clinical intervention based upon today's knowledge and technique. And disagreement about the meaning of individual flourishing and the common good captured in opponents' claims of narrow reductionism and perfectionism are ongoing. While eugenics programs were renounced for reasons sufficient unto the day, questions about whether policy-makers might endorse in some form some interventions to influence human heredity remain open. These three intertwined histories at the intersection of bioscientific and biotechnological advance with the complexity of human life systems and with procreation suggest that the debate about IGM will have some familiar aspects.

In these brief historical sketches, we catch a glimpse of a midpoint, not an endpoint, in the sorting out of cultural emanations from two scientific revolutions: the Darwinian revolution and the revolution in molecular biology, including the powerful reductionist techniques associated with the latter. As the Copernican revolution wrenched the earth from the center of the celestial orbs, forcing subsequent generations to reconstruct cultural creations founded on a geocentric conception of the heavens, so these twin biological revolutions wrenched humans from their unique status among the phenomena of life – and our cultural reconstruction project is ongoing. These twin revolutions invite us to see ourselves from two perspectives: as matter in motion, molecular biological products of a complex developmental process influenced by genes, and as the products of natural selection, our characteristics a set of responses to challenges posed over evolutionary time and implemented from the molecular level on up. They challenge us to see ourselves as more or different from the sum of these perspectives and to reconcile any such alternative perspective with what we have learned and accomplished in the wake of these two richly fruitful scientific revolutions in life science.

Eugenicists were precocious in pursuing the cultural implications of the twin biological revolutions, although they suffered early defeat in part because of three of the hallmarks of precocity: the substitution of overweening coercion for thoughtful persuasion; insufficient knowledge and inadequate technique to support their ambitions; and failure to recognize the persistent appeal of alternative perspectives on human life captured in opponents' objections to eugenic reductionism and perfectionism. Eugenicists asked important questions that we will soon revisit, in updated form, in the IGM debates. They asked first: what if our newly developed powers of medicine and improved standards of living disrupt the operation of the law of natural selection, thereby increasing the incidence of disease and disability – should we not then engage eugenic science and technique to correct for this and thus realign ourselves with the laws of nature? Justice Holmes approved the application of eugenic science and primitive reproductive technology, the scalpel, as reform measures aimed at bringing our social world into conformity with Darwinian evolution. Some eugenicists asked an even more ambitious question: after we have mastered the intricacies of the developmental process, should we not reach beyond this corrective by selecting for or even designing the features we want rather than accepting the features bequeathed us by the blind force of natural selection? Muller worried about the corruption to the gene pool wrought by modern medicine among other causes, but he also aspired to perfect humankind through selection for the best features, although his germinal-selection project foundered on his inability to articulate what features those might be.

We can see in the questions that eugenicists pursued the precursors of questions we will face when IGM becomes technically feasible: should we not press the powers of modern medicine beyond after-the-fact efforts to rescue and cure, and into the realm of prevention opened up by the new genomic science and technology, since the latter holds the potential to reduce disease and disability beyond the greatest efforts of the former? If we can prevent commonly recognized disease and disability, should we not also strive to correct any conditions that cause suffering or that yield below-average functionality or less-than-optimal functionality?

The debate about these and other questions will depend in part on whether or how coercion or persuasion might be employed and on risk—benefit assessments of the science and technique available to us. Coercion is widely viewed as fundamentally inconsistent with the practice of procreation and parenting and no one views interventions in which the risks outweigh the potential benefits as contributions to personal health, procreation and parenting, or public health. But judgments about whether a particular IGM policy would advance individual flourishing or the common good may turn on other aspects of our conceptions of personal well-being, procreation and parenting, and public health – aspects about which there is more disagreement.

We can see how eugenicists, drawing on the Darwinian and molecular perspectives, poured content into these components of individual flourishing and the common good. Personal well-being was conceived in terms of achieving fitness, procreation and parenting concerned the production of fit children, and public health consisted of the maximized fitness of the population. "Fitness" was measured against a yardstick constructed by the eugenic science of the day that was seen as objective and neutral as to point of view. The yardstick aimed to capture either what Darwinian evolution would have wrought or what were objectively superior features in light of our modern environment, and whether we measured up was understood to be very significantly influenced by hereditary molecular genetic influences.

To the extent genetic medicine is concerned with genetic influences and relies on the reductionist methods and technological innovation that brought great advances in science and clinical medicine beginning in the nineteenth century, it bears similarities to eugenics. But its historical focus on curing and relieving suffering, both in individual patients and in the population, infuse different meaning into the components of individual flourishing and the common good. Personal well-being is not viewed as a matter of measuring up to an ideal of "fitness" established by reference to an evolutionary process or any other standard. From the invention of antibiotics to efforts to develop SCGT, the focus has been on the patient – her illness and suffering as concerns in her life – with medicine serving as an ally in coping with them for her benefit. While facts about diseases may be seen as objective and neutral, and reductionist methods are recognized as effective in understanding and coping with diseases, the significance of these facts for individuals and their lives could vary; personal well-being and public health are advanced when patients and members of the populace are helped by their own lights, not when fitness is achieved by the lights of an abstract measure applied to an individual or across a population.

Similarly, if reproductive medicine and counseling are centered on informing potential parents and facilitating their choices, there may be overlap with eugenic practices, but there will be conflicts with eugenic aims as well. It is not simply that reproductive medicine and counseling now honor the choices of clients rather than imposing decisions on them by coercion, it is that they now embrace nuanced, complex, and diverse decisions based on the circumstances and values of each individual client and reject a single standard of fitness, abstracted from the context and values of individual lives, as a basis for decision-making.

As these histories of genetic medicine, eugenics, and reproductive medicine and counseling suggest, IGM policy-making will need to understand and cope with sometimes competing understandings of the content of individual flourishing and the common good despite widespread agreement that, generally, coercion and untoward risk are inconsistent with these. To illustrate in more concrete terms the tensions that may arise and the difficult choices policy-makers will face, consider once again the imagined future scenarios involving IGM.

13.4.2   Looking forward

Successful IGM for HD would appear to advance nearly any conception of personal well-being, procreation and parenting, and public health. Yet, as policy-makers contemplate how to craft a regulatory framework that could best realize these benefits, different understandings that could complicate the task might emerge.

If, for example, the medical aims of curing and relieving suffering inform the content of personal well-being and public health, then IGM or cures that were effective in children or adults might be preferred to choices that require the discarding of affected pre-embryos or the abortion of affected fetuses, in that the latter might be viewed as failures to achieve cures for particular future individuals, whether or not these acts were viewed as the destruction of present "persons." Individual flourishing and the common good informed by eugenic aims, in contrast, might best be vindicated by policy-making that encouraged the most cost-effective approaches to eliminating HD so as to improve fitness, regardless of the particular future individuals who might benefit from this. If the aims of reproductive medicine and counseling informed the meaning of procreation and parenting, this might lead policy-makers to craft the regulatory framework to ensure that a range of choices were available to parents rather than that any particular choice was favored – even if this failed to reduce the incidence of HD in the population.

In the case of HD – and, we might hypothesize, other deadly genetic conditions – policy-makers may not need to worry about conflicts of this sort because of the universal practical commitment to reducing the incidence of HD and, accordingly, the likelihood that practical compromises will be found for doing so. But in the case of deafness, it appears quite likely that they will need to worry.

Personal well-being and public health informed by the aims of genetic medicine need not be understood as requiring cures for patients who do not believe themselves to be ill or suffering. Policy-makers might conclude that it is our circumstances and values that determine whether we consider a condition, such as deafness, to detract from or contribute to our well-being, regardless of whether or not there is some sense in which deafness, as an objective matter, constitutes a disability. Thus, parents would be in the best position to choose what is best for their children's well-being and should be permitted to do so as an exercise of procreative and parenting choice, especially given that the costs to public health in accommodating deafness are trivial.

In the alternative, policy-makers might conclude that, while well-being is indeed a matter of values and interests and not simply a scientific fact-of-the-matter,

IGM should be encouraged, and perhaps subsidized, because it would hold open a broader range of opportunities for the child to realize personal well-being, however that child might understand it, than would a parental choice not to engage in IGM. Furthermore, the public health costs if parents failed to engage in IGM would be significant, if deprivation of this range of opportunities were included as a cost.

Individual flourishing and the common good informed by the eugenic understanding of "fitness" could not abide understandings that varied according to the beliefs of patients or the circumstances and values of parents; fitness, on the eugenic account, has an objective scientific meaning that is neutral as to point of view. Policy-makers might conclude that deafness constitutes, as an objective matter, a disability that is inconsistent with personal well-being and the public health – we could improve the well-being of many and apply scarce public health resources to purposes other than accommodating deafness if we reduced its incidence – and that it should be discouraged as a choice in procreation and parenting.

The case of IGM for extreme shyness raises questions that will carry policy-makers deeper into the thicket surrounding our beliefs about the meaning of well-being, the practices of procreation and parenting, and public health. That we are social animals is undeniable, and there is no doubt that certain characteristics – generally at the extremes of the distribution of temperamental, physical, and intellectual characteristics – are likely to make our social lives more difficult. We can hardly expect to change the attitudes, institutions, and practices of the world; the instinctive reactions to the strange or different underlying these are so widespread and persistent that we might fairly conclude that they are deep-seated features of our nature. We are not purely instinctive beings, of course, and most of us manage to treat others properly most of the time and subdue instincts that, if they were important to our survival in evolutionary time, are more destructive than helpful now. But there are enough of us who fail to do so on enough occasions that those whose characteristics fall at the extremes are at constant risk of internalizing negative views about themselves or of withdrawing from a social world littered with enough potholes to discourage efforts to negotiate it. Hence the wide appeal of growth hormones for short stature, cosmetic surgical procedures for facial features, various treatments for baldness, and, perhaps one day, IGM for conditions that parents can accurately predict would make it likely that the lives of their children would be more difficult.

Doctors might fairly conclude that the anticipated suffering of an extremely short man is a reason to provide growth hormone to the boy or IGM to the zygote, regardless of the absence of any objectively determined pituitary disease. While this might divert resources from treating objectively determined diseases, the real test for purposes of public health would count the diminution in suffering, not the diminution in objectively determined disease. And reproductive medicine and counseling also could honor the circumstances and values of parents that lead them to this choice. Thus it might be the ironic result that, in honoring the aims of medicine as well as procreational and parenting choice, the dreams of eugenicists (founded on unsound science that categorized many minority characteristics as if they were objectively determined disease) might be realized.

Doctors do not, however, respond to every complaint with a remedy that reduces discomfort or makes life go more smoothly for their patients; sometimes therapeutic exercise is required to recover, and sometimes the experience of some difficulty (in work, social settings, parenting) is necessary for growth into greater maturity and strength that expand the capacity of the person to cope and thrive, and achieve greater personal well-being. The aims of medicine include a recognition that curing and the relief from suffering pertain to the well-being of the whole person – a biological, intentional, and social being leading a life through time – not just the immediate discomforts of the biological being. If this were not so, doctors would merely dispense drugs that relieve discomfort to patients with complaints. Not every significant deviation from the norm would threaten personal well-being on an understanding informed by the aims of genetic medicine.

Furthermore, many persons with extreme features take pride in their distinctiveness and find their way to private communities that value them. To engage in IGM to eliminate their features would "do harm" to these individuals rather than advance their well-being, squandering resources that could be better allocated to advance public health. As it seems unlikely that we could predict in advance which individuals with extreme features would suffer and which would thrive, policy-makers might conclude that this sort of IGM should be discouraged in favor of the development and application of remedies that treat the child or adult, when assessment of the aptness of remedies would be far better informed.

An understanding of individual flourishing and public health with respect to extreme shyness and other extreme features that is informed by eugenic aims would be more difficult to construct. The task would bring eugenics back to part of its unfinished business growing out of the Darwinian and molecular revolutions. Part of the eugenic ambition has been to align the outcomes of human procreation with Darwinian evolution – to correct for the distortions in natural selection generated by human culture, including improved living conditions, modern medicine, and the use of nuclear devices that generate radiation. But another part of the ambition has been to do better – to work on perfecting what we have inherited from the blind operation of the law of natural selection through breeding practices or, thanks to the insight and technologies generated by the molecular revolution and successor research programs, to redesign ourselves from the molecular level up.

This might involve formulating a uniform conception of the characteristics of an improved human based on our knowledge and experience to date; perhaps extreme shyness would not "make the cut," given its general tendency to make life more difficult for those who have it. Or it might involve relying on a free market-place of parental choices, each exploring the possibilities, until a superior model emerged from future knowledge and experience. Or the uniform conception might consist in the realization of diverse designers' visions. On all of these conceptions, public health would be advanced to the extent individuals chose to advance the personal well-being of their children by implementing these choices. Coercion, no doubt, would be rejected as counterproductive, so policy-makers' primary responsibility in designing the regulatory framework would be to promote the research necessary to making choices available, and to uphold a regime of procreative and parenting choice.

13.5 Bioethically informed politics: a navigational approach

If, as I have argued, bioethics can inform politics about the questions posed by IGM in a way that illuminates and sharpens the contested issues at the core of the mission of the political community, then a bioethically-informed approach to policy-making, if it is to succeed in its mission, will need to be competent to make good use of this information in crafting the regulatory framework. What sort of policy-making approach would be competent to do so?

13.5.1 Utilitarianism

Utilitarian political philosophy[66] and its close cousin in policy analysis, welfare economics, are dedicated to maximizing welfare, conceived variously as pleasure or happiness or satisfaction of preferences, giving impartial weight in the maximization calculus to each person's welfare interests. The core commitment of utilitarianism to universal benevolence, to making the world a better place in the sense that welfare is maximized, lends it commonsensical appeal. The sophisticated instruments of modern policy analysis make its application to policy issues plausible. Objections to utilitarianism as a guide to *individual* action include the implausibility of demanding impartiality in calculating welfare maximization from humans who are, by nature, highly partial to family and friends; the difficulties of specifying what is meant by "welfare" and how it can be measured; the inadequacy of any conception of welfare in capturing important human values, such as preserving the integrity of one's life plan regardless of its value to others or appreciating the intrinsic value of relationships and other goods; and the practical difficulties of requiring calculation of welfare maximization in advance of every act or of requiring compliance with welfare-maximizing rules on occasions when compliance would not be welfare maximizing.

Utilitarianism as a guide to policy-making for the political community arguably retains its commonsensical appeal, enables policy-makers to wield the powerful tools of policy analysis, and avoids these objections to utilitarianism as a guide to individual action.[67] The exercise of impartiality by policy-makers seems both realistic, as a matter of human psychology, and virtuous, as a matter of what we expect of government officials. Reductionist approaches to the content of welfare, such as expressions of preferences by word or deed, seem unavoidable and apt in making the sorts of community-wide choices about the limited range of issues with which policy-makers are concerned: encouraging prosperity, preserving the peace, and so on. Policy-makers have access to data gathering, and analytic and statistical tools that make it possible to measure welfare conceived in a sufficiently accurate reductionist way. And calculation of welfare maximization in conjunction with policy choice also seems apt and feasible since policy-making consists in making calculated proactive choices for the community over a limited range of issues after study and deliberation.

Jonathan Glover has developed a generally utilitarian treatment of the policy issues surrounding IGM, but with modifications to allow for consideration of a richer array of values than standard welfare-maximizing accounts allow.[68] Glover frames the policy issues as fundamentally a matter of characterizing and assessing risks and benefits. While there would be risks that parents would unintentionally create people "who turn out worse than expected"[69] or that parents might choose poorly – overvaluing talents and abilities, for example, and undervaluing "a sense of humour" or "emotional warmth"[70] – there would be potential benefits as well, as would be most obvious in the case of therapeutic IGM.[71] And we should consider that there might be risks in refraining from IGM – the assessment of risks and benefits of proceeding or refraining should be framed in the same way as cases of "other possibly hazardous technology, or … large-scale social changes."[72] Glover argues that parents should not be permitted to diminish the abilities of their future children nor to eliminate features that contribute to key human capacities for "self-development and self-expression," forming "relationships," and developing "consciousness and understanding."[73] In other respects, they should not be bound by the natural as normative. Proceeding cautiously in light of the potential for unintended negative consequences, we should consider permitting enhancements for intelligence, so that our descendants might transcend the current limitations of our capacity to understand the world "because our growing understanding of the world is so central a part of why it is good to be human."[74] We might also consider revisions to human nature to reduce aggression, given the current threat to our survival posed by this formerly adaptive feature. Glover favors a regulated free market in IGM as the best approach to effectuating these policy positions.[75]

Utilitarianism as a public philosophy, even as modified by Glover's approach, is ill suited to coping with the problems posed by IGM technologies. A reductionist account of welfare interests cannot capture the variety and complexity of the values at stake in competing conceptions of individual flourishing and the common good, and indeed we see in Glover's modifications to a standard

utilitarian account an understandable resistance to reducing the issues surrounding IGM to a single measure of value, such as the exercise of preferences
in the marketplace. The interests at stake, such as those surrounding IGM for
deafness or extreme shyness, defy reduction to data and analysis concerning
risks and benefits that, after impartial weighing of the interests of all, could
yield policies that advance the mission of the political community; there are
competing conceptions of individual flourishing and the common good that
cannot be illuminated or addressed by this approach. Glover identifies a set of
human features that he argues are of prime importance, and, hence, should be
preserved or enhanced by a policy-making approach that advances a more
sophisticated conception of welfare than that of a simple maximization of preferences achieved in a marketplace. While this approach admits the possibility of
a richer conversation about the values at stake, it does not supply a process by
which more foundational questions might be contested: to advance personal
well-being and public health, should we adopt a set of preferred human features
as normative and encourage choices that approach that norm? Or should IGM
policy instead embrace a patient-focused conception of these components of
individual flourishing and the common good in which particular choices
might reflect diverse interests and values?

13.5.2   Deontology

Deontological approaches to policy-making assess the rightness of acts according to conformity with certain principles rather than according to their
welfare-maximizing effect or other consequences. Difficulties with deontological approaches include both arriving at and justifying a particular set of principles and determining how to apply them in particular cases. Could deontology
as a public philosophy succeed in making good use of the information supplied
by bioethics in devising IGM policy?

Provisions in international declarations, charters, and conventions invoke
neo-Kantian deontological principles centered on respect for persons, including
honoring their freedom and dignity, in prohibiting certain manipulations of the
human genome. The 1997 Universal Declaration on the Human Genome and
Human Rights, adopted by the General Conference of the United Nations'
Educational, Scientific, and Cultural Organization (UNESCO), bans "practices
which are contrary to human dignity," including human reproductive cloning.[76]
Similarly, the 2000 Charter of Fundamental Rights of the European Union
declares that "Human dignity is inviolable. It must be respected and protected,"[77]
and bans human reproductive cloning.[78] The 1997 Convention on Human
Rights and Biomedicine of the Council of Europe resolves to take necessary
measures "to safeguard human dignity and the fundamental rights and freedoms
of the individual with regard to the application of biology and medicine"[79] and
permits intervention in the human genome only if "undertaken for preventive,

diagnostic or therapeutic purposes, and only if its aim is not to introduce any modification in the genome of any descendants."[80] Roberto Andorno describes the reasoning behind bans on enhancement engineering in international law, drawing on neo-Kantian concepts of freedom and dignity:

In the case of germ-line interventions for enhancement purposes, the objections are ... based on the idea that we do not have the right to predetermine the characteristics of future individuals. That means that people should be free to develop their potentialities without being biologically conditioned by the particular conceptions of 'good' and 'bad' human traits that were dominant at the time of those who preceded them. In other words, genetics should not become the instrument for a kind of intergenerational tyranny. A second objection is that the procedure would profoundly affect our own self-perception as 'subjects': that is, as autonomous beings, which might lead us to consider ourselves as mere 'objects' or biological artifacts designed by others.[81]

In contrast, however, deontologist Ronald Dworkin, drawing on a set of principles developed in his political theory, argues that it should not only be permissible for parents to engage in IGM, it should be incumbent on them to do so when it can improve the lives of their children. Dworkin argues that the two principles of "ethical individualism" – the objectively equal importance of every life and each individual's ultimate responsibility for the success of her own life[82] – should lead us to "play God" to try to improve humankind and to refrain from restrictions on those who pursue the improvement:

There is nothing in itself wrong with the detached ambition to make the lives of future generations of human beings longer and more full of talent and hence achievement. On the contrary, if playing God means struggling to improve our species, bringing into our conscious designs a resolution to improve what God deliberately or nature blindly has evolved over eons, then the first principle of ethical individualism commands that struggle, and its second principle forbids, in the absence of positive evidence of danger, hobbling the scientists and doctors who volunteer to lead it.[83]

On Dworkin's account, worries about safety and the distribution of access to IGM can be addressed by regulatory and social policies.[84] While loss of human diversity may be a concern, there would be scientific limits on our capacity to engineer ideal social types and most parents likely would be interested only in correcting for major defects, so it is not a worry that should preclude proceeding.[85] And uniformity would be desirable with respect to eliminating serious disease and achieving superior abilities in future generations:

To some degree, of course, greater uniformity is unambiguously desirable: there is no value, aesthetic or otherwise, in the fact that some people are doomed to a disfigured and short life ... Presumably all parents, if given a choice, would wish their children to have the level of intelligence and other skills that we now regard as normal, or even that we now believe superior. But we cannot regard that as undesirable: it is, after all, the object of education, ordinary as well as remedial, to improve intelligence and skill levels across the board.[86]

As these examples illustrate, deontological approaches can and do yield conflicting principles. In the absence of consensus on a set of principles, or consensus as to what would justify choosing one set of principles over another so that members of a political community might engage in fruitful debate about them, it will be difficult to invoke a set of principles to resolve novel, complex, and potentially divisive issues of the sort raised by IGM. Sustained consensus, in any event, is quite unlikely within and across modern pluralistic political communities; while consensus might prevail for a time, it is likely to collapse just as the issues grow more pressing and the implications more concrete. For example, after the 1997 cloning of Dolly the sheep, President Clinton asked the National Bioethics Advisory Commission (NBAC) to study and prepare a report on human reproductive cloning. NBAC members agreed that the procedure would, at that time, be unsafe, but were unable to achieve a consensus on any other principle that should guide national policy on human cloning.[87]

The application of an agreed-upon set of principles will be open to dispute as well. While freedom and dignity may require refraining from enhancement engineering for some, others will compare genetic enhancement to selecting a mate or a gamete donor with desirable heritable characteristics or taking prenatal vitamins, and will find no offense to the principles of freedom and dignity in any of these practices. And while some may agree with Dworkin that a principle of equality generates a duty to equalize talents where possible, others will argue that it requires recognizing inherent equality in humans of varying dispositions, appearance, and talents, and that the drive to equalize talents would capture a narrow, parochial view of the good life rather than the true implications of the principle.

Deontology is unlikely to yield principles or applications that are widely agreeable to members of diverse political communities; if it could, it is unlikely that we would need to worry about the advent of IGM. Debates citing deontological principles and their applications, as we have seen in many of the most fruitless of current debates surrounding morally fraught issues, tend to recapitulate underlying disputes about the content of individual flourishing and the common good without illuminating them or sharpening the debate in a way that might be productive of increased understanding or facilitative of practical coping by the political community.

13.5.3   A navigational approach

The navigational approach that I recommend for IGM policy-making will listen to bioethics and proceed incrementally, responding to additional information about the emerging past and future in an ongoing, iterative process. I recommend it as well suited to IGM policy-making in particular because of its superior capacity to cope with novel, complex, and potentially divisive issues. I contrast it with the foregoing examples of utilitarian and deontological approaches to policy-making because those approaches are widely invoked and, I believe, ill suited to the sorts of issues that arise at the intersection of bioscientific and biotechnological innovation with the complexity of human life systems and with morally fraught practices such as those surrounding procreation. By listening to bioethics, a discipline that spends much of its time at this intersection, as it excavates and reflects on the past, and imagines and contemplates the future, politics can become better acquainted with the varied, nuanced, and difficult issues that arise there – a start on coping well with them.

A navigational approach to policy-making bears a kinship to common law decision-making in that no single principle, such as welfare maximization, or set of principles, such as freedom and dignity or equality and responsibility, is taken to be foundational to the decision-making process. Instead, the approach consists in an ongoing engagement of practical reasoners with problems that arise in experience and that implicate the mission of the political community. The goal, first, is to understand in concrete, contextualized detail the implications of one resolution or another of these problems for different conceptions of individual flourishing and the common good as they have emerged from our historical experience in similar cases. In contested cases decided at common law, the parties to a current controversy argue about the implications of one resolution or another for competing conceptions of individual flourishing and the common good that are embedded in our historical experience. In the case of proactive IGM policy-making, the parties to the debate will invoke future imaginings in place of current controversies, but much of their remaining work will be the same.

The resolutions captured in regulatory frameworks, as is oftentimes the case with resolutions of contested cases at common law, will not necessarily endorse in its entirety one conception over another. Diversity in values and conceptions built upon them is a fact of pluralistic societies, and accommodation of diversity, where possible, is a longstanding practice of policy-makers. Even when one conception is rejected, whether by a consensus achieved after the issues have been fully considered or by the procedural mechanism of a vote, a navigational approach holds the door open to reconsideration after more experience and further debate. To the extent that principles are at stake, they will be multiple and diverse; to the extent one is selected in favor of another, it is as a hypothesis subject to reconsideration on the evidence and reflection of experience and future cases, rather than as a timeless abstraction immune to revision.

A navigational approach does not concede that there is no correct set of practical principles capturing conceptions of individual flourishing and the common good that will emerge over time; instead, it captures the method of learning them and acknowledges that they may be numerous and limited in their range of application, given the complexity of the subject matter they address. It acknowledges that there is no authoritative source of all the practical principles that should guide our conduct as we encounter novel problems over time, but a collection of practical reasoners who develop these principles through engagement with experience and one another. The approach is risky for those who know resolutions to the questions of IGM in advance, but hopeful for those who do not know but want to.

NOTES

1 For explorations of the philosophical nature and implications of the complexity of human life systems, extending from the molecular to the social level, see Kenneth F. Schaffner, *Discovery and Explanation in Biology and Medicine*. Chicago: University of Chicago Press (1993); Philip Pettit, *The Common Mind: An Essay on Psychology, Society, and Politics*. New York: Oxford University Press (1996); Alexander Rosenberg, *Philosophy of Social Science*, 2nd edn, Boulder, CO: Westview Press (1995); and Alexander Rosenberg, *Instrumental Biology, or The Disunity of Science*. Chicago: University of Chicago Press (1994).

2 See Schaffner, *Discovery and Explanation in Biology and Medicine*, especially pp. 145–52. See also Roy Porter, *The Greatest Benefit to Mankind: A Medical History of Humanity*. New York: W.W. Norton (1997), especially pp. 337–41.

3 See discussion in Porter, *Greatest Benefit to Mankind*, pp. 431–45.

4 See discussion of the contributions of Liebig to the development of organic chemistry and Ludwig to the development of physiology in Porter, *Greatest Benefit to Mankind*, pp. 324–9; and of Virchow's contributions to the development of cell theory, pp. 330–3. See also discussion of Liebig in Timothy Lenoir, *The Strategy of Life: Teleology and Mechanics in Nineteenth-Century German Biology*. Chicago: University of Chicago Press (1989), pp. 158–68; of Ludwig, pp. 217–9; and of Virchow, pp. 14, 114, 195, 219, 225, 229, and 241.

5 For a history of medicine from ancient times through the twentieth century, see Porter, *Greatest Benefit to Mankind*. For an account of the development of modern medicine centered on the professionalization of the medical profession in the United States, see Paul Starr, *The Social Transformation of American Medicine*. New York: Basic Books (1982).

6 See Kim Sterelny and Paul E. Griffiths, *Sex and Death: An Introduction to Philosophy of Biology, Science and Its Conceptual Foundations Series*. Chicago: University of Chicago Press (1999), pp. 31–51. See generally Jane Maienschein and Michael Ruse (eds.), *Biology and the Foundation of Ethics*. Cambridge: Cambridge University Press (1999); and Alexander Rosenberg, *Darwinism in Philosophy, Social Science and Policy*, Cambridge Studies in Philosophy and Biology. Cambridge: Cambridge University Press (2000).

7 Robert Bud, *The Uses of Life: A History of Biotechnology*. Cambridge: Cambridge University Press (1993), pp. 164, 174; Daniel J. Kevles, *In the Name of Eugenics: Genetics and the Uses of Human Heredity*. Cambridge: Harvard University Press (1995), p. 267.

8 Bud, *Uses of Life*, pp. 177–8.

9 *Diamond v. Chakrabarty* (1980), 447 U.S. 303.

10 See discussion in Ryan M.T. Iwasaka, From Chakrabarty to chimeras: the growing need for evolutionary biology in patent law, *Yale Law Journal* 109 (2000), 1505–28. See also Bud, *Uses of Life*, pp. 215–6.

11 Kevles, *In the Name of Eugenics* (the next three paragraphs draw on this text for historical background).

12 See generally Robert Cook-Deegan, *The Gene Wars: Science, Politics, and the Human Genome*. New York: W.W. Norton (1995); Daniel J. Kevles and Leroy Hood (eds.), *The Code of Codes: Scientific and Social Issues in the Human Genome Project*. Cambridge: Harvard University Press (1992).

13 Cook-Deegan, *The Gene Wars*, p. 346.

14 See Bud, *Uses of Life*, pp. 177–88; and LeRoy Walters and Julie G. Palmer, *The Ethics of Human Gene Therapy*. New York: Oxford University Press (1997), pp. 17–59. See also National Institutes of Health, *Report and Recommendations of the Panel to Assess the NIH Investment in Research on Gene Therapy*, Stuart H. Orkin and Arno G. Motulsky, co-chairs, 7 December 1995, http://www.nih.gov/news/panelrep.html (last accessed 31 March 2005); Nathan Seppa, "Bubble" babies thrive on gene therapy, *Science News* 157, (29 April, 2000), 277; Nathan Seppa, Genetically altered cells ease hemophilia, *Science News* 159, (9 June, 2001), 357; Department of Health and Human Services, Public Health Service, Office of Biotechnology Activities, National Institutes of Health (NIH), Serious adverse event in a study of gene transfer in X-linked severe combined immunodeficiency, fact sheet, 14 January 2003, http://www4.od.nih.gov/OBA/RAC/Fact_Sheet.pdf (last accessed 31 March 2005).

15 See NIH, Advisory Committee to the Director, Working Group on NIH Oversight of Clinical Gene Transfer Research, Enhancing the protection of human subjects in gene transfer research at the National Institutes of Health, 12 July 2000, http://www.nih.gov/about/director/07122000.htm#exec (last accessed 31 March 2005).

16 Sheryl G. Stolberg, Despite ferment, gene therapy progresses, *New York Times*, 6 June 2000.

17 See generally John H. Evans, *Playing God? Human Genetic Engineering and the Rationalization of Public Bioethical Debate*. Chicago: University of Chicago Press (2002), pp. 45–71; Kevles, *In the Name of Eugenics*, pp. 3–147; and Diane B. Paul, *Controlling Human Heredity: 1865 to the Present*. Amherst, NY: Humanity Books (1998), pp. 30–114.

18 For discussion focused primarily on American eugenic thought and programs, see Kevles, *In the Name of Eugenics*; Evans, *Playing God?*; Paul, *Controlling Human Heredity*; Roberta M. Berry, From involuntary sterilization to genetic enhancement: the unsettled legacy of *Buck v. Bell*, *Notre Dame Journal of Law, Ethics and Public Policy* 12 (1998), 401–48; Mark H. Haller, *Eugenics: Hereditarian Attitudes in American Thought*. New Brunswick, NJ: Rutgers University Press (1963); and Kenneth M. Ludmerer, *Genetics and American Society: A Historical Appraisal*. Baltimore: Johns Hopkins University Press (1972).

19 Stephen Jay Gould, Carrie Buck's daughter, *Natural History* 93 (July 1984), 14, 16.

20 *Buck v. Bell* (1927), 274 U.S. 200, 207.

21 See Oliver Wendell Holmes, Law in science and science in law, *Harvard Law Review* 12 (1899), 443, 462; see also Oliver Wendell Holmes, The path of the law, *Harvard Law Review* 10 (1897), 457, 469; Philip P. Wiener, *Evolution and the Founders of Pragmatism*. Philadelphia: University of Pennsylvania Press (1972), pp. 174–5; Berry, *From Involuntary Sterilization to Genetic Enhancement*, pp. 432–8.

22 Berry, *From Involuntary Sterilization To Genetic Enhancement*, p. 438.

23 "Oliver Wendell Holmes to Harold J. Laski, May 12 1927," In: Mark De Wolfe Howe (ed.), *Holmes–Laski Letters: The Correspondence of Mr. Justice Holmes and Harold J. Laski, 1916–1935*, vol. 2. Cambridge: Harvard University Press (1953), p. 942.

24 Gould, Carrie Buck's daughter, p. 14; Kevles, *In the Name of Eugenics*, p. 275. There is ongoing debate surrounding contemporary statutes and practices regarding non-consensual sterilization of the mentally disabled when it is claimed to be in their best interests. See, e.g., Roger B. Dworkin, *Limits: The Role of the Law in Bioethical Decision Making*. Bloomington: Indiana University Press (1996), pp. 54–60; Robert L. Hayman, Jr., Presumptions of justice: law, politics, and the mentally retarded parent, *Harvard Law Review* 103 (1990), 1207–72; and Joe Zumpano-Canto, Nonconsensual sterilization of the mentally disabled in North Carolina: an ethics critique of the statutory standard and its judicial interpretation, *Journal of Contemporary Health Law and Policy* 13 (1996), 79–112.

25 Regarding the connections among American eugenic programs and eugenics programs of the Nazi era, see also Kevles, *In the Name of Eugenics*, pp. 116–8; Paul, *Controlling Human Heredity*, pp. 84–91.

26 Kevles, *In the Name of Eugenics*, p. 118.

27 See discussion of the views of Julian Huxley, Hermann Muller, and Theodosius Dobzhansky in Evans, *Playing God?* pp. 51–2.

28 Kevles, *In the Name of Eugenics*, pp. 122–8, 164–92; Paul, *Controlling Human Heredity*, pp. 117–21; Evans, *Playing God?* pp. 49–57.

29 See generally Kevles, *In the Name of Eugenics*, pp. 113–211; Paul, *Controlling Human Heredity*, pp. 117–21.

30 See Kevles, *In the Name of Eugenics*, pp. 176–8.

31 See *ibid.*, pp. 184–6.

32 Kevles, *In the Name of Eugenics*, p. 184 (citation omitted), see generally pp. 184–92.

33 Regarding the eugenics program of Nazi Germany, see Robert Proctor, *Racial Hygiene: Medicine under the Nazis*. Cambridge: Harvard University Press (1988); see also Kevles, *In the Name of Eugenics*, pp. 116–8, 169.

34 See Kevles, *In the Name of Eugenics*, pp. 251–90; Evans, *Playing God?* pp. 45–71.

35 Paul, *Controlling Human Heredity*, p. 121.

36 Kevles, *In the Name of Eugenics*, pp. 186–7.

37 Hermann J. Muller, Progress and prospects in human genetics: a preface to this journal, *American Journal of Human Genetics* 1 (1949), 1.

38 Muller, *Progress and Prospects in Human Genetics*, pp. 16–7.

39 Kevles, *In the Name of Eugenics*, pp. 259–60.

40 As quoted in Kevles, *In the Name of Eugenics*, pp. 260–1.

41 Kevles, *In the Name of Eugenics*, pp. 263–4. After Muller's death, a sperm bank was established by a former collaborator, pp. 262–3.

42 See Evans, *Playing God?* pp. 61–9; Kevles, *In the Name of Eugenics*, p. 289.

43 Kevles, *In the Name of Eugenics*, p. 251.

44 *Ibid.*, pp. 253–4; Paul, *Controlling Human Heredity*, pp. 122–9.

45 Kevles, *In the Name of Eugenics*, pp. 255–6.

46 *Roe v. Wade* (1973), 410 U.S. 113.

47 See discussion in John A. Robertson, Genetic selection of offspring characteristics, *Boston University Law Review* 76 (June 1996), 433–48.

48 See discussion in Jeffrey R. Botkin, Ethical issues and practical problems in pre-implantation genetic diagnosis, *Journal of Law, Medicine and Ethics* 26 (1998) 17–28; and Robertson, *Genetic Selection Of Offspring Characteristics*, 439–52.

49 Kevles, *In the Name of Eugenics*, pp. 253–8; Paul, *Controlling Human Heredity*, pp. 125–35.

50 See Charles Cantor, The challenges to technology and informatics. In: Kevles and Hood (eds.), *Code of Codes*, p. 105; Leroy Hood, Biology and medicine in the twenty-first century. In: Kevles and Hood (eds.), *Code of Codes*, p. 159; Evelyn Fox Keller, Nature, nurture, and the Human Genome Project. In: Kevles and Hood (eds.), *Code of Codes*, pp. 281, 295–6.

51 Paul, *Controlling Human Heredity*, pp. 125–9.

52 *Ibid.*, pp. 130–2.

53 Kevles, *In the Name of Eugenics*, p. 258; Paul, *Controlling Human Heredity*, pp. 125–9; see also Joan A. Scott, Inheritable genetic modification: clinical applications and genetic counseling considerations (Chapter 12, this volume).

54 Paul, *Controlling Human Heredity*, pp. 129–32. See also Kevles, *In the Name of Eugenics*, pp. 253–8; Thomas H. Murray, *The Worth of a Child*. Berkeley: University of California Press (1996), pp. 118–41.

55 See, e.g., remarks of Dena Davis, Glenn McGee and John A. Robertson 1999 symposium remarks: panel on pre-pregnancy gender selection, *Texas Journal of Women and the Law* 8 (1999), 267–83; and Mary Anne Warren, The ethics of sex preselection. In: Kenneth D. Alpern (ed.), *The Ethics of Reproductive Technology*. New York: Oxford University Press (1992). See also Robertson, *Genetic Selection Of Offspring Characteristics*; and Murray, *Worth of a Child*, pp. 118–41.

56 Paul, *Controlling Human Heredity*, p. 132 (citations omitted).

57 *Ibid.*, pp. 132–3.

58 Daniel J. Kevles, The ghost of Galton: eugenics past, present, and future. In: Michael A. Signer (ed.), *Humanity at the Limit: The Impact of the Holocaust Experience on Jews and Christians*. Bloomington: Indiana University Press (2000), p. 195.

59 See, e.g., *Poe v. Ullman* (1961), 367 U.S. 497, in which the U.S. Supreme Court dismissed a challenge to a Connecticut statute banning the use of contraceptives, which was overturned a few years later in *Griswold v. Connecticut* (1965), 381 U.S. 479.

In *Griswold*, the state of Connecticut had arrested a group of persons under the statute, and these persons challenged its constitutionality; but in *Poe*, no one had been arrested and there was no evidence that the statute had ever been enforced. In dismissing the challenge, Justice Frankfurter wrote of its "abstract character" (p. 501) and lack of "immediacy which is an indispensable condition of constitutional adjudication" (p. 508).

60 Friedrich Vogel and Arno G. Motulsky, *Human Genetics: Problems and Approaches*, 3rd edn, Berlin: Springer-Verlag (1997), pp. 106, 132.

61 Vogel and Motulsky, *Human Genetics*, pp. 130–2.

62 *Ibid.*, p. 132.

63 See also Rosemarie Tong, Traditional and feminist bioethical perspectives on gene transfer: is inheritable genetic modification really *the* problem? (Chapter 9, this volume), and Jackie Leach Scully, Inheritable genetic modification and disability: normality and identity (Chapter 10, this volume).

64 Vogel and Motulsky, *Human Genetics*, p. 549.

65 Associated Press, Bashful kids may be born that way, CBSNews.com, SciTech, section front, 19 June 2003, http://www.cbsnews.com/stories/2003/06/19/tech/main559442.shtml (last accessed 24 August 2004).

66 For discussion of the issues summarized in this paragraph, see Samuel Scheffler (ed.), *Consequentialism and Its Critics*. Oxford: Oxford University Press (1988); and Jonathan Glover (ed.), *Utilitarianism and Its Critics*. New York: Macmillan (1990).

67 The summary set forth in this paragraph relies largely on the arguments set forth in Robert E. Goodin, *Utilitarianism as a Public Philosophy*. Cambridge: Cambridge University Press (1995), pp. 7–11, 61–5.

68 Jonathan Glover, *What Sort of People Should There Be? Genetic Engineering, Brain Control and Their Impact on Our Future World*. Harmondsworth, England: Penguin (1984).

69 Glover, *What Sort of People Should There Be?* p. 42.

70 *Ibid.*, p. 52.

71 *Ibid.*, p. 42.

72 *Ibid.*, pp. 43–4.

73 *Ibid.*, pp. 157–61; 136.

74 *Ibid.*, pp. 180–1.

75 *Ibid.*, pp. 47–51; see also Peter Singer, Shopping at the genetic supermarket (Foreword, this volume).

76 UNESCO, *Universal Declaration on the Human Genome and Human Rights* (1997), Article 11.

77 European Union, *Charter of Fundamental Rights of the European Union* (2000), Article 1.

78 European Union, *Charter of Fundamental Rights*, Article 3.

79 Council of Europe, *Convention for the Protection of Human Rights and Dignity of the Human Being with regard to the Application of Biology and Medicine: Convention on Human Rights and Biomedicine* (1997), preamble.

80 Council of Europe, *Convention on Human Rights and Biomedicine*, Article 13; see also Eric T. Juengst, "Alter-ing" the human species? misplaced essentialism in science policy (Chapter 8, this volume).

81 Roberto Andorno, Biomedicine and international human rights law: in search of a global consensus, *Bulletin of the World Health Organization* 80 (2002), 959–63, p. 961 (citations omitted).

82 Ronald Dworkin, *Sovereign Virtue: The Theory and Practice of Equality*. Cambridge: Harvard University Press (2000), pp. 5–6, 447–8.

83 Dworkin, *Sovereign Virtue*, p. 452.

84 *Ibid.*, p. 440.

85 *Ibid.*, p. 442.

86 *Ibid.*, p. 441.

87 National Bioethics Advisory Commission, *Cloning Human Beings: Report and Recommendations of the National Bioethics Advisory Commission*. Rockville, MD: GEM Publications (1997).

Glossary of scientific terms[1]

John E.J. Rasko, Gabrielle M. O'Sullivan, and Rachel A. Ankeny

Achondroplasia   An inherited condition that results in unusually short stature. It is caused by a *mutation* in a *gene* that affects cartilage formation. The effect of the mutated gene is *dominant*.

Adeno-associated virus (AAV) vector   An adeno-associated virus that has been genetically engineered for use as a vehicle (*vector*) for introducing *gene*s into host cells, tissues, or organisms. The naturally occurring adeno-associated virus has a *genome* made of single-stranded *DNA*, is non-pathogenic, and is widespread in humans. It requires help from natural adenovirus to replicate. The currently available genetically-engineered vector has two major disadvantages: it accommodates small genes and has lost its site-specific integration ability, which results in random integration into human chromosomes and raises the possibility that the functions of normal genes might be disrupted (see *insertional mutagenesis*). However, its non-pathogenicity, its persistence in tissues over time, and its ability to infect non-dividing cells make it an attractive vector candidate for human *gene transfer*. It has been used as a vector in many human trials of gene transfer into brain, liver, skeletal muscle, and blood.

Adenosine deaminase (ADA)   An enzyme that is involved in the metabolism of adenosine, a *nucleoside* that is present in *DNA* and *RNA* and can also exist separately in an energetic form that has phosphate molecules attached to it. A deficiency of ADA leads to an accumulation of specific *nucleotides* (subunits of DNA) which are toxic to lymphoid *stem cells*. See *severe combined immune deficiency (SCID)*.

Adenoviral (AV) vector   An adenovirus that has been genetically engineered for use as a vehicle (*vector*) for introducing *gene*s into host cells, tissues, or organisms. Adenoviruses have double-stranded linear *DNA* as their *genome*. Their advantages as vectors are that they can carry large genes and can infect non-dividing cells. Their major disadvantages are that they can stimulate strong host immune responses and cannot integrate within the host genome, causing a loss of effectiveness over time. These vectors have been used in about a quarter of clinical *gene transfer* trials (e.g., in *cystic fibrosis* and cancer trials).

Adult stem cell   A *stem cell* that is found in body (somatic) tissues and can develop into the specialized cell types of that tissue. It is also known as a *somatic stem cell*. The term is not used to refer to a *gamete* or to stem cells found in an *embryo*. An example is the *hematopoietic stem cell* (i.e., blood forming), which is found in the bone marrow and, through rounds of division and *differentiation*, develops into the white and red blood cells of the body.

Albinism   A group of rare inherited conditions characterized by a lack of pigment (melanin) in skin, hair, or eyes. There are a number of different types of albinism caused by *mutations* in different *genes*. Usually the albinism-causing effect of the mutated gene is *recessive*.

Allele   One of the different forms of the same *gene*. In a cell there are two copies of each *chromosome*, one inherited from the father and one inherited from the mother. There is one copy of each gene located at the same position (*locus*) on each chromosome. If one gene copy differs from the other gene copy in an individual, each gene copy is known as an allele, and the individual is said to be *heterozygous* for that gene. If both gene copies are the same allele inherited from the father and mother, the individual is said to be *homozygous* for that gene.

Alzheimer disease   The most common form of dementia in elderly people. It is caused by the deposition of proteins known as beta amyloid and tau in the brain. Multiple genetic, and possibly environmental, factors are involved.

Amino acid   A basic structural unit of proteins. There are 20 commonly occurring amino acids.

Amniocentesis   A procedure for obtaining amniotic fluid (the liquid in the uterus that the developing *embryo* is suspended in) for prenatal diagnosis. The procedure is usually carried out in the 14–18th week of pregnancy.

Antibody   A molecule produced by *B cells* that recognizes and specifically binds to proteins, carbohydrates, or fatty substances and mediates specific immune responses to them.

Antibody depletion   The removal of antibodies from a substance, or the removal of substances or cells using antibodies. Antibodies that recognize and bind specific molecules on the substances or cells to be removed are added to a mixture of these substances or cells. The antibodies can be tagged in various ways to allow them (and the materials bound to them) to be selected and isolated from the mixture. Specific types of cell populations are obtained in the laboratory by this method.

Antisense   A *DNA* or *RNA* sequence that is *complementary* to a sequence of *messenger RNA*. When antisense DNA or RNA is added to a cell, it binds to a specific (sense) messenger RNA molecule and inactivates it.

Artificial chromosomes   *Chromosomes* that are made in the laboratory for the purpose of delivering *genes* into cells. They are designed to reside inside the cell and to be stable and self-replicating. If they were to be introduced early enough in development to be replicated in the *germ cells*, their introduction would be a type of *inheritable genetic modification*. Artificial chromosomes that could be experimentally manipulated were first made in yeast in 1987. Since then there have been attempts to make human artificial chromosomes by either paring down an existing functional chromosome to minimal *DNA* sequences, or by building up basic functional elements in yeast artificial chromosomes. A functional artificial chromosome has been inheritably transmitted in mice.[2]

Asexual reproduction   Reproduction that does not involve the union of *egg* and *sperm*. All, or almost all, the offspring's genetic material comes from a single ancestor and the offspring is a *clone* of this ancestor.

Autosome   Any *chromosome* that is not a *sex chromosome* (i.e., it is not an *X* or *Y chromosome*). In humans, they are numbered from the largest (chromosome 1) to the smallest (chromosome 22).

B cell   A type of *lymphocyte* that matures in the bone marrow and produces antibodies to foreign substances. B cells form part of the body's specific (acquired) immune system.

Beckwith–Wiedemann syndrome   A syndrome characterized by large organ and body size and, in infants, low blood sugar and an increased incidence of tumor development. It can be associated with a mutation in chromosome 11 or with *imprinted gene* errors.

Blastocyst   The name applied to an *embryo* at a very early stage in its development. A human embryo reaches this stage 4 days after conception. It consists of a spherical ball of cells surrounding a cavity in the center (blastocele or blastocoele). The cells are composed of an inner mass of cells (embryoblast) that will become the fetus and an outer layer of cells (trophoblast) that will become part of the placenta.

Cell therapy   The administration of cells into a patient to treat a disease.

Chimera   An organism or tissue containing two or more genetically distinct cell types. An individual composed of such tissues – such as occurs in recipients of bone marrow transplants from unrelated donors – is described as chimeric. See *mosaic*.

Chorionic villus sampling (CVS)   A procedure for obtaining cells from the chorion for prenatal testing of the early *fetus* for specific abnormalities. The chorion is the outer membrane enclosing the *embryo* that develops into the placenta and has cells of the same genetic composition as the embryo. CVS is usually carried out in the 10–12th week of pregnancy.

Chromatin   The material that *chromosomes* are composed of. It is a complex of *DNA* and proteins.

Chromosome   A long piece of *DNA* and its associated proteins (*chromatin*) that is found in the *nucleus* of a cell and contains a fixed linear sequence of *genes*. Higher organisms, such as humans and animals, have two sets of chromosomes in each cell of the body (except in secondary *germ cells* and the *gametes*): one set is inherited from the organism's father and the other is inherited from the organism's mother. Chromosomes are duplicated with the cell during cell division so that they can be passed on to each successive generation of cells (see *mitosis*). During the formation of gametes (*gametogenesis*), they undergo limited exchange of genetic material with each other and are assorted into different gametes to ensure that there is genetic variation between different offspring resulting from *fertilization* (see *meiosis*).

Clone   A group of *genes*, cells, or organisms that is derived from, and identical to, a single ancestor. Cloning is the deliberate replication of the genetic makeup of an individual by the use of an *asexual reproduction* technique, such as *somatic cell nuclear transfer*.

Cloned embryo   An *embryo* created by the use of an *asexual reproduction* technique known as *somatic cell nuclear transfer*. This involves the transfer of the *nucleus* of an adult body cell into a *fertilized egg* that has had its own nucleus removed from it, followed by stimulation of the hybrid cell to grow into an embryo (see *parthenogenesis*). Such an embryo might be created for the purpose of generating tissues for cellular and molecular research or for the purpose of producing an organism, including (potentially) a human child. Cloned animals usually develop abnormally because the nucleus from an adult body cell is not in the correct programming state to direct the development of a normal embryo: it is configured for the requirements of an adult cell and would have to be "reprogrammed" to meet the developmental requirements of an embryonic cell (see *imprinted genes*). Reprogramming is not yet feasible. It has been suggested that a cloned embryo is so distinct in composition and creative intent from an embryo formed by *sexual reproduction*, that its earliest form should be termed a "clonote"[3] to distinguish it from the earliest form of a sexually-produced embryo, which is termed a *zygote*. The first time that cloning led to the production of a fully-developed living animal was with the cloning of a sheep known as "Dolly."[4] Since then many other fully-developed animals have been cloned. Although there is a worldwide ban on cloning humans, there have been some claims that it has been achieved (e.g., by the Raelians). See *epigenetic reprogramming* and *epigenetic modification*.

Complementarity   A property of *DNA* whereby each *nitrogenous base* in a single strand of DNA pairs with a particular nitrogenous base in another single strand of DNA according to the rules: A with T and G with C. If two complementary single strands of DNA have sequences along their length that enable their bases to pair up, they will form a double helix structure. If a single DNA strand aligns with a single strand of *RNA* the base pairing follows the same rules except that A pairs with U (which replaces T in RNA).

Conditional gene targeting system   Or, conditional targeted mutagenesis system; a system for genetically modifying cells, tissues, or organisms that allows control over the timing, cell type, and tissue specificity of *gene* expression, or repression, during defined developmental stages.

Congenital   Present at birth.

Cryopreservation   A process for storing biological materials safely (e.g., frozen *embryos*) at extremely low temperatures (usually in liquid nitrogen) for use at a later date.

Cumulus cell   A type of *somatic cell* surrounding developing *egg* cells.

Cystic fibrosis (CF)   A condition that affects many organs, whereby abnormal body secretions lead to respiratory problems, incomplete digestion of food, and increased salt loss from sweat glands. It is caused by a *mutation* in a *gene* on chromosome 7 that makes a salt transport protein. The effect of the mutated gene is *recessive*.

Cytoplasm   The contents of a cell, not including its *nucleus*.

Differentiation   The process of a cell developing (i.e., maturing) from a state of being less specialized (i.e., less committed to a specific cell function) in terms of its morphology and functions to a state of being more specialized. The differentiation state of a cell describes the extent to which the morphology and functions of a cell have become specialized.

Diploid   Of organisms and cells, having two sets of *chromosomes* in each cell. One set is inherited from the organism's father and the other is inherited from the organism's mother. The non-reproductive (*somatic*) cells of humans, most animals, and many plants are diploid. Diploid is twice the *haploid* number of chromosomes that are found in the *gametes* of sexually reproducing higher organisms. Diploid is abbreviated as 2n.

DNA   Deoxyribonucleic acid (DNA) is the chemical substance that *genes* and *chromosomes* are made of. It consists of two chains of chemicals known as *nucleotides* that run alongside each other to form a double helix shape. A nucleotide consists of a sugar, a phosphate group, and a *nitrogenous base*. There are only four different kinds of nitrogenous bases in DNA (A, T, G, and C). It is the complementary pairing of each nitrogenous base in one chain with another particular base in the other chain (see *complementarity*) that enables the chains to form the double helix structure and the DNA to be replicated. Nucleotides are organized in groups of different combinations of three (triplets) along the length of each chain. It is the sequence of different triplets (called codons) along the length of the chain organised into genes that contains the genetic instructions (the "genetic code"). A cell has mechanisms for translating this genetic information into functional products (proteins) and for replicating the genetic information so that it can be passed on from one generation of cells to another.

DNA methylation   Reversible modification of *DNA* by the attachment of chemicals, known as methyl groups, to one of DNA's own constituent chemicals, known as *nucleotides*. This affects the way in which *genes* are expressed: usually, genes that have methyl groups attached to them are not expressed and genes that do not have methyl groups attached to them are expressed.[5] This is one form of *epigenetic modification* of genes.

DNA microinjection   The direct introduction of *DNA* into cells, tissues, and organisms using a very fine needle. DNA microinjection into *fertilized eggs* is the technique currently used to create transgenic animals. The technique is very inefficient and multiple *gene* copies are integrated randomly into the host *genome*, posing risks of disrupting the function of host genes and affecting the level of gene expression. The first generation offspring are *chimeras* (organisms in which only some cells carry the introduced gene) and a special breeding program must be implemented to obtain non-*chimeric* animals.

Dominant   In reference to observable traits (characteristics) that are determined by particular *genes*, a dominant trait is manifested by the presence of one gene copy rather than two (see *recessive*).

Down syndrome   A condition that affects intellectual, behavioral, and physical development and is associated with typical facial characteristics. It is caused by the presence of an extra *chromosome* (number 21) and is not inherited in most cases, but arises randomly during *gametogenesis*.

Egg   A reproductive cell of a female animal that carries one set of *chromosomes* (*haploid*). In normal sexual reproduction an egg is fertilized by a *sperm* cell to produce an *embryo*. Alternative terms are female *gamete* and *ovum*.

Embryo   A developing organism from the time of *fertilization* (conception) until (in humans) about 8 weeks later. After this stage the developing human becomes known as a *fetus*. Embryogenesis describes the formation, development, and growth of an *embryo*.

Embryoid body   An aggregate of cells derived from *embryonic stem cells* that undergoes a limited form of embryonic development.

Embryonic germ (EG) cell   A *stem cell* that is found in the part of an *embryo* known as the gonadal ridge and that eventually, normally, develops into mature *gametes*.

Embryonic stem (ES) cell   A *stem cell* found in the *embryo* that has the potential to produce an entire organism or, if appropriately stimulated, specific tissues or cell types. ES cells are said to be totipotent, denoting an ability to give rise to all cells of the body and to transmit genetic information to future generations.

Enucleated egg   An unfertilized *egg* from which the *nucleus* has been removed or destroyed.

Epigenetic modification   The modification of *genes* (e.g., by *DNA methylation*) during cell development (particularly when cells are developing specialized functions) that changes the way in which the genes are expressed in response to changing environmental circumstances. The modifications "program" the genes of the cells to be expressed in a developmental stage-appropriate way that is unlikely to suit other stages of cell development. *Cloning* has shown that many of the modifications present in the genes of mature body cells are not suited to support the development of normal *embryos*. Essentially, epigenetic modification is a mechanism for regulating gene expression that does not depend on *DNA* sequence.

Epigenetic reprogramming   The process of removing *epigenetic modifications* of *DNA*, so that *genes*, whose expression was turned "off" during cell and embryonic development, become active again. See *DNA methylation*.

Episomal DNA   *DNA* that is additional to the host cell's normal *genome*. In the autonomous state, which is often referred to as the "episomal state," it usually takes the form of circular double stranded DNA that will replicate and be transferred independently of the host genome.

Eugenics   An organized attempt to "improve" the genetic constitution of future generations through directed breeding, selective culling, or (potentially) *inheritable genetic modification*.

Familial adenomatous polyposis (FAP)   An inherited condition that leads to bowel cancer. It is due to a mutation in the adenomatous polyposis coli (APC) gene on chromosome 5 that is involved in the suppression of tumor formation. The effect of the mutated gene is *dominant*.

Fertilization   The union of an *egg* and a *sperm* cell to form a *zygote*, or *fertilized egg*.

Fetus   The product of conception after the *embryo* stage until the moment of birth. In humans the fetal stage begins 7–8 weeks after *fertilization*.

Fibroblast   A versatile type of cell that makes the chemical components of connective tissue. A fibroblast *stem cell*, called a mesenchymal stem cell, can give rise to other types of cells which comprise muscle, bone, and fat.

Founder selection   A selective breeding strategy to obtain parent (i.e., founder) animals that can be bred further to generate offspring (known as a "line") with the desired *genotype* and/or *phenotype*.

Gamete   A reproductive cell (*egg* in females and *sperm* in males) of an animal that carries one set of *chromosome*s (i.e., it is *haploid*). In normal sexual reproduction a gamete from each gender unites to produce a fertilized egg (see *zygote*), which produces an *embryo*. The term is sometimes used synonymously with *germ cell*. However, these terms are not always interchangeable as gamete refers specifically to the sperm or egg and not to the tissues that give rise to them, whereas germ cell refers to egg, sperm, and the tissues that give rise to them. Gametes are the products of germ cells.

Gametogenesis   The maturation of *germ cell*s and the process of *gamete* development in animals. Gametogenesis is known as *oogenesis* in females and as *spermatogenesis* in males. The resulting gametes are *egg*s in females and *sperm* in males. Gametogenesis involves cell division of maturing germ cells by *meiosis* to ensure that each gamete produced has only one set of *chromosome*s (i.e., is *haploid*). In normal *sexual reproduction* a gamete from each gender unites to produce an *embryo* in which all the cells (except the germ cells) have two sets of *chromosome*s (i.e., are *diploid*).

Gastrulation   A phase in *embryo* development when the first *germ cell*s are laid down.

Gene   Genetic information in the form of a segment of *DNA* that directs the formation of a specific product (usually a protein) by a cell and can be transmitted from one generation to the next. A gene is the fundamental physical and functional unit of heredity. The coordinated action of many genes and the influence of environmental factors determine the observable characteristics of an organism. See *chromosome*, *genotype*, and *phenotype*.

Gene delivery system   A system for introducing *gene*s into cells, tissues, or organisms. It may consist of injecting the genes directly into the cells or tissue (see *DNA microinjection* and *repair mechanisms*) or a more complex system might consist of using genetic material from another source, such as a virus or an artificially made *chromosome*, as a vehicle (*vector*) to carry the genes into the cells or tissue (see *viral vector* and *artificial chromosome*). Chemicals, such as *liposome*s, can also be used to increase the likelihood that *DNA* is taken up by a cell.

Gene expression   The process by which the information in *genes* (*DNA*) is converted into functional molecules such as proteins in cells.

Gene knockout organism A type of genetically modified organism created using the technique of *gene targeting*, whereby a *gene* is removed (deleted), or "knocked out," by an introduced external gene, which is usually an inactive or mutated form of the host organism's gene. *DNA* is introduced into *embryonic stem cells* that are allowed to multiply. The introduced DNA will become incorporated into the stem cell's own chromosomes by *homologous recombination* provided it has enough sequences that are similar to sequences in the stem cell's chromosomal DNA. Embryonic stem cells that have undergone homologous recombination are selected and injected into an *embryo* at a very early stage of development (*blastocyst*) and allowed to develop in the uterus of a receptive female (foster mother-to-be). The resulting offspring is *heterozygous* and chimeric. A *chimera* that has a high percentage of cells are deleted for one copy of the gene is mated with a normal animal to produce a second generation of animals that are also heterozygous. The second generation offspring are mated with each other to produce a percentage of third generation offspring that are *homozygous* for the deleted gene. These animals do not have the targeted gene in their *germ cells* and so this *genotype* is available for transmission to subsequent generations. The use of "knock out" technology has provided some of the most decisive insights in biology as it uses a whole organism approach to answer the question: "what happens if this particular gene is absent?"

Gene repair The correction of faults in *DNA* sequences. The term is often used to refer to corrections made by the process of *homologous recombination* or the technique of *gene targeting*. Gene repair refers to genetic modifications that can replace one gene with another gene, which is distinct from other kinds of genetic modifications (e.g., *gene transfer*) that add "new" genes into cells without replacing faulty genes.

Gene repair mechanism A set of natural processes in cells that corrects faults in *DNA* sequences, including mechanisms such as *homologous recombination*. This innate mechanism is harnessed in the laboratory to artificially incorporate new *gene*s into an organism's *genome*. It holds great promise for gene modification generally, especially *inheritable genetic modification*, because it could be used to replace faulty genes with corrected genes, thus obviating the problems encountered in *gene transfer* with gene expression and random integration. An example of a gene repair technology that has emerged from increased understanding of natural gene repair mechanisms is *oligonucleotide site directed gene repair*.

Gene targeting The application of a *gene repair* technique that harnesses the natural *gene repair mechanism* in cells known as *homologous recombination* to replace one gene with another. It can be used to replace a faulty gene with a correct gene as a form of therapy, or to replace a correct gene with a "silent" gene that will not be expressed, to produce a *gene knockout organism*. Gene targeting is used as another name for *targeted gene replacement*.

Gene therapy   *Gene transfer* into a patient's cells or tissues with the intention of treating a disease.

Gene transfer   The introduction of new *DNA* into an organism's cells using a variety of chemical, physical, or biological techniques. This term is frequently used to refer to the addition of *genes* (*transgenes*) to cells or tissues using a *vector* such as a genetically-modified virus. In this context, with the present technology, the introduced genetic material does not integrate within the host organism's *genome* at a predetermined target site, but inserts randomly into the host organism's genome or exists as *episomal DNA*. This highlights one of the risks of this technology for therapy, as the functions of normal genes in the host's genome might be disrupted by random integration of the introduced genes. Another limitation is the fact that the transferred (e.g., correct) genes do not replace (e.g., faulty) genes in host cell *chromosomes*. If a faulty gene produces a toxic product, addition of the normal functioning transgene will not prevent production of the toxin.

Genetic ablation   A genetic modification that disrupts the activity of an individual *gene* or drives the expression of drug sensitivity or the production of a cytotoxic protein that can be used to selectively suppress the growth of a predetermined cell population in a living organism.

Genome   All the genetic information in a cell or an organelle. In animals and plants most of this information is held in *chromosomes*, which usually reside in the *nucleus* of a cell. Additional genomic material is stored in *mitochondria*.

Genomics   The study of all the sequences in the *genomes* of organisms and the uses that organisms make of them.

Genotype   A description of the genetic information in an organism. It could encompass one or many *genes*.

Germ cell   A *gamete*-forming cell (i.e., an oogonium or an *oocyte* in females; a spermatogonium or a spermatocyte in males) and its cell products, the *gametes* (i.e., *eggs* in females and *sperm* in males). Germ cells are the reproductive cells of the body. The term *primordial germ cell* is sometimes used as an alternative to "germ cell."

Germ line   A term that has more than one connotation depending on its use. In the biological sciences it is used to refer to the reproductive cells of an organism (i.e., *germ cells* including their products, *gametes*) that can transmit genetic information from one generation to the next. In this context it refers to a cell line that in early embryonic development undergoes *differentiation* to become distinctly different to another cell line that gives rise to *somatic cells*, in that it has the potential to undergo *meiosis* and form *gametes*. In popular discourse, "germ line" is often used synonymously with "blood line" to refer to heritable characteristics (traits) and connections in families. In this context, it is frequently applied to characteristics that are passed from generation to generation by means that involve non-genetic factors (e.g., business acumen). "Germ line" can also connote a vehicle or breeding ground for inheritable gene defects, if such defects are perceived to be kinds of "infectious agents" (somewhat like viruses). In this context, transmission through the germ line might be conceived of as a kind of "vertical infection."

In some discussions the term "germ line" can be conflated with "embryo." For example, Eric T. Juengst and Erik Parens note "that in many discussions 'germ-line gene therapy' is initially defined as interventions directed at the 'germ cells' (e.g., the sperm and the egg), but then described in terms of strategies that involve transforming embryos," and that using the terminology in this way frames the discussions in a "less ominous" manner than using the language of embryo engineering.[6]

Germ-line gene therapy   An early term for inheritable genetic modification with the ultimate aim of treating a disease. The term *inheritable genetic modification (IGM)* is preferred by some commentators because they consider that the technology, and the theoretical basis from which to proceed towards its implementation, is too experimental at this stage to be associated with the term "therapy." An additional problem with this term is that the technology it seeks to describe does not aim to treat an already existing individual, but rather to prevent a genetic condition in a (potential) future individual.

Germ-line gene transfer (GLGT)   Also called germ-line engineering, germ-line genetic modification, and germ-line modification, all of which are variably used to refer to *inheritable genetic modification (IGM)*. But the term "germ-line gene transfer," and its synonyms, are not necessarily synonymous with IGM. The aims of IGM could be quite different to the aims of GLGT. For example, one might wish to implement GLGT with the aim of introducing a genetic change into every cell of an individual (while controlling tissue-specific expression) without wishing for the change to be inherited by his or her progeny, if this could be prevented.

Germ plasm   A term first used by August Weisman in 1893 in his theory of heredity. This theory held that, unlike *somatic cells*, the *nucleus* of a *germ cell* is composed of a heritable complex substance, which he named "germ plasm," that comprises ancestral germ plasms and remains qualitatively identical to that of the *zygote* from which the individual developed. This is the origin of the *germ-line*/somatic cell distinction that has pervaded biology until quite recently – despite the knowledge that *genes* are the units of hereditary and are present in both somatic and germ cells. Today the term is used to refer to complex (sometimes undefined) components in the germ cells that contribute to their function, such as the protoplasm, which consists of the *nucleus* and the body of *cytoplasm* with which it interacts. It is also sometimes used to refer to *genes*, or to the *germ cells* themselves, or their *cytoplasm*.

Haploid   Having one set of *chromosome*s in a cell. The *gamete*s of sexually-reproducing higher organisms are haploid. Haploid is half the *diploid* number of chromosomes that are found in the non-reproductive (*somatic*) cells of humans, most animals, and many plants. Haploid is abbreviated as n.

Hematopoietic stem cells (HSC)   *Stem cell*s in the bone marrow and fetal liver that give rise to mature blood cells. HSC are also found in the peripheral blood and blood obtained from umbilical cord. The two main features of HSC are their abilities to self-renew and to be multipotential (i.e., they are capable of producing differing blood cell lineages including red cells, white cells, and platelets). HSC are capable of being transplanted from oneself (autologous), or a relative or an unrelated immune matched donor (allogeneic) as therapy for diseases such as lymphomas (lymphoid tissue malignancies) and *leukemia*s. Genetic manipulation of HSC offers the possibility of treatments for diverse diseases such as thalassemia (an inherited blood disorder due to mutations in hemo-globin genes) and *severe combined immune deficiency (SCID)*.

Hemophilia   An *X-chromosome* linked disease due to non-functioning, or absent, blood clotting factors (e.g., Factor VIII or Factor IX). The severe form of hemophilia leads to life-threatening bleeding and therapy is currently based on intravenous administration of the relevant clotting factor.

Heritable genetic modification   Synonymous with *inheritable genetic modification*.

Heteroplasmy   The existence in an organism or cell of genetic heterogeneity within the populations of *mitochondria*.[7]

Heterozygosity   The state in which two *allele*s at a particular *gene locus* on each *chromosome* of a chromosome pair are different.

Homologous recombination   The swapping of *DNA* fragments between paired *chromosome*s. This is the normal *gene repair mechanism* by which cells correct breaks or faults in their DNA during cell replication. It has been harnessed to genetically modify cells in the laboratory (especially *embryonic stem cell*s). By this process, DNA that is introduced into actively dividing cells, such as mouse embryonic stem cells, will become incorporated into the chromosomes of the cells, provided it has enough sequences that are similar to sequences in the chromosomal DNA of the cells. Genetic modification by this method is safer than current *gene transfer* methods, as it excludes the possibility of producing organisms with genes whose functions are disrupted by the random insertion of new genes into the host *genome*. The term "homologous recombination" is used as another name for *gene targeting* or *gene repair*. See *gene knockout organism*.

Homologous sequences   *DNA* sequences which are very similar to each other. For example, in an organism the matching *chromosome*s (one from each parent of the organism) in each chromosome pair in a cell share significant sequence similarity (homology) across their entire length, and thus typically contain the same sequence of genes.

Homozygosity   The state in which both *alleles* at a particular gene *locus* on each chromosome of a chromosome pair are the same.

Huntington disease (HD)   A late onset, neurodegenerative condition that can affect males or females and is caused by a mutation on chromosome 4. The effect of the mutated gene is *dominant*.

Hybridization   The process of aligning two *complementary* strands of *DNA* or one each of DNA and *RNA* to form a double-stranded molecule.

Imprinted genes   For most *genes*, both copies, the one inherited from father and the one inherited from mother, are expressed. In contrast, for some genes, only one of the two copies – either the one from the mother or the one from the father – is expressed. These genes are known as imprinted genes. For imprinted genes the two copies are distinguished from each other by special marks, known as *DNA methylation* marks, that are imposed on them during the development of *eggs* in females (maternally-imprinted genes) or *sperm* in males (paternally-imprinted genes). The imposition of these marks is known as *epigenetic modification*. When the *egg* and *sperm* unite all the cells in the developing *embryo* bear the two copies of the imprinted genes that are epigenetically different to each other and remain so in all the *somatic cells* throughout adulthood. These marks distinguish the two copies and cause only one copy to be expressed whereas the other copy remains silent. It is estimated that only a small fraction of all genes are imprinted. Disturbances to normal imprinted gene expression leads to growth abnormalities during fetal life and can be the cause of major diseases in later life.[8]

Inheritable genetic modification (IGM)   A biomedical technical intervention (molecular, genetic, or cellular) that modifies the set of *genes* that a subject has available to transmit to his or her offspring. It includes all interventions made at a stage in an organism's development that is early enough to have inheritable effects on its *germ cells* (*gametes* and *gamete*-forming tissues). This book focuses mainly on intentional IGM by the application of techniques such as the use of *artificial chromosomes*, *viral vectors*, *oligonucleotides*, cell fusion, and subcellular component transplantation (e.g., *mitochondria*). Other potentially powerful mediators of IGM such as social and cultural practices, alteration of the environment (e.g., by nuclear radiation), and side effects of non-genetic treatments for infertility or other diseases (e.g., by chemotherapeutic agents) are not considered. *Germ cell* and *embryonic stem cell* modification constitute major IGM subtypes. The term *germ-line modification* is variably used as a synonym for IGM. The term *heritable genetic modification* is a synonym for IGM.[9]

Insertional mutagenesis   The alteration of the *DNA* sequence of a *gene* that is caused by the introduction of foreign DNA sequences into it. This may occur spontaneously in nature or be intentionally, or unintentionally, experimentally induced. With current clinically directed *gene transfer* techniques, there is no control over where the foreign DNA might integrate into the host cell's DNA (i.e., it is randomly inserted), leading to a fear that normal genes will be disrupted, perhaps causing unregulated cell growth and tumor formation.

Interleukin   A type of protein that mediates immune and inflammatory responses.

***In utero* gene therapy**   Genetic modification of an *embryo* in the uterus to treat a genetic disease. It would most likely be applied as therapy for a diseased embryo. If applied at an early stage of embryonic development *inheritable genetic modification* might result. *In utero* gene therapy is sometimes called *in utero gene transfer*.

***In vitro* fertilization (IVF)**   The union of an *egg* and *sperm* in an artificial environment outside the body. IVF is used as a technique to assist reproduction.

***In vitro* oocyte nuclear transplantation (or transfer) (IVONT)**   This is a technique that involves removing the *nucleus* from an unfertilized *egg* cell and placing it in the intact *cytoplasm* of another unfertilized egg that has had its own nucleus removed from it (i.e., an *enucleated egg*). The resulting hybrid egg is then fertilized with *sperm* in the laboratory before being implanted into the uterus of a receptive female. This technique might be used to treat genetic defects in *mitochondria* by transferring the nucleus from an egg of a woman with a mitochondrial defect to an enucleated egg from another woman who has healthy mitochondria. Once fertilized the hybrid egg would contain nuclear *DNA* from the mother to be, mitochondrial DNA from the woman who donated the enucleated egg, and nuclear DNA from the man who donated the sperm. Such an intervention can lead to *heteroplasmy*. See also *ooplasm transfer*.

Lesch–Nyhan syndrome   An inheritable condition in males due to mutations in a gene on the *X chromosome* that encodes for an enzyme known as hypoxanthine guanine phosphoribosyltransferase (HPRT) that is involved in the production of components of *DNA* and *RNA* known as *nitrogenous bases*.

Leukemia   A blood cell malignancy.

Liposome   An artificial fatty vesicle that encapsulates *DNA* and can therefore be used as a vehicle (*vector*) for transferring *genes* to cells, tissues, and organisms. Their current disadvantages are that they are unable to target to specific tissues; are rapidly cleared by the body; are susceptible to being ingested by cells; are less efficient than virus mediated approaches; and have a short half life. Their advantages are that they can accommodate large amounts of DNA and may not stimulate the immune system. They may have a role in the clinical application of *artificial chromosomes* and *oligonucleotides*.

Locus   The position of a *gene* or a genetic marker on a *chromosome*.

Lymphocyte   A type of white blood cell that arises from *stem cells* in the bone marrow and is found in blood, lymphoid, and most tissues. Lymphocytes mediate immune responses by expressing complex molecules (receptors) on their cell surfaces that bind protein molecules (peptide antigens) that are appropriately presented to them. *T cells*, *B cells*, and *natural killer cells* are all types of lymphocytes.

Major histocompatibility complex (MHC)   A large *gene locus* that encodes the molecules on cells (known as MHC molecules) that display catabolized protein molecules (peptides) to *T cells* for recognition and initiation of specific immune responses.

Marfan syndrome   An inherited connective tissue disorder that is caused by a *mutation* in a *gene* on chromosome 15 that encodes a protein called fibrillin, which is essential for the formation of elastic fibers. The effect of the mutated gene is *dominant*.

Meiosis   The process of cell division that a *diploid germ cell* undergoes during *gametogenesis* to produce *gametes*, each of which contains half the number of *chromosomes* (*haploid*) as in the original germ cell. This process is necessary to prevent *fertilization* doubling the number of chromosomes in every generation. Before meiosis begins, the two sets of chromosomes (one from the mother and one from the father) in the original diploid germ cell (2n) duplicate themselves to become four sets (4n): two from the mother which are paired together for each chromosome (a homologue pair) and two from the father which are paired together for each chromosome (a homologue pair). Meiosis has two parts: the first part (meiosis I) reduces the chromosome number per cell from 4n to 2n and the second part (meiosis II) reduces the chromosome number per cell from 2n to n. In meiosis I the homologue pairs for each chromosome align with each other in close proximity to allow some exchange of chromosomal material between them. This exchange allows the genetic variation that is seen between individual (outbred) offspring. The homologue pairs for each chromosome then move away from each other towards opposite sides of the cell, and a cell membrane that allows the cell to separate into two cells forms between them. In this way each of the two resulting cells contains one homologue pair (2n). In meiosis II, the individual chromosomes in a homologue pair move away from each other towards opposite sides of the cell, and a cell membrane that allows the cell to divide into two cells forms between them. In this way each of the two resulting gametes contains one set of chromosomes (n).

Messenger RNA (mRNA) A type of *RNA* that carries genetic information from the cell *nucleus* to the *cytoplasm*, where it acts as a template for protein synthesis. It is synthesized from a *DNA* template by a process called transcription.

Microarray analysis/technology The detection of the genetic make up of cells by exposing their contents to a microchip that contains tens of thousands of pieces of genetic material (*DNA, RNA*) that act as probes for particular *genes*. Any gene that binds to a probe stimulates a signal (fluorescence) that is detected using a scanner. The microchips are also known as biochips, or GeneChips (an Affymetrix trademark).

Mitochondria Small energy producing organelles found in the *cytoplasm* of cells. Mitochondria give rise to other mitochondria by copying their small piece of mitochondrial *DNA* (mtDNA) and passing one copy of the DNA along to each of the two resulting mitochondria. They are normally inherited through female *germ cells*.

Mitosis The process of cell division that a *somatic cell* undergoes that produces cells with identical numbers of *chromosomes* as the original cell (*diploid*). Before mitosis begins, the two sets of chromosomes (one from the mother and one from the father) in the original cell (2n) duplicate themselves to become four sets (4n): two from the mother and two from the father. In mitosis two of the sets (one from the mother and one from the father) move away from the other two sets (also one from the mother and one from the father) towards opposite sides of the cell, and a cell membrane forms between them, allowing the dividing cell to separate into two cells. In this way each of the two resulting cells (known as "daughter" cells) has two sets of chromosomes.

Monogenic Caused by a single *gene*.

Mosaic An animal or tissue containing two or more genetically distinct cell types. Mosaics, which are actually common in mammals, arise from a single *zygote*, in contrast to *chimeras*.

Multiple sclerosis (MS) A disease thought to be caused by the body's immune system attacking the protein and fat insulating material (myelin) that covers its own nerves. Myelin is important for the conduction of impulses along the nerves. In MS muscular weakness, loss of coordination, and speech and visual disturbances occur over time. It is thought that inherited and environmental factors are involved in its causation.

Mutation A change in *DNA* sequence (typically of a *gene*). In organisms, the change may be perceived of as a fault at the physiological level (see *phenotype*), or it may have no apparent effect, in which case it is said to be a "silent" mutation.

Myeloid Pertaining to non-*lymphocyte* white blood cells such as monocytes and granulocytes and the bone marrow progenitors that give rise to them.

Natural killer (NK) cell   A type of *lymphocyte* that attacks infected or malignant cells and is a part of the body's natural (innate) immune system.

Nitrogenous base   A basic constituent of *DNA* and *RNA*. There are five types: adenine (A), thymine (T), guanine (G), cytosine (C), and uracil (U). DNA has A, T, G, and C. RNA has A, U, G, and C (but no T).

Nuclear transfer   Nuclear transfer is the removal of the *nucleus* from a cell (donor) and its introduction to another cell (recipient), which has had its own nucleus removed (enucleated). The recipient cell is usually an *enucleated egg*. The type of nuclear transfer is determined by the type of donor cell used. If the donor cell is a *somatic cell*, the transfer is known as *somatic cell nuclear transfer (SCNT)*; if the donor cell is from an *embryo*, the transfer is known as embryo cell nuclear transfer (ECNT); and if the donor cell is from an unfertilized egg, the transfer is known as *in vitro oocyte nuclear transplantation (IVONT)*. The first two are forms of *cloning*.

Nucleoside   A *nitrogenous base* linked to a sugar molecule that is a basic constituent of *DNA* and *RNA*.

Nucleotide   A *nucleoside* linked to a phosphate group that is a basic constituent of *DNA* and *RNA*.

Nucleus   An organelle, present in most types of cells, which contains the *chromosomes*.

Oligonucleotide   A short strand of *DNA*.

Oligonucleotide site-directed gene repair   A *gene repair* strategy that involves artificially provoking the innate ability of cells to repair *mutations* (particularly those that cause disease) in their *DNA*. *Oligonucleotide*s that have similar DNA sequences to (i.e., are *homologous* with) sequences surrounding the mutation in the host cell *genome* – but different to the mutation itself – are introduced into the cell, typically without the use of a *vector*. Once there, they are transported to the *nucleus*, where they bind to the host cell's genetic material. Non-homology between the oligonucleotide and the host genome at the host mutation site causes a disruption in the binding. Disrupted DNA structures are recognized as a site for repair by the cell's naturally present DNA repair enzymes. This and the actual event of the oligonucleotide binding to the host's genetic material initiates repair, and thus corrects the mutation in the host cell's genetic material. The risks usually associated with *gene transfer* and the use of *viral vector*s are reduced because neither is employed. The advantages are that the gene correction would be highly specific and the oligonucleotides may not stimulate an immune response because they do not persist in tissues. However, the efficiency of oligonucleotide delivery is low and improvements may require some kind of a vector that might introduce other risks. Potential harms of the repair process operating on a physiological scale, especially in a developing *embryo*, are not yet known. A related technology to oligonucleotide site-directed gene repair is oligonucleotide-induced exon skipping which is being developed to ameliorate specific diseases such as muscular dystrophy.

Oocyte   A reproductive cell of a female organism that undergoes *meiosis* to produce an *egg*.

Oogenesis   The maturation of *germ cell*s and the process of *egg* production in female animals.

Ooplasm (or ooplasmic) transfer (or transplantation)   A technique whereby *cytoplasm* from one *egg* (the donor) is transferred into another egg (the recipient). Offspring produced as a result of *fertilization* would have nuclear *DNA* from the mother, *mitochondrial* DNA from the woman who donated the cytoplasm, and nuclear DNA from the father. See also *in vitro oocyte nuclear transplantation (IVONT)* and *heteroplasmy*.

Organelle   A structure within a cell, such as a *mitochondrion*, that performs a specific function.

Ovum   A term synonymous with *egg*.

Parthenogenesis   A form of *asexual reproduction* in which *egg*s are subjected to electrical shock or chemical treatment in order to initiate cell division and embryonic development.

Phenome   The comprehensive phenotypic characterization of a single species or organism.[10]

Phenotype   A description of the observable traits (characteristics) of an organism. It is often used to describe a specific physical or metabolic characteristic that is associated with a particular *genotype*.

Phenylketonuria (PKU)   A *recessive* inherited disorder in which the body lacks an enzyme that converts a chemical component of proteins known as phenylalanine (which is obtained in the diet) to another chemical component of proteins known as tyrosine. Left untreated, the disorder can cause intellectual impairment as a result of the accumulation of phenylalanine. The disorder can be detected through neonatal genetic testing, and the effects of the disorder can largely be avoided by adhering to a phenylalanine-free diet.

Pluripotent   A cell that can develop into many different types of specialized cells. The term "pluripotent" is usually interchangeable with the term "multipotent."

Polygenic   Caused by many different *gene*s acting together.

Polyomavirus JC   A double-stranded *DNA* virus that is found in all human populations worldwide. It has sequences that are specific to different geographic areas. The virus may have co-evolved with human ancestors.

Prader–Willi syndrome   A syndrome characterized by obesity, decreased muscle tone, and slower than normal intellectual development. It is caused by a gene imprinting error on chromosome 15 and is inherited.

Pre-implantation genetic diagnosis (PGD or PIGD)   The detection of genetic abnormalities or characteristics in *embryos* before they are implanted in the uterus. PGD techniques are usually used to select embryos created by the technique of *in vitro fertilization*. PGD can be used to determine the sex of an embryo.

Prenatal genetic diagnosis   The detection of fetal genetic abnormalities during pregnancy.

Primordial germ cell   A reproductive cell that gives rise to *eggs* in females and *sperm* in males. Often used synonymously with *germ cell*.

Pronucleus   The *nucleus* of the *egg* or *sperm* after *fertilization*, before the *chromosomes* from each have fused together to form the nucleus of the *zygote*.

Recessive   In reference to observable traits (characteristics) that are determined by particular *genes*, the manifestation of a recessive trait requires that both copies of the (abnormal) gene are expressed (see *dominant*).

Recombinant DNA   *DNA* that has been artificially manipulated in a laboratory.

Reproductive cloning   *Cloning* with the intention of producing a living organism.

Retroviral vector   A retrovirus that has been genetically engineered for use as a vehicle (*vector*) for introducing *genes* into cells, tissues, or organisms. Retroviruses encode their *genome* in ribonucleic acid (*RNA*). They have an enzyme known as reverse transcriptase that copies the single stranded RNA into *DNA*, which once duplicated is then integrated into the host cell's DNA. These vectors have been used in one quarter of the clinical *gene transfer* trials to date. They enter, but do not replicate in, host cells, thereby limiting their spread to other cells in the body. Their advantages are that they do not markedly stimulate the immune system and they integrate stably into the host cell's DNA. Their disadvantages are that they only infect dividing cells; they integrate into the host genome randomly; and they cannot accommodate large genes. Examples are murine Moloney Leukemia Virus (MuLV) and lentiviruses such as human immunodeficiency virus (HIV). Lentiviruses can enter non-dividing cells (such as *stem cells*), but their use has raised safety concerns due to a possibility that they might potentially result in the production of pathogenic viruses.

Rhodopsin   A light sensitive pigment found in the eye.

RNA   Ribonucleic acid (RNA). A similar molecule to *DNA* but with a slightly different structure. It plays an intermediary role in converting the information contained in DNA into proteins. RNA carries the genetic information from DNA to those parts of the cell where proteins are made.[11] See *messenger RNA*.

Severe combined immune deficiency (SCID)   A life-threatening disorder of the immune system in which the body lacks functional *T cells* and *B cells* to resist infection. It is caused by a mutation in any one of at least eight genes, such as the gene for *adenosine deaminase*. This disease was a focus for media attention in the 1970's through the "Bubble Boy," who lived in an isolation unit to reduce the chance of infection. In 2000, the first clear evidence of successful gene therapy for any human disease was reported by French scientists treating SCID. Subsequently some of the treated children developed *leukemia* due to *insertional mutagenesis*. The term also appears as "severe combined immunodeficiency."

Sex chromosome   A *chromosome* (*X* or *Y*) that determines the sex of an individual. Mammals generally have two sex chromosomes: males have one X and one Y and females have two X chromosomes.

Sex-linked gene   A gene carried by a *sex chromosome*. A number of diseases (e.g., *hemophilia*), which affect males only, are due to *X chromosome* gene faults owing to the fact that (XY) males, unlike (XX) females, lack a second non-faulty X chromosome that would be protective if present.

Sexual reproduction   Reproduction that involves the union of *egg* and *sperm* to form a fertilized egg (*zygote*).

Sickle cell anemia   A condition whereby the number and function of red blood cells in the body is reduced because of a *mutation* in a hemoglobin gene that causes abnormal hemoglobin to be produced and the red blood cells to be fragile. The disease-causing effect of the mutated gene is *recessive*.

Small interfering RNA (siRNA)   Specific *oligonucleotides* that are used as a promising technology for reducing the expression of specific target *genes*.

Somatic cell   Any cell in an organism that is not a reproductive cell (i.e., not a *gamete* or a gamete forming cell [*germ cell*]). The genes in a somatic cell cannot be passed on to future generations by normal *sexual reproduction*; but they can be passed on by the application of a *cloning* technique such as *somatic cell nuclear transfer*. A somatic cell contains two sets of *chromosomes* (*diploid*).

Somatic cell gene transfer (SCGT)   The introduction of *DNA* into the non-reproductive body cells (*somatic cells*) of an organism using a variety of chemical, physical, or biological techniques (see *gene transfer*). Currently, SCGT refers to *gene* addition rather than *gene repair* (correction), whereby the effects of a faulty gene are masked by the addition of a correct gene to the cell or tissue. To date it has been the predominant approach used in *gene therapy* and is potentially therapeutic for *recessive* loss of function genetic disorders. SCGT is not intended to modify *germ cells* (although this might be an unavoidable side effect of it). Somatic cell genetic modification (SCGM) is another term used to refer to *somatic cell gene transfer*.

Somatic cell nuclear transfer (SCNT)   A method by which the *nucleus* from a *somatic cell* (donor) is removed and introduced into an *enucleated egg* (recipient) to produce a *cloned embryo*. This method is not likely to be used to create a child (reproductive cloning) because it has considerable ethical and biosafety limitations. It could be used to create an *embryonic stem cell* line for therapeutic transplantation into an organism to treat a disease or injury (*therapeutic cloning*). It is controversial because the derivation of the *embryonic stem cell* line from a cloned embryo is an essential step that involves the destruction of the *embryo*, which some view as the loss of a potential human life.[12]

Somatic stem cell   A *somatic cell* that is a *stem cell*. It is also known as an *adult stem cell*.

Species   A unified species concept has not yet been achieved: instead there are various definitions. The first is known as the "biological species concept," whereby a species is defined as a group of organisms that are capable of interbreeding to produce fertile offspring. Another definition is the "evolutionary species concept," whereby it is the continuity of a group of organisms throughout evolutionary history that defines it as a species. The last is the "homeostatic property cluster concept," whereby a species is characterized by a cluster of properties no one of which, and no specific set of which, must be exhibited by any individual member of that species, but some set of which must be possessed by all individual members of that species.[13]

Sperm   A reproductive cell of a male animal that carries one set of *chromosomes* (*haploid*). In normal sexual reproduction a sperm fertilizes an *egg* to produce an *embryo*. Alternative terms are male *gamete* or spermatozoon.

Spermatogenesis   The maturation of *germ cells* and the process of *sperm* production in male animals.

Spermatogonial cells   *Germ cells* in the testis of male animals that give rise to cells, known as spermatocytes, which in turn give rise to *sperm*. They are *diploid*. An alternative term is "spermatogonia" (singular: spermatogonium).

Stem cell   An unspecialized cell that is capable of giving rise to new stem cells as well as to specialized cells of body tissues (see *differentiation*). There are many different kinds of stem cells and they are named after the tissue in which they are found (e.g., *embryonic stem cell*, *embryonic germ cell*, and *adult stem cell*).

Susceptibility gene   A mutated *gene* that increases the probability that an individual will be affected by a certain condition.

Targeted gene replacement   Another term for *gene targeting.*

Tay–Sachs disease   A fatal disease in which fatty substances known as gangliosides accumulate in the brain because of a deficiency of the enzyme (hexosaminidase A) that breaks them down. It is cause by a *mutation* in the hexosaminidase A gene located on chromosome 15. The effect of the mutated gene is *recessive.*

T cell   A type of *lymphocyte* that matures in the thymus. It attacks infected or malignant cells and is part of the body's specific (acquired) immune system.

Teratogen   An agent, such as a virus (e.g., rubella), a drug (e.g., thalidomide), or radiation, that interferes with normal embryonic development and causes a disorder in the *embryo* or *fetus.*

Therapeutic cloning   *Cloning* with the intention of producing cells (especially *stem cells*) that can be expanded outside the body and transplanted into an organism for the purpose of treating a disease.

Transgene   Any *DNA* sequence or combination of sequences that is transplanted (transplant *gene*) into the *genome* of an organism or cell (known as the host). Prior to transplantation the transgene of interest is often embedded into a larger genetic construct (*vector*) that assists the manufacture and subsequent integration and expression of the transgene within the host's genome when transplanted.

Transgenesis   The process of transplanting a *DNA* sequence or combination of sequences (a *transgene*) from one *genome* (known as the donor) into another genome (known as the recipient or host).

Transgenic organism   An organism that has a *transgene* stably integrated into its *genome*. The term is usually applied to an organism in which the transgene is integrated randomly into its *genome* because the *transgenesis* technique used did not allow the *gene* to be targeted to a predetermined site. This type of transgenic organism is created by injecting *DNA* into one (usually the male) of the two nuclei (each is known as a *pronucleus*) that are present in a *fertilized egg* prior to them fusing to become one *nucleus* in the developing *zygote*. The modified zygote is then implanted in the uterus of a receptive female (foster mother-to-be) and allowed to develop. In this way multiple copies of the transgene become randomly integrated in the zygote genome. Random integration can disrupt normal gene function in the zygote. This approach does not correct faulty genes but simply adds correct copies of the gene to the defective host genome: the faulty gene is still retained. Hence, it is an additive and untargeted approach. The offspring generated is *heterozygous* for the added gene and may be *chimeric*. By contrast, a "gene knock in" organism is a special kind of transgenic organism that is created by taking a *gene targeting* approach, in which a correction, or a new gene, can be introduced into the original faulty gene.

Tyrosinase   An enzyme that promotes the oxidation of an amino-acid known as tyrosine and thereby initiates the production of melanin, the dark pigment in skin, eyes, and hair. A deficiency of tyrosinase causes *albinism*.

Vector   An agent that can carry and introduce a *transgene* into a target host cell. It usually refers to a genetically-engineered virus, but it could also refer to a non-viral agent, such as a sequence of *DNA*. See *viral vector*, *artificial chromosome*, and *liposome*.

Viral vector   A virus that has been genetically engineered for use as a vehicle for introducing *genes* into cells, tissues, or organisms. Many kinds of viruses have been genetically engineered for this purpose including retroviruses, adenoviruses, adeno-associated viruses, and engineered hybrid viruses that exploit the advantages, and reduce the disadvantages, associated with individual viruses. See *retroviral vectors*, *adenoviral vectors*, and *adeno-associated viral vectors*.

X chromosome   A *sex chromosome* that is present in both sexes: males carry one copy and females carry two copies.

Xenotransplantation   The grafting of an organ or tissue from another species.

X-linked gene   A gene carried on the *X chromosome* and not on the *Y chromosome*.

Y chromosome   A *sex chromosome* that is present in males and not in females. Males have one Y chromosome and one *X chromosome*.

Zygote   The single cell that results from the *fertilization* of an *egg* by a *sperm*. It has a complete set of paired *chromosomes* (*diploid*). Zygote is another term for *fertilized egg*.

NOTES

1 The resources consulted during the compilation of this glossary include: Access Excellence Resources Centre Gene Testing Glossary, http://www.accessexcellence. org/AE/AEPC/NIH/gene27.html; Answers.com, http://www.answers.com/; Biotech Life Science Directory, http://biotech.icmb.utexas.edu/search/dict-search.html; Centre for Genetics Education, http://www.genetics.com.au/conditions/default. htm#; Gene Ontology Consortium, http://www.geneontology.org/, Helios, The University of Edinburgh, http://helios.bto.ed.ac.uk/bto/glossary/ab.htm#a; Mouse Genome Informatics Glossary, http://www.informatics.jax.org/javawi2/servlet/WIFetch?page= glossaryIndex&print=no#R; National Institutes of Health Stem Cell Information

Resources, http://stemcells.nih.gov/index.asp; and Wikipedia, http://en.wikipedia.org/wiki/Main_Page (all sites last accessed 29 March 2005).

2 Deborah O. Co, Anita H. Borowski, Joseph D. Leung, *et al.*, Generation of transgenic mice and germline transmission of a mammalian artificial chromosome introduced into embryos by pronuclear microinjection, *Chromosome Research* 8 (2000), 183–91.

3 A term attributed to Dr Paul McHugh in Stephen S. Hall, Specter of cloning may prove a mirage, *New York Times* 17 February 2004, http://www.genetics-and-society.org/resources/items/20040217_nytimes_hall.html (last accessed 29 April 2005).

4 Ian Wilmut, Angelika E. Schnieke, Jim McWhir, *et al.*, Viable offspring derived from fetal and adult mammalian cells, *Nature* 385 (1997), 810–13.

5 Rudolf Jaenisch, Nuclear cloning, embryonic stem cells and gene transfer (Chapter 3, this volume), Note 10.

6 Eric Juengst and Erik Parens, Germ-line dancing in Audrey R. Chapman and Mark S. Frankel (eds.), *Designing Our Descendents: The Promises and Perils of Genetic Modification*. Baltimore: John Hopkins University Press (2003), 20–36.

7 http://helios.bto.ed.ac.uk/bto/glossary/gh.htm (last accessed 29 March 2005).

8 Jaenisch, Nuclear cloning, embryonic stem cells and gene transfer.

9 See Audrey R. Chapman and Mark S. Frankel, Framing the issues. In Audrey R. Chapman and Mark S. Frankel (eds.), *Designing Our Descendents: The Promises and Perils of Genetic Modification*. Baltimore: John Hopkins University Press, (2003), 5–6.

10 Norberto de la Cruz *et al.*, The Rat Genome Database (RGD): developments towards a phenome database, *Nucleic Acids Research* 33 (2005), database issue D485– D491. http://nar.oupjournals.org/cgi/content/full/33/suppl_1/D485 (last accessed 29 March 2005).

11 National Centre for Biotechnology Education, The University of Reading, http://www.ncbe.reading.ac.uk/NCBE/GMFOOD/igdglossary.html (last accessed 29 March 2005).

12 Jaenisch, Nuclear cloning, embryonic stem cells and gene transfer.

13 Jason Scott Robert and Françoise Baylis, Crossing species boundaries, *The American Journal of Bioethics* 3 (2003), 3.

Index

abortion
    as a lesser question than genetic
       modification, 182, 185
    Down syndrome, xv
    IGM as alternative to, 96, 176, 182,
       185, 194
    IQ, xxiv
    justification for, xvi, xix
    opposition to, xvi, 96
    prenatal diagnosis/screening and, xv,
       xix–xxi, xxiv–xxv, 160, 164–7,
       182, 185, 225, 253
    selective, xiv–xv, xix–xx, xxiii, 182,
       185, 189, 193–4, 202, 225, 253
    and disability discrimination, 182–3,
       186–7
    Roe v. Wade, xvi, 253
achondroplasia, xv, 179, 181–2, 234–5
acquired traits, 136–7
adenosine deaminase (ADA), xxxiii, 131,
    195, 279, 298
    deficiency, 131, 195
adenoviral (AV) vector (*see* gene
    transfer, vectors)
African–Americans, 138, 168
Albinism, 280, 301
alcoholism, 178, 201
alternatives to IGM
    adoption, 139, 224–5, 230, 256
    as a basis for arguing for IGM, 96,
       163, 176
    in vitro fertilization (IVF) (*see also in
       vitro* fertilization (main entry)),
       172*n36*, 194, 225, 230, 253

    preimplantation genetic diagnosis
       (PGD), 180, 194, 202, 211,
       225–6, 230, 233, 253, 256
    prenatal diagnosis, 160, 182–3, 225–6,
       230, 238
    SCGT, 160, 231
    termination, 160, 182–4, 202, 225–6,
       253, 256, 263
    use of donor egg or sperm, 139, 180,
       225, 230
Alzheimer disease, 108, 162, 280
American Association for the
    Advancement of Science
    (AAAS), 108, 223–4
American Eugenics Society, 251
American Journal of Human Genetics,
    251
American Society of Human Genetics,
    236, 251
amniocentesis, 193, 202, 253, 280
ancestry/genealogical research,
    137–9, 142
Anderson, W. French, 195
ANDi, 107, 141
Andorno, Roberto, 269
animal experimentation
    as alternative to embryo research, 109
    cost–benefit assessments, 116–20
    for therapeutic development, 107
    justification for, 114
    public support for, 113–4
    regulation, 105, 107, 109, 121–2*n3–10*,
       124*n26*
    welfare issues, 11, 103–29

Printed in the United States
by Baker & Taylor Publisher Services